Bariatric Surgical Practice Guide

Editor-in-Chief
Praveen Raj Palanivelu

Saravana Kumar • Rachel Maria Gomes
Editors

Bariatric Surgical Practice Guide

Recommendations

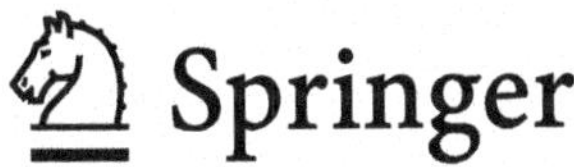

Editor-in-chief
Praveen Raj Palanivelu
GEM Hospitals Group
GEM Obesity and Diabetes Surgery Centre
Bariatric Division, Upper Gastrointestinal
Surgery and Minimal Access Surgery Unit
GEM Hospital and Research Centre
Coimbatore
Tamil Nadu
India

Editors
Saravana Kumar
Bariatric Division, Upper Gastrointestinal
Surgery and Minimal Access Surgery Unit
GEM Hospital and Research Centre
Coimbatore
Tamil Nadu
India

Rachel Maria Gomes
Bariatric Division, Upper Gastrointestinal
Surgery and Minimal Access Surgery Unit
GEM Hospital and Research Centre
Coimbatore
Tamil Nadu
India

ISBN 978-981-10-9687-7 ISBN 978-981-10-2705-5 (eBook)
DOI 10.1007/978-981-10-2705-5

Printed on acid-free paper

This Springer imprint is published by Springer Nature
The registered company is Springer Nature Singapore Pte Ltd.
The registered company address is 152 Beach Road, #21-01/04 Gateway East, Singapore 189721, Singapore

Foreword I

The obesity pandemic continues to invade our planet. In an effort to improve survival, basic scientists and clinicians carry on their quest to better understand, prevent and treat this devastating disease. The introduction of optoelectronic instrumentation, parenteral nutrition, sophisticated staplers, critical care, and anesthesia techniques have contributed to the evolution of bariatric surgery in the last 50 years, becoming one of the safest surgical disciplines with mortalities under 0.3 %. The introduction of sleeve gastrectomy has resulted in a revolution with a significant decline in the number of gastric bypass and the fall of the adjustable gastric banding being performed worldwide. The low morbidity and technical simplicity of sleeve gastrectomy resonates with patients and bariatric surgeons and has become the most common procedure and the platform for bariatric patients to get started with.

I commend the editors of this book Drs. Praveen Raj, Saravana Kumar, and Rachel Maria Gomes for an outstanding contribution. *Bariatric Surgical Practice Guide* has been planned to cover all the practical aspects in bariatric surgical practice with simple evidence recommendations at the end of each chapter. This book covers not only surgical but also complex medical situations that severely obese patients and surgeons will face before and after surgery.

At times when delivering healthcare has become more oriented towards higher quality, better outcomes, and rapid recovery strategies to shorten hospital stay and decrease costs, the evidence-based recommendations at the end of each chapter should help clinicians make the best decisions.

I thank the authors for the privilege to write this foreword and wish all bariatric surgeons and integrated health members best of luck and success in their practices.

Raul J. Rosenthal MD FACS FASMBS
President, American Society of Metabolic and Bariatric Surgeons
Professor of Surgery and Chairman
Department of General Surgery and
The Bariatric and Metabolic Institute
Cleveland Clinic, Weston, Florida

Foreword II

Obesity and type 2 diabetes mellitus are now among the most common chronic, debilitating diseases worldwide. Bariatric surgical approaches are not only successful in achieving and maintaining long-term weight loss in severe obese patients, but also in achieving pronounced metabolic effects, especially remission of type 2 diabetes mellitus. To incorporate bariatric/metabolic surgery into current treatments of obesity and type 2 diabetes mellitus and to select appropriate patients require cooperative work between surgeons and multi-discipline team members. Optimal outcomes for weight reduction and co-morbidities remission after bariatric/metabolic surgery will occur if the best performance is provided by a cooperative team and patients best suited for the surgery are selected, while those who will predictably have a poor result are excluded.

In this book, Dr. Praveen Raj and his colleagues have provided a practical clinical book for bariatric/metabolic surgeons after an extensive paper review. The content is not only useful and up to date but also supported by strong medical evidence. I would like to wholeheartedly recommend this book to all bariatric/metabolic surgeons and allied health colleagues.

Wei-Jei Lee, M.D., Ph.D.
Professor of Surgery, Min-Sheng General Hospital,
National Taiwan University, Taiwan
Founding President of Asia Pacific Metabolic
and Bariatric Surgery Society (APMBSS)

Foreword III

The evolution of bariatric surgery is one of the biggest revolutions in the field of surgery. As the world is getting lesser invasive, with many newer modalities emerging for the treatment of so-called surgical diseases like gastroesophageal reflux disease, achalasia cardia, etc., interestingly, we are now seeing surgery as a treatment of medical diseases like type 2 diabetes, dyslipidemia, non-alcoholic fatty liver disease, etc., in the form of metabolic surgery. With tremendously increasing rates of obesity and type 2 diabetes, the need for bariatric surgery too is increasing with increasing numbers of surgeons now taking up the speciality. But what we lack is a regulated curriculum or established clinical practice guidelines for a more unified treatment approach. Many reasons could be attributed to this including varied outcomes of different procedures amongst different patient population, cultural issues integral to specific communities, varied experience amongst surgeons, differing surgical background with differing principles amongst surgeons, lack of evidence-based guidelines, etc. But we cannot let it go long.

The editors of this book Dr. Praveen Raj, Dr. Saravana Kumar and Dr. Rachel Maria Gomes have taken great effort in bringing in all the important practical issues together with a review of existing literature in a form applicable to everyday clinical practice. Each chapter has been structured in a way that makes it easier for a surgeon to understand the principles without any controversy.

As the saying by Franz Kafka goes "A book must be the axe for the frozen sea within us", this book will definitely uncover all controversial issues amongst bariatric surgeons with a much better clarity.

C. Palanivelu, MS, FRCS (Hon), FACS, PhD
Chairman, Gem Hospital and Research Centre, Coimbatore, India
Founding President-Association of Minimal Access Surgeons of India
Past President-Association of Surgeons of India

Preface

Bariatric surgery is the most effective method of treatment for morbid obesity. The number of bariatric procedures performed each year is growing continuously. The field of bariatrics has slowly developed over time into a new subspecialty in the field of surgery. But as in any developing field, there still remain many unanswered questions and controversial issues. Surgeons are left with many questions in their day-to-day practice. "Which patient should I select for bariatric surgery?", "Can I predict the outcomes of my bariatric procedure?", "Should specific circumstances change the choice of my procedure?", "How can I perform my procedure safely and successfully?", "How do I manage my patient after surgery?", "How can I avoid complications?", "What do I do in case of complications?", "How do I nutritionally care for my patient?", "What procedure do I choose in those who require a re-do surgery?", etc. These questions can be very confusing for the bariatric surgeon, especially at the beginning of his career. However even with experience, bariatric surgeons will continue to ponder over these questions throughout their entire career. This textbook on bariatric surgery is aimed to provide both practical and evidence-based answers to these questions. It is meant to be a quick-reference book that provides easy access information on a day-to-day basis with detailed explanations for the same.

The first section of this book deals with the selection of patients for bariatric surgery. Several bariatric procedures have been tried in several populations over time. We are now clear as to who will benefit from these bariatric procedures. In the first chapter, we review existing BMI guidelines used to select bariatric procedures in adults. Existing guidelines in adolescents are looked into in the next chapter. The subsequent chapters cover certain special situations in bariatric surgery and preoperative evaluation pathways. The second section of this book deals with the predictors of outcomes after bariatric procedures with the first chapter dedicated on defining success and failure followed by two detailed chapters summarizing the predictors of weight loss and diabetes mellitus remission after bariatric surgery. In the third section, the two standard bariatric procedures of sleeve gastrectomy and roux-en-Y gastric bypass are reviewed with evidence-based support for each step of the technique. The several variants of duodenal switch and the technique of gastric plication are reviewed in the subsequent chapters in the section. The fourth section of this book details on specific situations of gastroesophageal reflux, ventral hernia, polycystic ovarian disease, pregnancy, nonalcoholic fatty liver disease, diabetic microvascular complications, and end-organ failure and were discussed in the context of bariatric surgery. Postoperative pathways are discussed in detail in the fifth section with a summary on enhanced recovery after surgery and common complications after bariatric surgery are reviewed in the section six. Section seven deals in detail with revisional options after laparoscopic adjustable gastric banding, laparoscopic sleeve gastrectomy, and laparoscopic roux-en-Y gastric bypass. Bariatric surgery candidates are susceptible to the development of nutritional deficiencies, and the section on nutrition covers these issues in detail and their management strategies. In each chapter, we have arrived at recommendation statements based on current available evidence.

Through this format, a first of its kind, we hope to provide our readers with a thorough understanding of the subject and answers for all practical steps involved in bariatric surgical practice, hence the title *Bariatric Surgery Practice Guide*.

Praveen Raj Palanivelu, MS, DNB, DNB(SGE), FALS, FMAS
Director, GEM Hospital Groups
Head, GEM Obesity and Diabetes Surgery Centre
President of the Indian chapter of the
International Excellence Federation of Bariatric Surgery

Contents

About the Editors

Praveen Raj Palanivelu completed his graduate medical training with honors from the PSG Institute of Medical Sciences, Coimbatore, India and his general surgical training, and Masters in General Surgery from the prestigious Sri Ramachandra University, Chennai, India. He also secured his Masters in Surgery and Surgical Gastroenterology from the Diplomate of the National Board (DNB) of India. He has been conferred with the Honorary Fellow in Advanced Laparoscopy (FALS) by the Indian Association for Gastrointestinal Endosurgeons (IAGES). Currently, he is Director at the GEM Hospital Group and heads the GEM Obesity and Diabetes Surgery Centre and the Bariatric division of the Upper Gastrointestinal Surgery and Minimal Access Surgery unit at GEM hospital and research center, Coimbatore, India. He is a Senior Consultant Bariatric Surgeon and his center is recognized by the Tamil Nadu Dr. MGR Medical University for conducting a 2-year fellowship program in bariatric surgery. Through his biannual training program, he has trained more than 150 surgeons in the field of bariatric surgery. He has also instituted international fellowship programs where physicians from abroad train with him in India.

Dr. Praveen Raj is currently the President of the Indian chapter of the International Excellence Federation of Bariatric Surgery and an active member of the Obesity and Metabolic Surgery Society of India and the International Federation for Surgery of Obesity and Metabolic disorders. He and his center were the first in South India to be accredited as an International Center of Excellence by the Surgical Review Corporation, USA. He has authored several papers on laparoscopic and bariatric surgery and presents frequently at conferences. His recently completed the NASHOST trial, aimed to study the influence of bariatric surgery on nonalcoholic fatty liver disease which is the first registered clinical trial on bariatric surgery in the country. He has also commenced a trial on lower BMI metabolic surgery for the treatment of type 2 diabetes mellitus, which when completed will be the first of its kind in the world. He has also instituted international fellowship programs where surgeons train with him in India.

Saravana Kumar graduated and completed his general surgical training from the Madurai Medical College, India. He later acquired his laparoscopic skills at the renowned Gem Hospital & Research Centre, Coimbatore, under Professor C. Palanivelu. He is currently a Senior Consultant Bariatric Surgeon in the Bariatric division of the Upper Gastrointestinal Surgery and Minimal Access Surgery unit at the same Institute. He has many international publications in the field of bariatric surgery and, along with Dr. Praveen Raj and Professor C. Palanivelu, is actively involved in training of surgeons. He is a member of the Association of Minimal Access Surgeons of India, the Obesity and Metabolic Surgery Society of India, and the International Federation for Surgery of Obesity and Metabolic disorders.

Rachel Maria Gomes graduated and completed her general surgical training with accolades from the Goa Medical College under the Goa University of India. She then specialized in gastrointestinal and laparoscopic surgery at the Bhatia Hospital and the Jaslok Hospital at Mumbai, India. She is currently a Senior Consultant General and Laparoscopic Surgeon under the Directorate of Health Services, Goa, India and was recently associated with the Bariatric Division of the Upper Gastrointestinal Surgery and Minimal Access Surgery unit of GEM Hospital & Research Centre at Coimbatore, India. Her clinical and research interests include advanced laparoscopic gastrointestinal surgery, laparoscopic hernia repairs, anti-reflux surgery and bariatric surgery. She has to her credit over 50 peer-reviewed national and international publications and book chapters, and has delivered numerous presentations at national and international conferences with several awards for outstanding presentations. She is a member of the Association of Surgeons of India, the Indian Association of Surgical Gastroenterology, the Indian Association of Gastrointestinal and Endoscopic Surgeons, the Obesity and Metabolic Surgery Society of India and the International Federation for Surgery of Obesity and Metabolic disorders.

Part I

Selection of a Patient

Selection Guidelines for Bariatric Surgery

1

Narong Boonyakard and Suthep Udomsawaengsup

1.1 Introduction

Morbid obesity is becoming a serious public health problem worldwide. In Asian countries, the prevalence has increased many times over in the past few decades. Bariatric surgery has been shown to be the most effective treatment for these patients. The primary goal of bariatric surgery is to reduce the body weight or the body mass index (BMI). However, it is increasingly recognized that this surgery can also help several medical comorbidities associated with obesity such as type 2 diabetes mellitus (T2DM), dyslipidemia, obstructive sleep apnea etc.

Clinical guidelines for bariatric surgery were first suggested by the NIH (National Institutes of Health) in 1991 and over the past few decades, there have been many modifications introduced by many national and international societies. BMI cutoff points and co-morbidities are commonly used to define the indications for bariatric surgery. According to the world health organization (WHO) criteria, BMI cutoffs for obesity in Asian population are lower than the Western countries because obesity associated health risks tend to occur at a lower threshold of BMI in Asians.

This aim of this chapter was to review the indications for bariatric surgery from many guidelines worldwide, especially in Asian countries. The discussed guidelines include those by the National Institutes of Health, Asian Pacific Metabolic and Bariatric Surgery Society, Diabetes Surgery Summit, Obesity Surgery Society of Australia and New Zealand, Asian Consensus Meeting of Metabolic Surgery, Asian Diabetes Surgery Summit, The International Diabetes Federation, The International Federation for the Surgery of Obesity-Asia Pacific, American Society for Metabolic & Bariatric Surgery and the International Federation for the Surgery of Obesity-European guidelines.

N. Boonyakard • S. Udomsawaengsup, MD, FACS, FRCST (✉)
Chula Minimally Invasive Surgery Center, Chulalongkorn University, Bangkok, Thailand
e-mail: suthep.u@gmail.com

P.R. Palanivelu et al. (eds.), *Bariatric Surgical Practice Guide*,
DOI 10.1007/978-981-10-2705-5_1

1.2 Guidelines Recommendation

1.2.1 Western Guidelines

1.2.1.1 National Institute of Health (NIH 1991, Update 2011)

The indication for bariatric surgery in an adult is a BMI ≥40 or BMI ≥35 with a serious health problem linked to obesity. These guidelines were updated in 2011 for adolescents (age >13 for girls and >15 for boys) wherein the indication was BMI ≥40 with serious health problems linked to weight with failed attempt at weight loss with conservative measures like diet and exercise for at least 6 months. Also it stressed the fact that the patients need to be committed to a healthy and active lifestyle.

1.2.1.2 Obesity Surgery Society of Australia and New Zealand (OSSANZ: 2008)

The indication for bariatric surgery is a BMI ≥40 or BMI ≥35 in the presence of severe obesity-associated complications. Surgery is recommended for patients with an age of ≥15 years. This guideline recommends against bariatric surgery for adolescents under the age of 14 years, pregnant or breast-feeding adolescents, significant cognitive disabilities, untreated or untreatable psychiatric or psychological disorder and Prader-Willi syndrome and other similar hyperphagic conditions.

1.2.1.3 American Society for Metabolic and Bariatric Surgery (ASMBS: 2013)

The indication for bariatric surgery is a BMI ≥40 without coexisting medical problems or BMI ≥35 with one or more severe obesity-related comorbidities. In patients with BMI of 30–34.9 with diabetes or metabolic syndrome, bariatric procedure may also be offered.

1.2.1.4 International Federation for the Surgery of Obesity: European Chapter (IFSO-EC: 2014)

The indication for bariatric surgery is a BMI ≥40 or BMI 35–40 with co-morbidities. Surgery is recommended for patients with in the age groups from 18 to 60 years.

1.2.2 Asia-Specific Guidelines

1.2.2.1 Asia Pacific Metabolic and Bariatric Surgery Society (APMBSS: 2005)

The indication for bariatric surgery for Asian people is a BMI ≥37 or BMI ≥32 with T2DM or two significant obesity related co-morbidities. Surgery is recommended for patients with in the age groups of >18 years and <65 years.

1.2.2.2 Asian Consensus Meeting of Metabolic Surgery (ACMOMS: 2008)

The indication for bariatric surgery in people with Asian ethnicity are BMI ≥35 without comorbidities, BMI ≥32 with comorbidities and BMI ≥30 if they have central obesity with at least two of the additional criteria for metabolic syndrome.

1.2.2.3 International Federation for the Surgery of Obesity: Asia Pacific Chapter (IFSO-APC: 2011)

Bariatric surgery should be considered in patients with BMI ≥35 with or without co-morbidities and patients with BMI ≥30 with T2DM or metabolic syndrome. In patients with BMI ≥27.5 with inadequately controlled T2DM or metabolic syndrome, the surgical approach may be considered as a non-primary alternative to treat. The recommended procedures are laparoscopic roux-en-Y gastric bypass (LRYGB), laparoscopic sleeve gastrectomy (LSG), laparoscopic adjustable gastric banding (LAGB) and biliopancreatic diversion-duodenal switch (BPD/DS). Surgery is recommended for patients with in the age of >18 and <65 years.

1.2.3 Guidelines from Medical Association/Societies

1.2.3.1 The International Diabetes Federation (IDF: 2011)

Bariatric surgery is an accepted option for T2DM patients with BMI ≥35 and alternative treatment for patients with BMI 30–35 with inadequately controlled T2DM. In Asian population, BMI may be reduced by 2.5 points.

1.2.3.2 Diabetes Surgery Summit (DSS 2007)

Bariatric surgery should be considered for the treatment of T2DM in patients with BMI ≥35 inadequately controlled by lifestyle and medical therapy and may also be appropriate as a non-primary alternative in patients with BMI of 30–35. The recommended surgical option for diabetes treatment is LRYGB.

1.2.3.3 Asian Diabetes Surgery Summit (ADSS: 2010)

Bariatric surgery for Asian diabetes people should be considered in patients with BMI ≥37 or BMI ≥32 when T2DM is not well controlled (HbA1c >7.5 %) after intensive medical treatment. Bariatric surgery may be considered in patients with BMI ≥27 with many co-morbidities and when T2DM is not well controlled (HbA1c >7.5 %) after intensive medical treatment. Surgery is recommended for patients with in the age groups of >18 years and <70 years.

Tables 1.1, 1.2, and 1.3 summarizes each of the guidelines according to BMI cut offs, age and recommended bariatric procedures respectively.

Table 1.1 Indication for surgery

Guidelines	Without comorbidities	With comorbidities	Recommendations
Western guidelines			
National Institute of Health	BMI ≥40	BMI ≥35	Should be considered
Obesity Surgery Society of Australia and New Zealand	BMI >40	BMI ≥35	Should be considered
American Society for Metabolic & Bariatric Surgery	BMI ≥40	BMI ≥35 BMI ≥30	Should be considered May also be offered
International Federation for the Surgery of Obesity: European Chapter	BMI ≥40	BMI ≥35	Should be considered
Asian guidelines			
Asia Pacific Metabolic and Bariatric Surgery Society	BMI >37	BMI ≥32 with DM or two co-morbidities	Should be considered
Asian Consensus Meeting of Metabolic Surgery	BMI ≥35	BMI ≥32 BMI ≥30 Central obesity + 2 metabolic BMI <30 Strictly under study protocol	Should be considered Should be considered
International Federation for the Surgery of Obesity: Asia Pacific Chapter	BMI ≥35	BMI ≥30 BMI ≥27.5 with inadequately controlled DM BMI <27.5 with inadequately controlled DM Strictly under study protocol	Should be considered May be considered
Medical association guidelines			
The International Diabetes Federation	–	BMI ≥35 with DM **(Asian −2.5) BMI 30–35 with inadequately controlled DM Alternative treatment	Accepted option
Diabetes Surgery Summit	–	BMI ≥35 BMI 30–35	Should be considered May also be appropriate
Asian Diabetes Surgery Summit	BMI ≥37	BMI ≥32 with DM (HbA1c >7.5) BMI ≥27 with many co-morbidities May be considered	Should be considered

**In Asian population, BMI may be reduced by 2.5 points.

Table 1.2 Age recommendations

Guidelines	Age in years (adult)	Age in years (pediatric)
Western guidelines		
National Institute of Health	–	>13 for girls, >15 for boys
Obesity Surgery Society of Australia and New Zealand	≥15	Against: under the age of 14 years
American Society for Metabolic & Bariatric Surgery	–	–
International Federation for the Surgery of Obesity: European Chapter	>18 to <60	Skeletal and developmental maturity
Asian guidelines		
Asia Pacific Metabolic and Bariatric Surgery Society	>18 to <65	<18: under special circumstances
Asian Consensus Meeting of Metabolic Surgery	–	–
International Federation for the Surgery of Obesity: Asia Pacific Chapter	>18 to <65	–
Diabetic association guidelines		
The International Diabetes Federation	–	–
Diabetes Surgery Summit	–	
Asian Diabetes Surgery Summit	>18 to <70	–

Table 1.3 Procedure recommendation

Guidelines	Operation
Western guidelines	
National Institute of Health	LABG, LRYGB, LSG, BPD-DS
Obesity Surgery Society of Australia and New Zealand	LAGB, RYGB, BPD/DS
American Society for Metabolic & Bariatric Surgery	–
International Federation for the Surgery of Obesity: European Chapter	LRYGB, LSG, LAGB, BPD/DS
Asian guidelines	
Asia Pacific Metabolic and Bariatric Surgery Society	–
Asian Consensus Meeting of Metabolic Surgery	–
International Federation for the Surgery of Obesity: Asia Pacific Chapter	LRYGB, LSG, LAGB, BPD/DS
Diabetic association guidelines	
The International Diabetes Federation	LRYGB, LAGB, BPD, BPD-DS, LSG
Diabetes Surgery Summit	LRYGB, LAGB, BPD
Asian Diabetes Surgery Summit	–

LAGB laparoscopic adjustable gastric banding, *LSG* laparoscopic sleeve gastrectomy (LSG), *LRYGB* laparoscopic roux-en-Y gastric bypass, *BPD-DS* biliopancreatic diversion-duodenal switch

Conclusions

All Western clinical guidelines recommend that bariatric surgery should be considered for a BMI ≥40 without co-morbidities and a BMI ≥35 with comorbidities. Some suggest that bariatric surgery may be offered for a BMI ≥30. It needs to be also noted that all the guidelines stress the importance of failed weight loss attempts and the need for long term lifestyle change. Most Asia-specific guidelines recommend that bariatric surgery can be considered for a BMI ≥35–37 without co-morbidities and a BMI ≥30–32 with comorbidities. A recent consensus has also suggested that bariatric surgery can be considered for BMI ≥27.5 with inadequately controlled DM. Also bariatric surgery may be offered for BMI <27.5 with inadequately controlled DM strictly under study protocol. Most medical association clinical guidelines consider bariatric surgery as an accepted option with a BMI ≥35 (−2.5 points for Asians) with DM. They also consider bariatric surgery to be an alternative treatment for BMI 30–35 with inadequately controlled DM. Some suggest that bariatric surgery may be offered for BMI ≥27 with inadequately controlled DM. Most societies suggest that bariatric surgery is recommended for patients with an age of >18 years with less than this only in special circumstances. Patients above 65–70 years are usually not recommended for bariatric surgery. Standard recommended bariatric procedures are laparoscopic adjustable gastric banding, laparoscopic sleeve gastrectomy, laparoscopic roux-en-Y gastric bypass and biliopancreatic diversion-duodenal switch.

Recommendations

- BMI is a major factor for patient selection for bariatric surgery
- BMI cutoffs can be adjusted based on patient population and severity of co-morbidities
- Bariatric surgery may be offered outside existing guidelines in special circumstances

2 Bariatric Surgery in Adolescents

Simon Chapman, Martha Ford-Adams, and Ashish Desai

2.1 Introduction

The worldwide rise in obesity in the last 30 years is now well documented, and it places a significant burden of morbidity and mortality on adult populations across the globe. Comorbidities that accompany the rise in obesity affect all aspects of human physiology, and may even through epigenetic mechanisms affect our as yet unborn future generations.

A rising prevalence of obesity is also being seen in the paediatric population. Data from the national schools measurement programme suggested that 19.1 % of all children aged 11 years were obese in 2013–2014 in UK [1]. Of these approximately 2.9 % of girls and 3.9 % of boys have severe obesity [2] By adolescence, obesity is often well-established and difficult to reverse as behaviours and environment are often entrenched. This is exacerbated by physiology i.e. adolescence is a time of physiological relative insulin resistance driven by growth, and therefore a vulnerable time for the development of diabetes.

The management of obesity internationally has been to focus on the treatment of comorbidities whilst encouraging weight loss through lifestyle measures, reserving bariatric surgery for those situations when the medical comorbidities are intolerable or they outweigh the risks related to surgery. Given the widespread and popular success of bariatric surgery, it would follow therefore that a similar approach can be used to tackle the rise in childhood obesity – after all, it is known that obese children tend to become obese adults, will have lower attainment in education and training, will therefore be less productive in the work place and use more resources through

S. Chapman, BA, BM, FRCPCH • M. Ford-Adams, DCH, FRCPCH
Department of Pediatrics, Kings College Hospital, London, UK
e-mail: simon.chapman@nhs.net; martha.ford-adams@nhs.net

A. Desai, MCh, DNB, FRCS (✉)
Department of Pediatric Surgery, Kings College Hospital, London, UK
e-mail: ashishdesai@nhs.net

P.R. Palanivelu et al. (eds.), *Bariatric Surgical Practice Guide*,
DOI 10.1007/978-981-10-2705-5_2

treatment of their comorbidities [3–9]. Furthermore, children now experience similar comorbidities as adults at ever-earlier ages [10].

Whilst primary prevention of obesity is the obvious answer to this, community-based interventions have yet to demonstrate significant and lasting positive results. In the meantime, while we wait for political and national policies on obesity to have effect, we might consider surgery in children as an answer to those who cannot wait. However, compelling as this may sound, the use of bariatric surgery as secondary prevention in children should be approached with caution.

2.2 BMI Cut-offs Defining Obesity in Children

The definition of obesity in children is itself extrapolated from the adult definition. The main accepted surrogate measure of obesity and overweight in adults is adjusted weight for height, or the body mass index (BMI), calculated by dividing the square of the height in meters by the weight in kilograms. Based on mortality and morbidity data, BMI is associated with worse outcomes once it begins to rise above 25 kg/m^2 [11]. This has led to the World Health Organisation (WHO) definition of obesity based on BMI cut-offs (Table 2.1). In childhood, however, this mortality and morbidity data has never been collected, and therefore cut off values for obesity are merely extrapolated back from adults [12]. A BMI of 25, 30, 35 or 40 kg/m^2 in an adult patient equates to 1, 2, 3 and 4 standard deviations from the mean, cut-offs which can be applied further back on the growth charts of children. It is not yet clear if the relationship between complications or mortality and BMI in adults necessarily is the same in children. There are several reasons to suggest that children may be different to adults: height, weight and body composition all change markedly from birth, through childhood, to adolescence and finally adulthood. Furthermore childhood and adolescence (characterised by puberty) have markedly different effects on metabolism to adulthood, and therefore to managing the effects of excess adipose.

Table 2.1 World Health Organisation (WHO) classification of obesity based on BMI cut-offs.

	BMI (kg/m^2)	
Classification	Principal cut-off points	Additional cut-off points
Normal range	**18.50–24.99**	**18.50–22.99**
		23.00–24.99
Overweight	**≥25.00**	**≥25.00**
Pre-obese	25.00–29.99	25.00–27.49
		27.50–29.99
Obese	**≥30.00**	**≥30.00**
Obese class I	30.00–34.99	30.00–32.49
		32.50–34.99
Obese class II	35.00–39.99	35.00–37.49
		37.50–39.99
Obese class III	≥40.00	≥40.00

For example, HOMA-IR (Homeostatic model of assessment) scores, a measure of insulin resistance, doubles in puberty alone [13]. Whilst it is true that children get the same comorbidities as adults, and indeed particularly some of the metabolic and cardiovascular risk factors manifest as early as 10 years, the level of obesity at which these occur is still not known [10].

2.3 Rationale for Intervention

Evaluating the 'cost' of obesity is of great interest to governments planning health care for future generations. In 2007 the economic cost of obesity in the UK was placed at £15.8 billion per year, encompassing £4.2 billion in direct costs to the NHS, and taking into account other costs in loss of earnings and productivity in the wider economy [9]. In children these economic estimates have not been made but there is clearly a long-term economic cost when children drop out of education and training as a result of their obesity [14, 15].

2.4 Treatment Options and Patient Selection

2.4.1 Lifestyle Modifications

Dietetic and lifestyle interventions, together with treatment of medical comorbidities, form the cornerstone of obesity management particularly in the younger age group. In a growing child, weight maintenance could lead to significant reduction in BMI due to increasing height. This in turn is associated with an improvement in cardiovascular risk factors and comorbidities of obesity such as diabetes mellitus, non-alcoholic fatty liver disease and polycystic ovary syndrome. In particular, children aged 5–12 years and children who are overweight rather than obese profit from lifestyle interventions [16].

2.4.2 Bariatric Surgery

Bariatric surgery has been shown to be effective in achieving meaningful and sustained weight loss as well as resolution of obesity-related comorbidities in adults [17].

2.4.2.1 Patient Selection Guidelines

Indications for surgery in adolescents have evolved in recent years so that criteria for surgery are now more clearly defined. In the UK, NICE (National Institute for Health and Care Excellence) have provided guidance regarding appropriate patient selection for adolescent bariatric surgery. Adolescent bariatric surgery should be offered in exceptional circumstances to patients who have nearly completed puberty. Their BMI should be between 35 and 40 kg/m^2 if they have significant comorbidities or above 40 kg/m^2 without comorbidities. This should be performed in a multi-disciplinary team with paediatric expertise for preoperative and postoperative care. Similar guidelines were also approved by Scottish Intercollegiate Guidelines Network (SIGN) in 2010.

2.4.2.2 Why Surgery Should Be Avoided Before Puberty?

The average age of onset of puberty in the UK is 11.2 years in girls and 11.6 years in boys, with the onset of menarche now 13.06 years [18]. Several records from northern Europe from the 1860s show that menarche at that time was 16–17 years, and sporadic reports at periods since suggest a gradual reduction as body mass has increased [19]. Whilst improved nutrition has begun this process in train, several anthropometric and epidemiological studies and the discovery of leptin (1994) and kisspeptin (1996), all increasingly point towards the obesity epidemic as an important factor in this decline [20–22].

The process of puberty is a fascinating and remarkable stage of life. It is said that primates are the only species to experience it. During this time the skeleton changes, the brain remodels, and the infertile child develops over 2–3 years into the fertile adult. Puberty leads to changes in body composition too, with lean mass in boys increasing to form the 'android' shape, and fat mass redistributing in girls to form the 'gynaecoid' shape in preparation for child rearing. It is no mistake that evolution has chosen to tie the fates of nutrition and fertility together.

When assessing children and young people, therefore, it is critical to assess their obesity in the context of their stage of puberty. In 1948 Dr James Tanner, a paediatric endocrinologist began a project in Harpenden just to the north of London, studying growth in malnourished children. Over his career that followed, however, his observations led him to characterise the five discrete 'Tanner' stages of puberty, and importantly to link these directly to the growth chart. In girls, he noted, the growth spurt begins early in puberty, accompanying thelarche (development of the breast bud), whereas in boys it does not occur until later into puberty (Tanner IV). Clearly, obesity that is identified prior to puberty requires relatively less intervention than that found later on after most growth is complete, as the increase in stature counters the weight to some degree. One way to see this is in BMI; to calculate BMI one must first square the height before dividing it into the weight. This means that changes in height disproportionately affect BMI over changes in weight. Strategies to weight loss in small children with moderate obesity therefore may often seek to maintain weight, rather than actively to lose it until such time as the growth spurt has occurred and allowed the height to 'catch up' with the weight.

It must be emphasised that there is only a window of opportunity for this pubertal transformation to occur. In the same way that body composition changes, so too do the androgens and oestrogens that come in puberty causing the skeleton to grow and strengthen. Bone mineral accrual is at its peak at the same time as the growth spurt, though continues on into the third decade, long after epiphyses have fused. This process is uniquely sensitive to nutrition – as evidenced by the secular trend in increase in stature alongside improvements over the last century with sanitation and nutrition. Short stature and 'stunted' growth due to starvation in childhood is well described, indeed a key finding of James Tanner's work [23].

Given this, nutritional interventions in growing children must be carefully considered. Obesity is mistakenly thought of as the complication of excessively wealthy diets but this is undermined by the well-recognised knowledge that obesity is found in greatest prevalence amongst the more deprived groups in society, a finding seen across the world [24, 25]. In fact the cause of obesity is in large part down to diets rich in energy and poor in nutrient. Many children with obesity have very poor quality diets [1, 26]. Calorie restriction as part of a diet must go hand in hand with appropriate supplementation or this will lead to growth restriction. In the adult, calorie restriction typically causes a reduction in the metabolic rate, a switch in metabolism to catabolism (ketosis, lipolysis, proteolysis) and activation of a state of subfertility or infertility mediated through reduction in pulsatility in gonadotropin releasing hormone (GnRH) [27]. Clinically this manifests as bradycardia, hypothermia and hypotension, mood change and secondary amenorrhoea. Patients have muscle wasting and accompanying specific signs of coexisting nutritional deficiencies. In children, however, all this occurs but also growth is affected – starvation paradoxically causes an increase in growth hormone alongside growth hormone resistance and a decoupling of GH-IGF-1 interaction contributing to growth failure [28, 29]. Bone demineralisation occurs as a result of nutrient and vitamin D depletion, and muscle wasting which in turn reduces the strain on bones required for remodelling to occur.

It is for this reason that international centres that consider bariatric surgery in children do not intervene until growth is complete, lest the calorie restriction and metabolic changes that necessarily follow a bariatric procedure prejudice the growth and bone mineralisation in the growing child irreversibly.

2.4.2.3 Adolescent Bariatric Team

The adolescent bariatric team should consist of the following:

Paediatrician with special interest in obesity
Paediatric or adult surgeon with expertise in adolescent bariatric surgery
Paediatric dietician and
Child or adolescent psychologist and/or psychiatrist

It is desirable to also have a paediatric nurse practitioner and physical trainer. Expertise and referral pathways in child safeguarding are essential.

2.4.2.4 Surgical Outcomes and Effect on Comorbidities

Same surgeries are performed in adolescents as in adults with almost similar results. A meta-analysis of bariatric surgery in adolescents shows that there is moderate weight loss in all patients after surgery. Mean BMI loss at 12 months was −17.2 kg/m^2 for laparoscopic roux-en-y bypass (LRYGB), −14.5 kg/m^2 for laparoscopic sleeve gastrectomy (LSG) and −10.5 kg/m^2 for laparoscopic adjustable gastric banding (LAGB) [30]. In an interventional study comparing adolescents with adults, BMI loss was 32 % and 31 % respectively in adolescents and adults at 2 years follow up. LRYGB has also been shown to improve cardiovascular risks as well as improve quality of life [31]. Surgery is effective in improving obesity related comorbidities. LRYGB and LSG are both effective. Type 2 diabetes (T2DM) remissions occur in almost 95 % of participants while obstructive sleep apnoea improves in 99 % of patients [32]. LRYGB and LSG are also known to improve weight-related quality of life significantly [33]. However, studies have also showed increased risk of micronutrient deficiency with almost 57 % patients having hypoferritinaemia in one study. These patients need long term psychological support too as there is increased risk of addictive substance misuse and attempted suicides.

2.4.2.5 Bariatric Surgery and Capacity to Consent

As bariatric surgery gathers momentum and gains in popularity in adults, the pressure mounts to perform the same procedures on children [34]. The comorbidities of obesity now present at increasingly young ages. It is not uncommon to see small children as young as 2 years with obstructive sleep apnoea. As these cases present, clinicians increasingly resort to these operations at lower and lower ages. The youngest reported case is only 2.5 years of age [35]. In this age group however there is no published data on efficacy, safety or cost effectiveness. By contrast, in small children even with severe comorbidities there is evidence that confident parenting and multidisciplinary support over time can achieve good outcomes [36, 37]. This has led many to question the morality of such an approach given the epidemic nature of obesity across the world [38]. Far beyond the unanswered questions of outcome are also the unexplored ethical issues on whether this intervention respects the child's autonomy, or is performed with informed consent or assent.

2.4.2.6 Education and Training

Children with obesity are more likely to have depression, anxiety and poor self-esteem [39–44]. Obesity in children is associated with lower levels of socioeconomic status [39]. When compared with their normal weight peers, they miss more school and have poorer levels of educational attainment [14]. These are of course associations and not causal relationships, but in those cases where obesity is a significant contributory factor to young people falling out of education and training, bariatric surgery should be considered early on.

Conclusions

Whilst the evidence is available therefore in the adult population for BMI-related morbidity, the clear statistical relationship between obesity in childhood and associated illness has yet to be demonstrated. Clearly, overweight children are less healthy than 'normal' weight children, but the degree to which BMI is related to physical health risk has yet to be characterised. This is important when deciding whether to apply an intervention as serious and irreversible as bariatric surgery on a child – do the risks of surgery outweigh the risks of doing nothing? In these circumstances, whilst comorbidities can be demonstrated often in children, the absolute risk of not intervening is not known. This uncertainty is compounded by the fact that the comorbidities themselves are not static in a growing child, and may indeed improve if left alone.

Furthermore, bariatric surgery is as yet of unproven efficacy and safety in small children – there are key physiological, psychological and developmental differences between pre-pubertal or pubertal children and adults that should prevent the widespread use of this intervention until more is known about the longer term implications.

Recommendations

- Bariatric surgery can be offered to adolescents who have nearly completed puberty at a BMI cut-off of 35 kg/m^2 if they have significant comorbidities or above 40 kg/m^2 without comorbidities.
- Assessing the capacity of adolescents to make an informed decision regarding weight loss surgery and to comply with postoperative instructions is important. Parental support for bariatric surgery for their adolescent is also important.
- Laparoscopic adjustable gastric banding, laparoscopic sleeve gastrectomy and laparoscopic roux-en-y gastric bypass have comparable safety in adolescents.
- Bariatric surgery should be performed in a multi-disciplinary team with paediatric expertise for pre- and postoperative care.

References

1. Statistics on obesity, physical activity and diet, England – 2015 – Publications – GOV.UK [Internet]. [Cited 2016 Mar 19]. Available from: https://www.gov.uk/government/statistics/statistics-on-obesity-physical-activity-and-diet-england-2015.
2. Ells LJ, Hancock C, Copley VR, Mead E, Dinsdale H, Kinra S, et al. Prevalence of severe childhood obesity in England: 2006-2013. Arch Dis Child. 2015;100(7):631–6.
3. Singh AS, Mulder C, Twisk JWR, van Mechelen W, Chinapaw MJM. Tracking of childhood overweight into adulthood: a systematic review of the literature. Obes Rev Off J Int Assoc Study Obes. 2008;9(5):474–88.
4. Herman KM, Craig CL, Gauvin L, Katzmarzyk PT. Tracking of obesity and physical activity from childhood to adulthood: the Physical Activity Longitudinal Study. Int J Pediatr Obes IJPO Off J Int Assoc Study Obes. 2009;4(4):281–8.
5. Carey FR, Singh GK, Brown HS, Wilkinson AV. Educational outcomes associated with childhood obesity in the United States: cross-sectional results from the 2011-2012 National Survey of Children's Health. Int J Behav Nutr Phys Act. 2015;12 Suppl 1:S3.
6. Gortmaker SL, Must A, Perrin JM, Sobol AM, Dietz WH. Social and economic consequences of overweight in adolescence and young adulthood. N Engl J Med. 1993;329(14):1008–12.
7. Sargent JD, Blanchflower DG. Obesity and stature in adolescence and earnings in young adulthood. Analysis of a British birth cohort. Arch Pediatr Adolesc Med. 1994;148(7):681–7.
8. Viner RM, Cole TJ. Adult socioeconomic, educational, social, and psychological outcomes of childhood obesity: a national birth cohort study. BMJ. 2005;330(7504):1354.
9. Butland B, Jebb S, Kopelman P. Reducing obesity: future choices – Publications – GOV.UK [Internet]. [Cited 2016 Mar 19]. Available from: https://www.gov.uk/government/publications/reducing-obesity-future-choices.
10. Pulgarón ER. Childhood obesity: a review of increased risk for physical and psychological comorbidities. Clin Ther. 2013;35(1):A18–32.

11. Prospective Studies Collaboration, Whitlock G, Lewington S, Sherliker P, Clarke R, Emberson J, et al. Body-mass index and cause-specific mortality in 900 000 adults: collaborative analyses of 57 prospective studies. Lancet Lond Engl. 2009;373(9669):1083–96.
12. Cole TJ, Bellizzi MC, Flegal KM, Dietz WH. Establishing a standard definition for child overweight and obesity worldwide: international survey. BMJ. 2000;320(7244):1240–3.
13. Xu L, Li M, Yin J, Cheng H, Yu M, Zhao X, et al. Change of body composition and adipokines and their relationship with insulin resistance across pubertal development in obese and non-obese Chinese children: the BCAMS study. Int J Endocrinol. 2012;2012:389108.
14. Geier AB, Foster GD, Womble LG, McLaughlin J, Borradaile KE, Nachmani J, et al. The relationship between relative weight and school attendance among elementary schoolchildren. Obes Silver Spring Md. 2007;15(8):2157–61.
15. Must A. Morbidity and mortality associated with elevated body weight in children and adolescents. Am J Clin Nutr. 1996;63(3 Suppl):445S–7.
16. Reinehr T. Lifestyle intervention in childhood obesity: changes and challenges. Nat Rev Endocrinol. 2013;9(10):607–14.
17. Puzziferri N, Roshek TB, Mayo HG, Gallagher R, Belle SH, Livingston EH. Long-term follow-up after bariatric surgery: a systematic review. JAMA. 2014;312(9):934–42.
18. de Muinich Keizer SM, Mul D. Trends in pubertal development in Europe. Hum Reprod Update. 2001;7(3):287–91.
19. Kaplowitz PB. Link between body fat and the timing of puberty. Pediatrics. 2008;121 Suppl 3:S208–17.
20. Kaplowitz PB, Slora EJ, Wasserman RC, Pedlow SE, Herman-Giddens ME. Earlier onset of puberty in girls: relation to increased body mass index and race. Pediatrics. 2001;108(2):347–53.
21. Zhang Y, Proenca R, Maffei M, Barone M, Leopold L, Friedman JM. Positional cloning of the mouse obese gene and its human homologue. Nature. 1994;372(6505):425–32.
22. Lee JH, Miele ME, Hicks DJ, Phillips KK, Trent JM, Weissman BE, et al. KiSS-1, a novel human malignant melanoma metastasis-suppressor gene. J Natl Cancer Inst. 1996;88(23):1731–7.
23. (mr) Web Master UK. Find data [Internet]. 2010 [cited 2016 Mar 19]. Available from: http://www.hscic.gov.uk/catalogue/PUB16988.
24. Zilanawala A, Davis-Kean P, Nazroo J, Sacker A, Simonton S, Kelly Y. Race/ethnic disparities in early childhood BMI, obesity and overweight in the United Kingdom and United States. Int J Obes (Lond) 2005. 2015;39(3):520–9.
25. King T, Kavanagh AM, Jolley D, Turrell G, Crawford D. Weight and place: a multilevel cross-sectional survey of area-level social disadvantage and overweight/obesity in Australia. Int J Obes (Lond) 2005. 2006;30(2):281–7.
26. National Diet and Nutrition Survey: results from years 1 to 4 (combined) of the rolling programme for 2008 and 2009 to 2011 and 2012 – Publications – GOV.UK [Internet]. [Cited 2016 Mar 19]. Available from: https://www.gov.uk/government/statistics/national-diet-and-nutrition-survey-results-from-years-1-to-4-combined-of-the-rolling-programme-for-2008-and-2009-to-2011-and-2012.
27. Keys A, Brožek J, Henschel A, Mickelsen O, Taylor LH. The biology of human starvation (2 vols), vol. xxxii. Oxford: University of Minnesota Press; 1950. 1385 p.
28. Merimee TJ, Fineberg SE. Growth hormone secretion in starvation: a reassessment. J Clin Endocrinol Metab. 1974;39(2):385–6.
29. Fazeli PK, Misra M, Goldstein M, Miller KK, Klibanski A. Fibroblast growth factor-21 may mediate growth hormone resistance in anorexia nervosa. J Clin Endocrinol Metab. 2010;95(1):369–74.
30. Black JA, White B, Viner RM, Simmons RK. Bariatric surgery for obese children and adolescents: a systematic review and meta-analysis. Obes Rev Off J Int Assoc Study Obes. 2013;14(8):634–44.

31. Olbers T, Gronowitz E, Werling M, Mårlid S, Flodmark C-E, Peltonen M, et al. Two-year outcome of laparoscopic Roux-en-Y gastric bypass in adolescents with severe obesity: results from a Swedish Nationwide Study (AMOS). Int J Obes (Lond) 2005. 2012;36(11):1388–95.
32. Inge TH, Courcoulas AP, Jenkins TM, Michalsky MP, Helmrath MA, Brandt ML, et al. Weight loss and health status 3 years after bariatric surgery in adolescents. N Engl J Med. 2016;374(2):113–23.
33. Alqahtani AR, Elahmedi MO, Al Qahtani A. Co-morbidity resolution in morbidly obese children and adolescents undergoing sleeve gastrectomy. Surg Obes Relat Dis Off J Am Soc Bariatr Surg. 2014;10(5):842–50.
34. Ibele AR, Mattar SG. Adolescent bariatric surgery. Surg Clin North Am. 2011;91(6):1339–51, x.
35. Mohaidly MA, Suliman A, Malawi H. Laparoscopic sleeve gastrectomy for a two-and half year old morbidly obese child. Int J Surg Case Rep. 2013;4(11):1057–60.
36. Golan M. Parenting and management of pediatric obesity. In: Clinical insights: obesity and childhood [Internet]. Future Medicine Ltd; 2014 [cited 2016 Mar 19]. p. 39–56. Available from: http://www.futuremedicine.com/doi/abs/10.2217/ebo.13.549.
37. Brown RE, Willis TA, Aspinall N, Candida H, George J, Rudolf MCJ. Preventing child obesity: a long-term evaluation of the HENRY approach. Community Pract J Community Pract Health Visit Assoc. 2013;86(7):23–7.
38. Hofmann B. Bariatric surgery for obese children and adolescents: a review of the moral challenges. BMC Med Ethics. 2013;14:18.
39. Bell LM, Curran JA, Byrne S, Roby H, Suriano K, Jones TW, et al. High incidence of obesity co-morbidities in young children: a cross-sectional study. J Paediatr Child Health. 2011;47(12):911–7.
40. Eschenbeck H, Kohlmann C-W, Dudey S, Schurholz T. Physician-diagnosed obesity in German 6- to 14-year-olds. Prevalence and comorbidity of internalising disorders, externalising disorders, and sleep disorders. Obes Facts. 2009;2(2):67–73.
41. Hillman JB, Dorn LD, Bin Huang. Association of anxiety and depressive symptoms and adiposity among adolescent females, using dual energy X-ray absorptiometry. Clin Pediatr (Phila). 2010;49(7):671–7.
42. Gibson LY, Byrne SM, Blair E, Davis EA, Jacoby P, Zubrick SR. Clustering of psychosocial symptoms in overweight children. Aust N Z J Psychiatry. 2008;42(2):118–25.
43. Datar A, Sturm R. Childhood overweight and parent- and teacher-reported behavior problems: evidence from a prospective study of kindergartners. Arch Pediatr Adolesc Med. 2004;158(8):804–10.
44. Anderson SE, Cohen P, Naumova EN, Must A. Association of depression and anxiety disorders with weight change in a prospective community-based study of children followed up into adulthood. Arch Pediatr Adolesc Med. 2006;160(3):285–91.

Selection of Bariatric Surgery Procedures in Special Circumstances

3

Praveen Raj Palanivelu

Bariatric surgery has evolved to be an excellent treatment modality for the treatment of obesity and related co-morbidities with standardization of guidelines for selection of the patient; however controversies still exist in certain situations in bariatric surgery. This not only includes the need for bariatric surgery, but also the choice of appropriate procedures. In this chapter, we have reviewed the existing literature on the role of bariatric surgery in the elderly, in the super obese and in those with pre-existing dyslipidemia.

3.1 Bariatric Surgery in the Super Obese

Bariatric surgery has provided the most consistent results in terms of weight loss and resolution of comorbidities [1]. It is also a known fact that morbidly obese patients are high risk candidates for any surgical intervention and this risk increases with increasing body mass index (BMI) [2, 3]. It has been shown that in terms of percentage of excess weight loss (%EWL), the results in morbidly obese patients have been inferior in the super obese [4, 5]. Considering these factors, selection of an appropriate bariatric procedure needs better understanding in this specific subset of patients. With no available guidelines, this subsection aims to understand the effectiveness of the various bariatric procedures available in this group of patients.

A BMI above 50 is referred as super obesity. A BMI more than 60 is referred to as super super obesity and a BMI over 70 is referred to as mega obesity. All different bariatric procedures have been described in this subset of patients including

P.R. Palanivelu, MS, DNB, DNB(SGE), FALS, FMAS
Bariatric Division, Upper Gastrointestinal Surgery and Minimal Access Surgery Unit, GEM Hospital and Research Centre, Coimbatore, India
e-mail: drraj@geminstitute.in

P.R. Palanivelu et al. (eds.), *Bariatric Surgical Practice Guide*,
DOI 10.1007/978-981-10-2705-5_3

laparoscopic sleeve gastrectomy (LSG), laparoscopic roux-en-Y gastric bypass (LRYGB), laparoscopic adjustable gastric banding (LAGB), laparoscopic minigastric bypass (LMGB), laparoscopic biliopancreatic diversion/duodenal switch (LBPD/DS) with variable success among them [6–16].

LSG was initially performed as a first stage procedure prior to LRYGB or LBPD/DS in super obese patients [17, 18]. With excellent outcomes, it has evolved into a primary stand alone procedure. This staged option is still the most preferred option in many centres. This is mainly due to the simplicity of LSG in these patients compared to the bypass procedures and the reasonable outcomes with the procedure [6–8]. Lemanu et al. had shown a better %EWL of 58.9 % in the superobese patients compared to non-super obese patients with no increase in the major complication rate [6]. Daigle et al. demonstrated a %EWL of 48.3 % with LSG in elderly super obese [8]. This was slightly lesser than the LRYGB group and significantly better that LAGB which has had a poorer result overall [12].

LRYGB has also been increasingly performed in the super and super super obese. Mehaffey et al. had shown that LRYGB was well tolerated with no significant differences in post-operative outcomes and complications [4]. Schwartz et al. had demonstrated a %EWL of 55 % at 2 years and concluded that LRYGB was effective in terms of weight loss, resolution of comorbidities and improvements in quality of life (QoL) as well [9]. Giodano et al. had shown that even when compared to LAGB, there was no difference in the early complication rate with a %EWL of 55 % at 1 year [10]. Similar results have been shown in the Asian population as well [11]. It has also been shown that construction of a longer roux limb LRYGB could be more efficient in super obese patients. But with only limited data available, no firm conclusions can be drawn [19].

LBPD/DS when compared to LRYGB had greater weight loss in this group of patients. But this was at the expense of more frequent gastrointestinal side effects, more nutritional complications requiring more closer follow up and supplementations [20]. Even distal RYGB has been reported to have high mortality rates in super obese patients [15].

This now leaves us with the option of LSG and LRYGB.As discussed above Daigle et al. has shown better weight loss outcomes with LRYGB compared to LSG [8]. Zerrweck et al. also had shown that amongst the two procedures LRYGB had a significantly better weight loss at 1 year (64 % vs 44 %) [21]. Similar results has been shown by a few others too [22, 23]. Considering the above results, both LRYGB and LSG can be safely done in the super obese and super-super obese patients. But when LSG is chosen, the possibility of requiring a second stage procedure is nearly 50 % [24]. This has to be discussed with the patients in advance in the decision making.

In mega obese patients, considering the high risk profiles and the higher complication rates with malabsorptive procedures, staged procedures in the form of first stage LSG followed by a second stage LRYGB or LBPD/DS is recommended [25]. Eldar et al. also had shown that staged procedures in patients with BMI between 70 and 125 had better weight loss outcomes compared to single stage LSG/LRYGB [26].

3.2 Bariatric Surgery in Elderly

The prevalence of morbid obesity is also rising sharply amongst the elderly patients. With the additional burden of co-morbidities in the elderly, quality of life deteriorates further. Bariatric surgery has evolved to be the primary treatment option for the morbidly obese who fail lifestyle interventions [27]. There is sufficient data on the efficacy of these surgical procedures on weight reduction and remission of the associated co-morbidities. Bariatric surgery in most centers is limited to patients <65 years of age for many reasons [27]. Concerns regarding increased perioperative complications had led to reluctance to offer bariatric surgery to older patients [28]. Scozzari et al. had reported age as an important prognostic factor in bariatric surgery and had recommended surgical indications in patients >50 years should be carefully weighed [29]. Age is considered to be an independent prognostic factor in addition to BMI, presence of diabetes mellitus and smoking in predicting postoperative mortality [30]. Santo et al. had reported increased incidence of postoperative thromboembolism in the elderly [31]. Further, increased post-operative morbidity and mortality rates in the elderly, as reported by Flum et al. and Livingston et al. has been a concern among surgeons on the safety of procedures in the elderly [28, 32].

With improvement in anesthetic techniques, standardization of surgical procedures and better patient selection, there's now sufficient data on the safety and efficacy of the bariatric surgical procedures in the elderly [33]. Ramirez et al. had shown bariatric surgeries can be safely performed even in patients >70 years of age with low rate of complications and acceptable improvement of co-morbidities [34]. Although the elderly patients (>65 years) have a slightly prolonged hospital stay, Dorman et al. had reported no increased morbidity or mortality compared to the younger population [35]. Willkomm et al. reported no differences in post-operative complications between patients above and less than 65 years of age [33]. A recent meta-analysis of 1206 elderly patients operated for morbid obesity had reported a mortality rate of 0.25 % which is comparable to the mortality rates published by the Longitudinal Assessment of Bariatric Surgery Consortium for a younger cohort of patients (0.3 %) [36]. Most of the available data on bariatric surgery for patients >50 year has been either for LRYGB or LAGB [37–48]. In the meta-analysis by Lynch et al., perioperative complication rates and mortality were higher in LRYGB group compared to LAGB group [36]. At the same time, they had also shown better weight loss at 6 and 12 months and significantly better co-morbidity resolution in the LRYGB group [27].

Since its inception, LSG has evolved to be an acceptable standalone procedure for morbid obesity. A randomized controlled trial by Andrei Keidar et al. had shown no difference in excess weight loss or resolution of co-morbidities compared to LRYGB [49]. Yaghoubian et al. had shown comparable morbidity and mortality and although insignificant, but better weight loss in the sleeve gastrectomy group [50]. Vidal et al. had shown similar short and midterm weight loss between the two procedures and more importantly reduced complications rates in the sleeve gastrectomy group [51]. The safety and efficacy of LSG has also been demonstrated in the elderly group also. The results of Van Rutte et al. and Soto et al. have shown LSG to be relatively safe and effective procedure in the terms of weight loss and co-morbidity resolution in the elderly [52, 53]. Considering the safety profile and better results, LSG has emerged to be a better alternative to LRYGB and LAGB, as suggested by Carlin et al. [54]. But the efficacy of LSG has been questioned by a few authors. A recent meta-analysis by Li et al. had shown LRYGB to be more effective to LSG, both in weight loss and also resolution of co-morbidities [55]. There exists very limited data on the comparison of these procedures in the patient groups over 50 years of age. We have retrospectively analyzed our patients over 50 year of age where LRYGB had a %EWL of 82.76 % at 12 months which was significantly better compared to LSG with %EWL of 60.19 % [55]. This result was similar to the results reported from many other centers [37, 39, 52, 53].

In conclusion, bariatric surgery is an effective procedure for weight loss and can be safely performed even in the elderly. Although LSG has emerged to be a standalone bariatric procedure with comparable results to LRYGB in the general population, LRYGB may offer better weight loss compared to LSG with no added morbidity.

3.3 Bariatric Surgery in Dyslipidemia

Bariatric surgery over the years has proven to be an effective treatment for all components of the metabolic syndrome. This also includes dyslipidemia along with resolution of diabetes and hypertension [56, 57]. A still unanswered question is whether this improvement in the lipid profile is merely weight-dependent or otherwise or whether its related to the inherent principles of the bariatric procedure itself [57]. This along with the predicting factors is still not very clear. With many varieties of bariatric procedures being performed, this sub-section aims to understand the effects of different bariatric procedures on the outcomes of different parameters of dyslipidemia.

Based on existing literature, it is now very clear that intestinal malabsorption has a significant role to play in improving all the parameters of dyslipidemia [58]. The same has also been shown by the Scopinaro procedure as well where intestinal malabsorption has significant impact of the improvement in lipid profiles [59]. A recent RCT had also shown that when laparoscopic duodenal switch (LDS) was compared to laparoscopic roux en Y gastric bypass (LRYGB), the reductions in total cholesterol (TC), low density lipoprotein (LDL) and triglycerides (TG) was significantly better when compared to the LRYGB group, but at the expense of more surgical, nutritional complications and gastrointestinal side-effects [60]. It is also clear that a purely restrictive procedure like a LDS, although has demonstrated some improvement especially with improvements in high density lipoprotein (HDL) and TG, it has been mainly related to weight loss [61]. With decreasing popularity of malabsorptive procedures, the focus of research has been mainly on outcomes of LRYGB and LSG.

Increasing reports are now proving LSG to be an effective alternative to LRYGB for treatment of obesity and type 2 diabetes, however its effects on dyslipidemia is hardly reported. It is now clear that the mechanisms of LSG on the resolution of type 2 diabetes is beyond just restriction like accelerated gastric emptying, increasing intestinal transit etc., which is expected to influence the outcomes of dyslipidemia as well [62, 63]. But it has been shown that the impact of LSG on lipid profile was related only to weight change and did not have a significant impact over the 5 year follow up [61, 64]. Others have reported significant improvement in all the parameters, at least in the short term, with the outcomes becoming better when combined with additional physical activity [65–68].

Two RCTs comparing LSG and RYGB have shown significant improvements in both the groups, with no differences between patients receiving a LSG or LRYGB [69, 70]. But the study populations in both these groups have been small. Except for these two trials, majority of the other authors have reported better improvements in lipid parameters among patients undergoing LRYGB procedure [6, 16–19]. A meta-analysis by Yang et al. also had shown that the outcomes after LRYGB was better compared to that of LSG. It was also noted that an age dependent trend towards better lipid improvements was noted in young patients after LSG [71].

It is also interesting to note that LSG has shown good impact in increasing HDL and reducing TG, but not in reducing total cholesterol and LDL levels [61, 66, 71–73]. Griffo et al. suggest that GLP-1 peak as the best predictor of LDL improvement, and that differential effects between the procedures could contribute the differences in LDL outcomes [72]. He had also suggested that the improvements in TG are related to improvements in insulin resistance and weight loss. Similar results were shown by Cunha et al. who had demonstrated weight loss to be major factor in this irrespective of the type of bariatric procedure [61]. This could be because obesity and insulin resistance are commonly associated with hypertriglyceridaemia and lower HDL due to an increase in hepatic very low-density lipoprotein (VLDL) cholesterol synthesis and a decreased peripheral clearance [74, 75].

Hence it can be concluded that all types of bariatric procedures have impact in improving the parameters of dyslipidemia with variable outcomes. Also more the malabsorption, the better the outcomes as shown with procedures like LBPD/DS. Amongst the more commonly performed LRYGB and LSG, LRYGB has shown better outcomes especially with the improvements in total cholesterol and LDL.

Recommendations

Bariatric surgery in superobese

- Both LSG and LRYGB can be safely performed in super obese and super super obese patients but when LSG is chosen the need for a second stage procedure is high which has to be counseled to the patient.
- In mega obese patients, considering the high risk profiles and the higher complication rates with malabsorptive procedures, staged procedures in the form of first stage LSG followed by a second stage LRYGB or LBPD/DS is recommended

Bariatric surgery in elderly

- Bariatric surgery is an effective procedure for weight loss and can be safely performed even in the elderly
- Both LSG and LRYGB can be safely performed. LRYGB may offer better weight loss with no added morbidity.

Bariatric surgery with dyslipidemia

- Bariatric surgery by direct and indirect mechanisms is very effective in improving all parameters of dyslipidemia.
- Malabsorptive procedures including LRYGB improve all parameters including total cholesterol, triglycerides, HDL and LDL.
- Laparoscopic sleeve gastrectomy is equally effective in reducing triglycerides and increasing HDL but not for reducing total cholesterol and LDL.

References

1. Sjöström L, Peltonen M, Jacobson P, Ahlin S, Andersson-Assarsson J, Anveden Å, et al. Association of bariatric surgery with long-term remission of type 2 diabetes and with microvascular and macrovascular complications. JAMA. 2014;311(22):2297–304.
2. Parkin L, Sweetland S, Balkwill A, Green J, Reeves G, Beral V, et al. Body mass index, surgery, and risk of venous thromboembolism in middle-aged women: a cohort study. Circulation. 2012;125(15):1897–904.
3. Yeh P-S, Lee Y-C, Lee W-J, Chen S-B, Ho S-J, Peng W-B, et al. Clinical predictors of obstructive sleep apnea in Asian bariatric patients. Obes Surg. 2010;20(1):30–5.

4. Mehaffey JH, LaPar DJ, Turrentine FE, Miller MS, Hallowell PT, Schirmer BD. Outcomes of laparoscopic Roux-en-Y gastric bypass in super-super-obese patients. Surg Obes Relat Dis Off J Am Soc Bariatr Surg. 2015;11(4):814–9.
5. Gould JC, Garren M, Boll V, Starling J. The impact of circular stapler diameter on the incidence of gastrojejunostomy stenosis and weight loss following laparoscopic Roux-en-Y gastric bypass. Surg Endosc. 2006;20(7):1017–20.
6. Lemanu DP, Srinivasa S, Singh PP, Hill AG, MacCormick AD. Laparoscopic sleeve gastrectomy: its place in bariatric surgery for the severely obese patient. N Z Med J. 2012;125(1359):41–9.
7. Mukherjee S, Devalia K, Rahman MG, Mannur KR. Sleeve gastrectomy as a bridge to a second bariatric procedure in superobese patients – a single institution experience. Surg Obes Relat Dis Off J Am Soc Bariatr Surg. 2012;8(2):140–4.
8. Daigle CR, Andalib A, Corcelles R, Cetin D, Schauer PR, Brethauer SA. Bariatric and metabolic outcomes in the super-obese elderly. Surg Obes Relat Dis Off J Am Soc Bariatr Surg. 2016;12(1):132–7.
9. Schwartz A, Etchechoury L, Collet D. Outcome after laparoscopic gastric bypass for super-super obese patients. J Visc Surg. 2013;150(2):145–9.
10. Giordano S, Tolonen P, Victorzon M. Comparision of linear versus circular stapling techniques in laparoscopic gastric bypass surgery – a pilot study. Scand J Surg SJS Off Organ Finn Surg Soc Scand Surg Soc. 2010;99(3):127–31.
11. Wang C, Yang W, Yang J. Surgical results of laparoscopic Roux-en-Y gastric bypass in super obese patients with BMI≥60 in China. Surg Laparosc Endosc Percutan Tech. 2014;24(6):e216–20.
12. Arapis K, Chosidow D, Lehmann M, Bado A, Polanco M, Kamoun-Zana S, et al. Long-term results of adjustable gastric banding in a cohort of 186 super-obese patients with a BMI≥ 50 kg/m2. J Visc Surg. 2012;149(2):e143–52.
13. Peraglie C. Laparoscopic mini-gastric bypass (LMGB) in the super-super obese: outcomes in 16 patients. Obes Surg. 2008;18(9):1126–9.
14. Rezvani M, Sucandy I, Klar A, Bonanni F, Antanavicius G. Is laparoscopic single-stage biliopancreatic diversion with duodenal switch safe in super morbidly obese patients? Surg Obes Relat Dis Off J Am Soc Bariatr Surg. 2014;10(3):427–30.
15. Kalfarentzos F, Skroubis G, Karamanakos S, Argentou M, Mead N, Kehagias I, et al. Biliopancreatic diversion with Roux-en-Y gastric bypass and long limbs: advances in surgical treatment for super-obesity. Obes Surg. 2011;21(12):1849–58.
16. Sundbom M. Open duodenal switch for treatment of super obesity – surgical technique. Scand J Surg SJS Off Organ Finn Surg Soc Scand Surg Soc. 2015;104(1):54–6.
17. Cottam DR, Fisher B, Sridhar V, Atkinson J, Dallal R. The effect of stoma size on weight loss after laparoscopic gastric bypass surgery: results of a blinded randomized controlled trial. Obes Surg. 2009;19(1):13–7.
18. Silecchia G, Rizzello M, Casella G, Fioriti M, Soricelli E, Basso N. Two-stage laparoscopic biliopancreatic diversion with duodenal switch as treatment of high-risk super-obese patients: analysis of complications. Surg Endosc. 2009;23(5):1032–7.
19. Orci L, Chilcott M, Huber O. Short versus long Roux-limb length in Roux-en-Y gastric bypass surgery for the treatment of morbid and super obesity: a systematic review of the literature. Obes Surg. 2011;21(6):797–804.
20. Laurenius A, Taha O, Maleckas A, Lönroth H, Olbers T. Laparoscopic biliopancreatic diversion/duodenal switch or laparoscopic Roux-en-Y gastric bypass for super-obesity-weight loss versus side effects. Surg Obes Relat Dis Off J Am Soc Bariatr Surg. 2010;6(4):408–14.
21. Zerrweck C, Sepúlveda EM, Maydón HG, Campos F, Spaventa AG, Pratti V, et al. Laparoscopic gastric bypass vs. sleeve gastrectomy in the super obese patient: early outcomes of an observational study. Obes Surg. 2014;24(5):712–7.
22. Thereaux J, Corigliano N, Poitou C, Oppert J-M, Czernichow S, Bouillot J-L. Comparison of results after one year between sleeve gastrectomy and gastric bypass in patients with BMI ≥ 50 kg/m^2. Surg Obes Relat Dis Off J Am Soc Bariatr Surg. 2015;11(4):785–90.

23. Gonzalez-Heredia R, Sanchez-Johnsen L, Valbuena VSM, Masrur M, Murphey M, Elli E. Surgical management of super-super obese patients: Roux-en-Y gastric bypass versus sleeve gastrectomy. Surg Endosc. 2016;30(5):2097–102.
24. Alexandrou A, Felekouras E, Giannopoulos A, Tsigris C, Diamantis T. What is the actual fate of super-morbid-obese patients who undergo laparoscopic sleeve gastrectomy as the first step of a two-stage weight-reduction operative strategy? Obes Surg. 2012;22(10):1623–8.
25. Spyropoulos C, Bakellas G, Skroubis G, Kehagias I, Mead N, Vagenas K, et al. A prospective evaluation of a variant of biliopancreatic diversion with Roux-en-Y reconstruction in mega-obese patients (BMI > or = 70 kg/m(2)). Obes Surg. 2008;18(7):803–9.
26. Eldar SM, Heneghan HM, Brethauer SA, Khwaja HA, Singh M, Rogula T, et al. Laparoscopic bariatric surgery for those with body mass index of 70–125 kg/m2. Surg Obes Relat Dis Off J Am Soc Bariatr Surg. 2012;8(6):736–40.
27. NIH conference. Gastrointestinal surgery for severe obesity. Consensus Development Conference Panel. Ann Intern Med. 1991;115(12):956–61.
28. Flum DR, Salem L, Elrod JAB, Dellinger EP, Cheadle A, Chan L. Early mortality among Medicare beneficiaries undergoing bariatric surgical procedures. JAMA. 2005;294(15):1903–8.
29. Scozzari G, Passera R, Benvenga R, Toppino M, Morino M. Age as a long-term prognostic factor in bariatric surgery. Ann Surg. 2012;256(5):724–8; discussion 728–9.
30. Padwal RS, Klarenbach SW, Wang X, Sharma AM, Karmali S, Birch DW, et al. A simple prediction rule for all-cause mortality in a cohort eligible for bariatric surgery. JAMA Surg. 2013;148(12):1109–15.
31. Santo MA, Pajecki D, Riccioppo D, Cleva R, Kawamoto F, Cecconello I. Early complications in bariatric surgery: incidence, diagnosis and treatment. Arq Gastroenterol. 2013;50(1):50–5.
32. Livingston EH, Langert J. The impact of age and Medicare status on bariatric surgical outcomes. Arch Surg Chic Ill 1960. 2006;141(11):1115–20; discussion 1121.
33. Willkomm CM, Fisher TL, Barnes GS, Kennedy CI, Kuhn JA. Surgical weight loss >65 years old: is it worth the risk? Surg Obes Relat Dis Off J Am Soc Bariatr Surg. 2010;6(5):491–6.
34. Ramirez A, Roy M, Hidalgo JE, Szomstein S, Rosenthal RJ. Outcomes of bariatric surgery in patients >70 years old. Surg Obes Relat Dis Off J Am Soc Bariatr Surg. 2012;8(4):458–62.
35. Dorman RB, Abraham AA, Al-Refaie WB, Parsons HM, Ikramuddin S, Habermann EB. Bariatric surgery outcomes in the elderly: an ACS NSQIP study. J Gastrointest Surg Off J Soc Surg Aliment Tract. 2012;16(1):35–44; discussion 44.
36. Lynch J, Belgaumkar A. Bariatric surgery is effective and safe in patients over 55: a systematic review and meta-analysis. Obes Surg. 2012;22(9):1507–16.
37. Fazylov R, Soto E, Merola S. Laparoscopic Roux-en-Y gastric bypass in morbidly obese patients > or =55 years old. Obes Surg. 2008;18(6):656–9.
38. Papasavas PK, Gagné DJ, Kelly J, Caushaj PF. Laparoscopic Roux-En-Y gastric bypass is a safe and effective operation for the treatment of morbid obesity in patients older than 55 years. Obes Surg. 2004;14(8):1056–61.
39. Sosa JL, Pombo H, Pallavicini H, Ruiz-Rodriguez M. Laparoscopic gastric bypass beyond age 60. Obes Surg. 2004;14(10):1398–401.
40. St Peter SD, Craft RO, Tiede JL, Swain JM. Impact of advanced age on weight loss and health benefits after laparoscopic gastric bypass. Arch Surg Chic Ill 1960. 2005;140(2):165–8.
41. Trieu HT, Gonzalvo JP, Szomstein S, Rosenthal R. Safety and outcomes of laparoscopic gastric bypass surgery in patients 60 years of age and older. Surg Obes Relat Dis Off J Am Soc Bariatr Surg. 2007;3(3):383–6.
42. Wittgrove AC, Martinez T. Laparoscopic gastric bypass in patients 60 years and older: early postoperative morbidity and resolution of comorbidities. Obes Surg. 2009;19(11):1472–6.
43. Busetto L, Angrisani L, Basso N, Favretti F, Furbetta F, Lorenzo M, et al. Safety and efficacy of laparoscopic adjustable gastric banding in the elderly. Obes Silver Spring Md. 2008;16(2):334–8.
44. Abu-Abeid S, Keidar A, Szold A. Resolution of chronic medical conditions after laparoscopic adjustable silicone gastric banding for the treatment of morbid obesity in the elderly. Surg Endosc. 2001;15(2):132–4.

45. Clough A, Layani L, Shah A, Wheatley L, Taylor C. Laparoscopic gastric banding in over 60s. Obes Surg. 2011;21(1):10–7.
46. Taylor CJ, Layani L. Laparoscopic adjustable gastric banding in patients >or =60 years old: is it worthwhile? Obes Surg. 2006;16(12):1579–83.
47. Frutos MD, Luján J, Hernández Q, Valero G, Parrilla P. Results of laparoscopic gastric bypass in patients > or =55 years old. Obes Surg. 2006;16(4):461–4.
48. Silecchia G, Greco F, Bacci V, Boru C, Pecchia A, Casella G, et al. Results after laparoscopic adjustable gastric banding in patients over 55 years of age. Obes Surg. 2005;15(3):351–6.
49. Keidar A, Hershkop KJ, Marko L, Schweiger C, Hecht L, Bartov N, et al. Roux-en-Y gastric bypass vs sleeve gastrectomy for obese patients with type 2 diabetes: a randomised trial. Diabetologia. 2013;56(9):1914–8.
50. Yaghoubian A, Tolan A, Stabile BE, Kaji AH, Belzberg G, Mun E, et al. Laparoscopic Roux-en-Y gastric bypass and sleeve gastrectomy achieve comparable weight loss at 1 year. Am Surg. 2012;78(12):1325–8.
51. Vidal P, Ramón JM, Goday A, Benaiges D, Trillo L, Parri A, et al. Laparoscopic gastric bypass versus laparoscopic sleeve gastrectomy as a definitive surgical procedure for morbid obesity. Mid-term results. Obes Surg. 2013;23(3):292–9.
52. van Rutte PWJ, Smulders JF, de Zoete JP, Nienhuijs SW. Sleeve gastrectomy in older obese patients. Surg Endosc. 2013;27(6):2014–9.
53. Soto FC, Gari V, de la Garza JR, Szomstein S, Rosenthal RJ. Sleeve gastrectomy in the elderly: a safe and effective procedure with minimal morbidity and mortality. Obes Surg. 2013;23(9):1445–9.
54. Carlin AM, Zeni TM, English WJ, Hawasli AA, Genaw JA, Krause KR, et al. The comparative effectiveness of sleeve gastrectomy, gastric bypass, and adjustable gastric banding procedures for the treatment of morbid obesity. Ann Surg. 2013;257(5):791–7.
55. Li J-F, Lai D-D, Ni B, Sun K-X. Comparison of laparoscopic Roux-en-Y gastric bypass with laparoscopic sleeve gastrectomy for morbid obesity or type 2 diabetes mellitus: a meta-analysis of randomized controlled trials. Can J Surg J Can Chir. 2013;56(6):E158–64.
56. Buchwald H, Williams SE. Bariatric surgery worldwide 2003. Obes Surg. 2004;14(9):1157–64.
57. Stefater MA, Wilson-Pérez HE, Chambers AP, Sandoval DA, Seeley RJ. All bariatric surgeries are not created equal: insights from mechanistic comparisons. Endocr Rev. 2012;33(4):595–622.
58. Benetti A, Del Puppo M, Crosignani A, Veronelli A, Masci E, Frigè F, et al. Cholesterol metabolism after bariatric surgery in grade 3 obesity: differences between malabsorptive and restrictive procedures. Diabetes Care. 2013;36(6):1443–7.
59. Vila M, Ruíz O, Belmonte M, Riesco M, Barceló A, Perez G, et al. Changes in lipid profile and insulin resistance in obese patients after Scopinaro biliopancreatic diversion. Obes Surg. 2009;19(3):299–306.
60. Risstad H, Søvik TT, Engström M, Aasheim ET, Fagerland MW, Olsén MF, et al. Five-year outcomes after laparoscopic gastric bypass and laparoscopic duodenal switch in patients with body mass index of 50 to 60: a randomized clinical trial. JAMA Surg. 2015;150(4):352–61.
61. Cunha FM, Oliveira J, Preto J, Saavedra A, Costa MM, Magalhães D, et al. The ffect of Bariatric Surgery Type on Lipid Profile: An Age, Sex, Body Mass Index and Excess Weight Loss Matched Study. Obes Surg. 2016;26(5):1041–7.
62. Chambers AP, Smith EP, Begg DP, Grayson BE, Sisley S, Greer T, et al. Regulation of gastric emptying rate and its role in nutrient-induced GLP-1 secretion in rats after vertical sleeve gastrectomy. Am J Physiol Endocrinol Metab. 2014;306(4):E424–32.
63. Melissas J, Leventi A, Klinaki I, Perisinakis K, Koukouraki S, de Bree E, et al. Alterations of global gastrointestinal motility after sleeve gastrectomy: a prospective study. Ann Surg. 2013;258(6):976–82.
64. Strain GW, Saif T, Ebel F, Dakin GF, Gagner M, Costa R, et al. Lipid profile changes in the severely obese after laparoscopic sleeve gastrectomy (LSG), 1, 3, and 5 years after surgery. Obes Surg. 2015;25(2):285–9.

65. Perathoner A, Weißenbacher A, Sucher R, Laimer E, Pratschke J, Mittermair R. Significant weight loss and rapid resolution of diabetes and dyslipidemia during short-term follow-up after laparoscopic sleeve gastrectomy. Obes Surg. 2013;23(12):1966–72.
66. Bužga M, Holéczy P, Svagera Z, Svorc P, Zavadilová V. Effects of sleeve gastrectomy on parameters of lipid and glucose metabolism in obese women - 6 months after operation. Wideochirurgia Inne Tech Małoinwazyjne Videosurg Miniinvasive Tech Kwart Pod Patronatem Sekc Wideochirurgii TChP Oraz Sekc Chir Bariatrycznej TChP. 2013;8(1):22–8.
67. Hady HR, Dadan J, Gołaszewski P, Safiejko K. Impact of laparoscopic sleeve gastrectomy on body mass index, ghrelin, insulin and lipid levels in 100 obese patients. Wideochirurgia Inne Tech Małoinwazyjne Videosurg Miniinvasive Tech Kwart Pod Patronatem Sekc Wideochirurgii TChP Oraz Sekc Chir Bariatrycznej TChP. 2012;7(4):251–9.
68. Ruiz-Tovar J, Zubiaga L, Llavero C, Diez M, Arroyo A, Calpena R. Serum cholesterol by morbidly obese patients after laparoscopic sleeve gastrectomy and additional physical activity. Obes Surg. 2014;24(3):385–9.
69. Yang J, Wang C, Cao G, Yang W, Yu S, Zhai H, et al. Long-term effects of laparoscopic sleeve gastrectomy versus roux-en-Y gastric bypass for the treatment of Chinese type 2 diabetes mellitus patients with body mass index 28–35 kg/m(2). BMC Surg. 2015;15:88.
70. de Barros F, Setúbal S, Martinho JM, Monteiro ABS. Early endocrine and metabolic changes after bariatric surgery in grade III morbidly obese patients: a randomized clinical trial comparing sleeve gastrectomy and gastric bypass. Metab Syndr Relat Disord. 2015;13(6):264–71.
71. Yang X, Yang G, Wang W, Chen G, Yang H. A meta-analysis: to compare the clinical results between gastric bypass and sleeve gastrectomy for the obese patients. Obes Surg. 2013;23(7):1001–10.
72. Griffo E, Cotugno M, Nosso G, Saldalamacchia G, Mangione A, Angrisani L, et al. Effects of sleeve gastrectomy and gastric bypass on postprandial lipid profile in obese type 2 diabetic patients: a 2-year follow-up. Obes Surg. 2016;26(6):1247–53.
73. Benaiges D, Flores-Le-Roux JA, Pedro-Botet J, Ramon JM, Parri A, Villatoro M, et al. Impact of restrictive (sleeve gastrectomy) vs hybrid bariatric surgery (Roux-en-Y gastric bypass) on lipid profile. Obes Surg. 2012;22(8):1268–75.
74. Taskinen M-R. Diabetic dyslipidemia. Atheroscler Suppl. 2002;3(1):47–51.
75. Kaur J. A comprehensive review on metabolic syndrome. Cardiol Res Pract. 2014;2014:943162.

Preoperative Evaluation and Contraindications to Bariatric Surgery

4

Saravana Kumar and Rachel Maria Gomes

4.1 Introduction

Bariatric surgery is the most effective treatment option for the morbidly obese patients who fail weight loss by lifestyle interventions [1]. In addition to weight loss, it results in resolution or improvement of obesity associated co-morbidities of diabetes, hypertension, dyslipidemia, obstructive sleep apnea, gastro-esophageal reflux etc. Improvement in long-term survival and overall quality of life has been demonstrated in several studies. It has been shown that morbidly obese patients are high risk candidates for any surgical intervention [2, 3]. They can have several potential perioperative and long term complications after surgical intervention. Hence any patient who needs to be subjected to bariatric surgery should be thoroughly evaluated and accordingly optimized prior to surgery.

The main objective of this chapter is to describe the preoperative evaluation of the bariatric patient and discuss the contraindications to bariatric surgery.

4.2 Patient Selection

The most important step of the preoperative process is patient selection. Body mass index (BMI) is still an important factor for patient selection for bariatric surgery and several medical and surgical associations have defined guidelines based on BMI for

S. Kumar, MS, FMAS (✉) • R.M. Gomes, MS, FMAS
Bariatric Division, Upper Gastrointestinal Surgery and Minimal Access Surgery Unit, GEM Hospital and Research Centre, Coimbatore, India
e-mail: drsakubariatric@gmail.com; dr.gomes@rediffmail.com

P.R. Palanivelu et al. (eds.), *Bariatric Surgical Practice Guide*,
DOI 10.1007/978-981-10-2705-5_4

selection of patients for bariatric surgery. These cut-offs can be adjusted in day to day practice based on patient population and severity of co-morbidities. Details regarding the patient selection based on existing guidelines have been discussed in detail in Chap. 1. Although BMI helps in identifying patients that may benefit from bariatric surgery, patient selection is a dynamic process over the course of preoperative evaluation and not a single time decision.

4.3 Preoperative Evaluation of a Bariatric Surgery Patient

4.3.1 Clinical Evaluation

The first step in preoperative evaluation involves eliciting an obesity focused history. Onset of weight gain has to be enquired. In majority of patients weight gain has a late onset secondary to a change in life events or stressful life events. These events commonly include change in marital status, change in occupation, severe illness, pregnancy, menopause, restricted mobility etc. Early onset obesity is identified by a history of childhood or adolescent obesity. Early onset of obesity is a predictor of severe obesity in adulthood [4]. Predisposing genetic background need to be assessed by enquiring for obesity in parents and/or siblings. Parental obesity more than doubles the risk of adult obesity [4].

Dietary intake has to be assessed in all patients. Eating disorders such binge eating disorder, bulimia, or night-eating syndrome etc need to be looked for. The calorie/protein intake of the patient should be assessed. Common preexisting nutritional deficiencies need to be looked for and corrected. A physical activity history is also to be assessed.

Determining a patient's motivation is also an important part of the initial evaluation. Firstly this involves assessment of the appropriateness of the patient's goals and expectations. An assessment of time availability and constraints, stressful life events, psychiatric status etc helps understand the likelihood of lifestyle change. Assessment of psychological and psychiatric history is to be routinely performed to confirm the patient's ability to incorporate nutritional and behavioral changes before and after bariatric surgery [6–8]. Physical examination in addition to a routine examination should look for stigmata of syndromes associated with obesity like dysmorphism, hypogonadism, purple abdominal striae etc. A system wise evaluation is covered in the subsequent sections.

4.3.2 Cardiac Evaluation

Obesity is associated with several cardiac co-morbidities including hypertension, arrhythmias, coronary artery disease, cardiac failure, cardiomyopathy etc [9]. Every patient should be evaluated with a cardiac specific history, history of coronary risk factors and a physical examination. General evaluation requires a 12-lead electrocardiogram (ECG) and echocardiogram. In case stress testing is deemed necessary a dobutamine stress echocardiogram is performed since exercise induced echocardiogram is usually not possible in obese patients [10]. Cardiac computed tomography angiogram can be used as a method to evaluate the coronary vasculature in patients prior to invasive imaging procedures. Invasive cardiac interventions if needed are performed based on the assessment and advice of a cardiologist.

The routine recommendation for hypertension is adequate control of blood pressure before the procedure [10]. In patients with cardiac disease close collaboration with the patient's cardiologist during the preoperative workup, intraoperatively and postoperatively is needed for optimal management. In patients who have undergone cardiac stenting antiplatelet therapy in the perioperative period often presents a controversy for the surgeons. Specific to bariatric surgery, it is recommended that patients with bare metal or drug eluting stents should not undergo surgery within the first year of stent placement. If, as determined by a cardiologist, the patient requires dual therapy longer than 1 year after stent placement, recommendation is to remain on antiplatelet therapy and this should not be discontinued.

4.3.3 Venous Evaluation

Obesity is a hypercoagulable state [11]. This leads to an increased risk of venous thromboembolism (VTE) in morbidly obese patients undergoing bariatric surgery. Venous thromboembolic events are a leading cause for mortality after bariatric surgery. The reported incidence of symptomatic VTE is <1 % for laparoscopic bariatric surgery. However common predisposing factors cited for an increased risk of VTE in obese patients are elderly patients, prior deep venous thrombosis (DVT), hypercoagulable states, superobesity, documented obesity hypoventilation and/or pulmonary hypertension. It is generally recommended that patients undergoing weight loss surgery receive VTE chemoprophylaxis in adjunct to mechanical methods during the perioperative period [12]. Details regarding peri-operative DVT prophylaxis after bariatric surgery have been discussed in detail in Chap. 19. Routine screening for deep venous thrombosis prior to bariatric surgery is controversial but may be advisable in high risk patients as outlined before. Also patients with suspicious limb findings or findings suggestive of venous insufficiency should be investigated for a preexisting thrombus. The preferred method for evaluation is venous duplex ultrasound. This study has a sensitivity and specificity of 97 % and 94 %, respectively, of diagnosing a lower extremity DVT [13].

4.3.4 Pulmonary Evaluation

Obesity related impairment of respiratory function is caused by deposition of fatty tissue in and around the upper airways by reducing oropharyngeal patency (resulting in obstructive sleep apnoae [OSA]) and increased adipose tissue resulting in mechanical restriction of adequate ventilation by reducing diaphragmatic excursion and chest wall expansion (resulting in obesity hypoventilation syndrome [OHS]).

Obesity is also a risk factor for airway disease and there is a 50 % higher incidence of severe asthma in obese patients when compared to normal controls [14, 15]. Details regarding OSA and OHS have been discussed in detail in Chap. 21.

Chest radiographs are ordered frequently as part of a routine preoperative evaluation. Spirometry has value in diagnosing obstructive lung disease and can be ordered if this is present or suspected. A reduction in the expiratory reserve volume (ERV) is the most commonly identified abnormality on spirometry in patients with obesity.

The definitive diagnosis of obstructive sleep apnea (OSA) is made with an overnight polysomnography (PSG). However an overnight PSG is expensive and inconvenient to use in all patients. The Epworth Sleepiness Score, the Berlin Questionnaire and the STOP-BANG Questionnaire are clinical screening tools designed to quickly assess if a patient should be assessed further for OSA by PSG. A PSG assesses the Apnoea/Hypnoea index (AHI). In general, an AHI of less than 5 is normal, 5–15 is mild sleep apnea, >15 is moderate sleep apnea and >30 severe sleep apnea. Obesity hypoventilation syndrome (OHS) manifests with daytime hypercapnia with $PaCO_2$ >44 mmHg or 6 kPa, elevated hematocrit, with sleep disordered breathing and needs an arterial blood gas analysis in addition to a PSG for diagnosis. Screening tests for deranged arterial blood gases can be done by pulse oximetry and serum bicarbonate levels. A room air saturation of <94 % is suspicious of a paO_2 <70 mmHg and a serum bicarbonate of >27 mEq/L is suspicious of elevated $paCO_2$ levels. If these tests are suggestive of derangement they should be followed by arterial blood gas analysis. Patients with moderate to severe apnea/OHS should be optimized with preoperative incentive spirometry and continuous positive airway pressure (CPAP) or bi-level positive airway pressure (Bi-PAP). Details regarding the perioperative management of OSA after bariatric surgery have been discussed in detail in Chap. 21.

Smoking is a common entity which significantly impacts pulmonary function. It has been identified as an independent factor associated with a greater incidence of acute respiratory failure after bariatric surgery and also shown to be an independent predictor of increased hospital length of stay [16]. Therefore smoking cessation at least for 3 weeks is an essential component of the preoperative assessment to prevent further morbidities.

4.3.5 Endocrine Evaluation

Obesity has been found to be associated with type 2 diabetes mellitus (T2DM) and hypothyroidism [17, 18]. Glycemic control in T2 DM should be assessed preoperatively by performing hemoglobin A1c (Hb A1c) levels in addition to fasting and postprandial glucose levels. Poor glycemic control is associated with lower rates of type 2 DM remission [19]. C-peptide levels need to assessed in patients with T2DM to know to measure beta cell function. Directly measuring insulin levels may be fallacious in those who are receiving insulin therapy. WJ Lee et al reported that a fasting C-peptide levels more than or equal to 3 nmol/l is the best prognostic marker of good remission after bariatric surgery [20]. He also reported that low C-peptide levels <1 nmol/l in severely obese T2DM indicated partial beta cell failure and predicted a markedly reduced chance of resolution of T2DM [21].

Hypothyroidism is a known cause of obesity; however, de novo thyroid dysfunction such as subclinical hypothyroidism is associated with obesity [18]. In some patients, the TSH level has been shown to return to normal levels after significant weight loss, however the outcome is not universal.

4.3.6 Gastrointestinal Evaluation

Obesity is a risk factor for gastroesophageal reflux disease, erosive esophagitis, and esophageal adenocarcinoma [22]. The rationale for performing an UGI endoscopy before bariatric surgery is to detect and treat UGI lesions that might cause symptoms or complications in the postoperative period or to detect lesions that may need a change in bariatric procedure performed. While some institutions routinely evaluate patients with preoperative UGI endoscopy prior to bariatric surgery, some suggest symptom-directed UGI endoscopy as in the general population [23]. In places where gastric and other upper gastrointestinal cancers are more prevalent, routine screening OGD is a must for all patients especially in procedures which exclude the stomach. It is also necessary in all patients undergoing revision surgery. Routine screening for H. pylori and eradication is indicated in high prevalence areas. Patients with normal findings or mild mucosal inflammatory lesions (mild to moderate esophagitis, gastritis, or duodenitis) or mild anatomical abnormalities (lax lower esophageal sphincter, small hiatal hernias) proceed with surgery as previously planned [24]. Patients with severe erosive gastritis or duodenitis or gastroduodenal ulcers require treatment with proton pump inhibitors for 4 weeks with reassessment to confirm mucosal healing [24]. Gastroesophageal reflux disease associated with hiatal hernias and Barrett's esophagus found preoperatively may require a change in planned bariatric procedure [24].

In morbidly obese patients from bariatric surgery series the incidence of non-alcoholic fatty liver disease is as high as 65–95 % and that of non-alcoholic steatohepatitis is around 30–40 % [25–30]. Obese patients are also at an increased risk for biliary disease with a prevalence of 13.6–47.9 % [31, 32]. Routine ultrasound of the abdomen and pelvis is performed to assess for evidence of fatty liver or parenchymal disease as well as the presence of gallstones and gall bladder wall thickening. A fatty infiltration of the liver of >30 % can be detected by imaging [33].

4.4 Contraindications to Bariatric Surgery

With improvement in anesthetic techniques, standardization of surgical procedures and good postoperative care, bariatric surgery can be safely performed with improved quality of life with benefits of sustained weight loss and resolution of co-morbidities. It can now be said that there is no absolute contraindication to bariatric surgery. Specific considerations are as discussed below.

4.4.1 Severe Medical Illness

A contraindication to bariatric surgery often cited is severe medical illness that will worsen despite treatment of severe obesity. Though this list commonly includes those with severe cardiopulmonary disease and other end organ failure, the benefits of bariatric surgery are now being increasingly reported in patients with end-organ disease which has been described in a pre-transplant/post-transplant setting and even as a combined procedure with transplantation. Bariatric surgery can be offered as a treatment option in experienced centers in those with end-organ failure. Details regarding benefits of bariatric surgery in end-organ disease have been discussed in detail in Chap. 18.

Malignancy is not an absolute contraindication for bariatric surgery. In patients with malignancy, those with metastatic disease or an inoperable primary are contraindications because of limited life expectancy. The exception also includes patients with esophageal cancer. A choice of bariatric surgery however can be made in carefully selected malignancy patients in remission with good prognosis and life expectancy.

Around 20% of HIV-infected patients receiving antiretroviral therapy (ART) progress to obesity because of antiretroviral lipodystrophy. With use of modern ART, life expectancy in HIV-infected patients has increased. Studies have shown that in selected HIV-infected patients with good response to ART, bariatric surgery is an effective treatment option without effect on virologic suppression [34].

4.4.2 Ability to Consent/Psychiatric Illness/Substance Abuse

Many studies have reported that the most common reasons for delaying or denying surgery were psychosis, bipolar disorder, untreated or undertreated depression, and lack of understanding about the risks and postoperative requirements of surgery [8].

Impaired intellectual capacity or the inability to comprehend the surgical intervention or poor motivation for surgery put patients at the risk of developing dangerous nutritional complications and poor outcomes. Thus patients unable to comply should be considered a contraindication to surgery. Eating disorders do not usually preclude bariatric surgery. However the only eating disorder that is a contraindication to bariatric surgery is active bulimia nervosa [5].

Successful bariatric surgery has been demonstrated with major depression, schizophrenia, and stable bipolar disorders. Active psychosis however warrants delaying surgery. Depression is commonly associated in patients presenting for bariatric surgery. Certain manifestations like recent suicidal attempts, suicidal ideation, untreated depression, stressful life events require postponement of surgery. Active drug or alcohol abuse is a contraindication to surgery and surgery should be deferred till de-addiction and rehabilitation.

4.4.3 Bariatric Surgery and Pregnancy

Patients who are pregnant should have any bariatric procedure deferred as rapid weight loss may be unhealthy for the mother and the baby. It is advisable to delay pregnancy for 12–18 months following the bariatric procedure to avoid nutritional deficiencies [35, 36].

4.4.4 Praeder Willi Syndrome or Malignant Hyperphagia

Prader-Willi Syndrome (PWS) is a multisystemic genetic disease characterized by hypothalamic hypogonadism, mental retardation and compulsive hyperphagia associated with early and severe obesity. Poor results have been reported after bariatric surgery in these patients but this may be offered as a last resort when severe obesity becomes life threatening.

4.4.5 Extremes of Age

Evidence shows that selected adolescents when treated with bariatric surgery have equivalent outcomes to adults [37]. However when offering bariatric surgery to adolescents it is important that obesity is assessed along with their stage of puberty. Bariatric surgery should be offered only to adolescents who have nearly completed puberty. Of importance is that the adolescent should be able to provide informed consent for bariatric surgery and follow postoperative instructions. They should also have parental support for bariatric surgery in the postoperative period. Details regarding bariatric surgery in adolescents have been discussed in detail in Chap. 2. Thus important contraindications in the younger cohort would be those who have not completed puberty, lack of understanding of the operation and lack of family support.

Several studies have reported increased post-operative morbidity and mortality rates in the elderly [38, 39]. This has led most centers to limit bariatric surgery to patients <65 years of age. However sufficient evidence has accumulated proving the safety and efficacy of bariatric surgery in the elderly [40]. A meta-analysis of 1206 elderly patients undergoing bariatric surgery reported a mortality rate of 0.25 % comparable to the general bariatric surgery population [41]. It has been shown that bariatric surgery can be safely performed even in patients >70 years of age with low rate of complications and acceptable improvement of co-morbidities [42]. Details regarding bariatric surgery in elderly have been discussed in detail in Chap. 3.

Conclusion

Selection of a patient for bariatric surgery is a dynamic process. Appropriate preoperative evaluation and optimization of patients prior to bariatric surgery helps in streamlining patient care and increasing safety of bariatric procedures.

Indications of bariatric surgery have expanded with advancements in anesthesia although certain factors need to be taken into consideration in special situations.

Recommendations

- The preoperative evaluation of the bariatric surgery patient requires a multidisciplinary approach, ultimately coordinated by the surgeon.
- There are many details to which attention must be paid including medical, nutritional and psychological aspects in an effort to fully evaluate the patient as a whole.

References

1. NIH conference. Gastrointestinal surgery for severe obesity. Consensus Development Conference Panel. Ann Intern Med. 1991;115(12):956–61.
2. Parkin L, Sweetland S, Balkwill A, Green J, Reeves G, Beral V, et al. Body mass index, surgery, and risk of venous thromboembolism in middle-aged women: a cohort study. Circulation. 2012;125(15):1897–904.
3. Yeh P-S, Lee Y-C, Lee W-J, Chen S-B, Ho S-J, Peng W-B, et al. Clinical predictors of obstructive sleep apnea in Asian bariatric patients. Obes Surg. 2010;20(1):30–5.
4. Whitaker RC, Wright JA, Pepe MS, Seidel KD, Dietz WH. Predicting obesity in young adulthood from childhood and parental obesity. N Engl J Med. 1997;337(13):869–73.
5. Snyder AG. Psychological assessment of the patient undergoing bariatric surgery. Ochsner J. 2009;9(3):144–8.
6. Greenberg I, Sogg S, M Perna F. Behavioral and psychological care in weight loss surgery: best practice update. Obes Silver Spring Md. 2009;17(5):880–4.
7. Goldstein N, Hadidi N. Impact of bariatric pre-operative education on patient knowledge and satisfaction with overall hospital experience. Bariatr Nurs Surg Patient Care. 2010;5(2):137–44.
8. Walfish S, Vance D, Fabricatore AN. Psychological evaluation of bariatric surgery applicants: procedures and reasons for delay or denial of surgery. Obes Surg. 2007;17(12):1578–83.
9. Zalesin KC, Franklin BA, Miller WM, Peterson ED, McCullough PA. Impact of obesity on cardiovascular disease. Med Clin North Am. 2011;95(5):919–37.
10. Fleisher LA, Beckman JA, Brown KA, Calkins H, Chaikof E, Fleischmann KE, et al. ACC/AHA 2007 guidelines on perioperative cardiovascular evaluation and care for noncardiac surgery: a report of the American College of Cardiology/American Heart Association Task Force on Practice Guidelines (Writing Committee to Revise the 2002 Guidelines on Perioperative Cardiovascular Evaluation for Noncardiac Surgery): developed in collaboration with the American Society of Echocardiography, American Society of Nuclear Cardiology, Heart Rhythm Society, Society of Cardiovascular Anesthesiologists, Society for Cardiovascular Angiography and Interventions, Society for Vascular Medicine and Biology, and Society for Vascular Surgery. Circulation. 2007;116(17):e418–99.
11. Mertens I, Van Gaal LF. Obesity, haemostasis and the fibrinolytic system. Obes Rev Off J Int Assoc Study Obes. 2002;3(2):85–101.
12. Kuruba R, Koche LS, Murr MM. Preoperative assessment and perioperative care of patients undergoing bariatric surgery. Med Clin North Am. 2007;91(3):339–51, ix.
13. Zierler BK. Ultrasonography and diagnosis of venous thromboembolism. Circulation. 2004;109(12 Suppl 1):I9–14.

14. Mosen DM, Schatz M, Magid DJ, Camargo CA. The relationship between obesity and asthma severity and control in adults. J Allergy Clin Immunol. 2008;122(3):507–11.e6.
15. Beuther DA, Sutherland ER. Overweight, obesity, and incident asthma: a meta-analysis of prospective epidemiologic studies. Am J Respir Crit Care Med. 2007;175(7):661–6.
16. Masoomi H, Reavis KM, Smith BR, Kim H, Stamos MJ, Nguyen NT. Risk factors for acute respiratory failure in bariatric surgery: data from the Nationwide Inpatient Sample, 2006-2008. Surg Obes Relat Dis Off J Am Soc Bariatr Surg. 2013;9(2):277–81.
17. Mechanick JI, Youdim A, Jones DB, Timothy Garvey W, Hurley DL, Molly McMahon M, et al. Clinical practice guidelines for the perioperative nutritional, metabolic, and nonsurgical support of the bariatric surgery patient – 2013 update: cosponsored by American Association of Clinical Endocrinologists, the Obesity Society, and American Society for Metabolic & Bariatric Surgery. Surg Obes Relat Dis Off J Am Soc Bariatr Surg. 2013;9(2):159–91.
18. Janković D, Wolf P, Anderwald C-H, Winhofer Y, Promintzer-Schifferl M, Hofer A, et al. Prevalence of endocrine disorders in morbidly obese patients and the effects of bariatric surgery on endocrine and metabolic parameters. Obes Surg. 2012;22(1):62–9.
19. Perna M, Romagnuolo J, Morgan K, Byrne TK, Baker M. Preoperative hemoglobin A1c and postoperative glucose control in outcomes after gastric bypass for obesity. Surg Obes Relat Dis Off J Am Soc Bariatr Surg. 2012;8(6):685–90.
20. Lee W-J, Ser K-H, Chong K, Lee Y-C, Chen S-C, Tsou J-J, et al. Laparoscopic sleeve gastrectomy for diabetes treatment in nonmorbidly obese patients: efficacy and change of insulin secretion. Surgery. 2010;147(5):664–9.
21. Lee W-J, Chong K, Ser K-H, Chen J-C, Lee Y-C, Chen S-C, et al. C-peptide predicts the remission of type 2 diabetes after bariatric surgery. Obes Surg. 2012;22(2):293–8.
22. Hampel H, Abraham NS, El-Serag HB. Meta-analysis: obesity and the risk for gastroesophageal reflux disease and its complications. Ann Intern Med. 2005;143(3):199–211.
23. Greenwald D. Preoperative gastrointestinal assessment before bariatric surgery. Gastroenterol Clin North Am. 2010;39(1):81–6.
24. Praveenraj P, Gomes RM, Kumar S, Senthilnathan P, Parathasarathi R, Rajapandian S, et al. Diagnostic yield and clinical implications of preoperative upper gastrointestinal endoscopy in morbidly obese patients undergoing bariatric surgery. J Laparoendosc Adv Surg Tech A. 2015;25(6):465–9.
25. Dixon JB, Bhathal PS, O'Brien PE. Nonalcoholic fatty liver disease: predictors of nonalcoholic steatohepatitis and liver fibrosis in the severely obese. Gastroenterology. 2001;121(1):91–100.
26. Beymer C, Kowdley KV, Larson A, Edmonson P, Dellinger EP, Flum DR. Prevalence and predictors of asymptomatic liver disease in patients undergoing gastric bypass surgery. Arch Surg Chic Ill 1960. 2003;138(11):1240–4.
27. Gholam PM, Kotler DP, Flancbaum LJ. Liver pathology in morbidly obese patients undergoing Roux-en-Y gastric bypass surgery. Obes Surg. 2002;12(1):49–51.
28. Ong JP, Elariny H, Collantes R, Younoszai A, Chandhoke V, Reines HD, et al. Predictors of nonalcoholic steatohepatitis and advanced fibrosis in morbidly obese patients. Obes Surg. 2005;15(3):310–5.
29. Praveenraj P, Gomes RM, Kumar S, Karthikeyan P, Shankar A, Parthasarathi R, et al. Prevalence and predictors of non-alcoholic fatty liver disease in morbidly obese South Indian patients undergoing bariatric surgery. Obes Surg. 2015;25(11):2078–87.
30. Praveen Raj P, Gomes RM, Kumar S, Senthilnathan P, Karthikeyan P, Shankar A, et al. The effect of surgically induced weight loss on nonalcoholic fatty liver disease in morbidly obese Indians: "NASHOST" prospective observational trial. Surg Obes Relat Dis Off J Am Soc Bariatr Surg. 2015;11(6):1315–22.
31. Fobi M, Lee H, Igwe D, Felahy B, James E, Stanczyk M, et al. Prophylactic cholecystectomy with gastric bypass operation: incidence of gallbladder disease. Obes Surg. 2002;12(3):350–3.
32. Dittrick GW, Thompson JS, Campos D, Bremers D, Sudan D. Gallbladder pathology in morbid obesity. Obes Surg. 2005;15(2):238–42.

33. Fris RJ. Preoperative low energy diet diminishes liver size. Obes Surg. 2004;14(9):1165–70.
34. Selke H, Norris S, Osterholzer D, Fife KH, DeRose B, Gupta SK. Bariatric surgery outcomes in HIV-infected subjects: a case series. AIDS Patient Care STDS. 2010;24(9):545–50.
35. Kanadys WM, Leszczyńska-Gorzelak B, Oleszczuk J. Obesity among women. Pregnancy after bariatric surgery: a qualitative review. Ginekol Pol. 2010;81(3):215–23.
36. Tan O, Carr BR. The impact of bariatric surgery on obesity-related infertility and in vitro fertilization outcomes. Semin Reprod Med. 2012;30(6):517–28.
37. Olbers T, Gronowitz E, Werling M, Mårlid S, Flodmark C-E, Peltonen M, et al. Two-year outcome of laparoscopic Roux-en-Y gastric bypass in adolescents with severe obesity: results from a Swedish Nationwide Study (AMOS). Int J Obes (Lond) 2005. 2012;36(11):1388–95.
38. Flum DR, Salem L, Elrod JAB, Dellinger EP, Cheadle A, Chan L. Early mortality among Medicare beneficiaries undergoing bariatric surgical procedures. JAMA. 2005;294(15):1903–8.
39. Livingston EH, Langert J. The impact of age and Medicare status on bariatric surgical outcomes. Arch Surg Chic Ill 1960. 2006;141(11):1115–20; discussion 1121.
40. Willkomm CM, Fisher TL, Barnes GS, Kennedy CI, Kuhn JA. Surgical weight loss >65 years old: is it worth the risk? Surg Obes Relat Dis Off J Am Soc Bariatr Surg. 2010;6(5):491–6.
41. Lynch J, Belgaumkar A. Bariatric surgery is effective and safe in patients over 55: a systematic review and meta-analysis. Obes Surg. 2012;22(9):1507–16.
42. Ramirez A, Roy M, Hidalgo JE, Szomstein S, Rosenthal RJ. Outcomes of bariatric surgery in patients >70 years old. Surg Obes Relat Dis Off J Am Soc Bariatr Surg. 2012;8(4):458–62.

Part II

Preoperative Predictors of Outcomes

Definition of Outcomes After Bariatric Surgery

5

Lilian Kow

5.1 Introduction

Bariatric surgery has been shown to be the most effective method of successful weight loss in the long term. However, with the number of bariatric surgeries being performed around the world, what defines the success of a bariatric procedure?

Traditionally, weight loss was used as the benchmark. The more weight a patient lost, the more successful the surgery. However, it is now better understood that obesity results in multisystemic diseases and that bariatric surgery has an impact on a large number of organs and systems. It also results in an improved quality of life. Hence just weight loss alone would be only one of many parameters to define the effectiveness of bariatric surgery. The complications of bariatric surgery are not insignificant and also need to be taken into consideration.

The aim of this chapter is to review the existing literature and provide guidance for reporting outcomes after bariatric surgery.

5.2 Weight Loss Outcomes

5.2.1 Weight Loss Measures

It was in 1981, when Reinhold first defined success of bariatric surgery based on a risk–benefit principle [1]. He used the then known correlation between absolute body weight and general health and expressed postoperative weight as multiples of the patient's ideal body weight (IBW), labeling 200 % IBW as failure, 150 % IBW as success, and 125 % IBW as excellent outcome. MacLean et al. modified the Reinhold classification in 1993, converting the cumbersome multiples of IBW into body mass

L. Kow, BMBS, PhD, FRACS
Adelaide Bariatric Centre, Adelaide, Australia
e-mail: lilian.kow@flinders.edu.au

P.R. Palanivelu et al. (eds.), *Bariatric Surgical Practice Guide*,
DOI 10.1007/978-981-10-2705-5_5

index (BMI) criteria: BMI 35 for success and BMI 30 for an excellent result [2]. However, the most widespread used definitions of bariatric failure and success became the 25 and 50 % excess weight loss (%EWL) marks (often mistaken for the Reinhold criteria). They were introduced by Oria in 1998 as part of an elaborate scoring system, but as single weight loss thresholds, they had no evidence-base correlation with either benefit or risk [3]. These BMI 35 and 50 % EWL marks are still used as bariatric weight loss criteria, implying a certain level of successful overall health improvement. However, just weight loss alone whether defined by BMI or %EWL is considered no longer adequate for defining success of bariatric surgery. Brethauer et al. suggested that weight loss measurements should include as follows [4]:

1. Mean initial BMI of the cohort
2. Change in BMI (ΔBMI):

$$\Delta\text{BMI} = \text{Initial BMI} - \text{Postoperative BMI}$$

3. Percentage of total weight loss (%TWL):

$$\%\text{TWL} = \frac{\text{Initial Weight} - \text{Postoperative Weight}}{\text{Initial Weight}} \times 100$$

4. Percentage of excess BMI loss (%EBMIL):

$$\%\text{EBMIL} = \frac{\Delta\text{BMI}}{(\text{Initial BMI} - 25)} \times 100$$

and/or

5. Percent excess weight loss (%EWL):

$$\%\text{EWL} = \frac{\text{Initial Weight} - \text{Postoperative Weight}}{(\text{Initial Weight} - \text{Ideal Body Weight})} \times 100$$

5.2.2 Percentile Charts

Van de Laar recommended percentile-based charts based on large numbers of patients from multiple surgeons and centres with essentially good follow-up data [5]. He implied that percentile charts are neutral and can be based on different characteristics such as gender, age or baseline BMI. However these percentile charts are scarcely found in the literature.

5.2.3 Body Fat Parameters

The relationship between BMI and mortality is U-shaped and hence believed that body fat mass is a better measurement of outcomes. The use of BMI as a proxy for the measurement of adiposity can be misleading as body weight is the sum of individual organs and tissues including adipose tissue, skeletal muscle mass and organ mass. In addition, BMI does not convey any information on fat distribution in the body [6].

Bioelectric Impedence Analysis (BIA) is one of the available direct measurements of body fat [7–9]. Clinical studies have validated foot-to-foot BIA technology for body composition analysis [10]. National norms for BIA differences between ethnic and racial groups based on NHANES111 have been published recently. Studies on fat mass show a direct linear relationship between body fat and all-cause mortality [11].

5.3 Co Morbidities Outcomes

The metabolic effects from weight loss should also be considered in defining success of bariatric surgery. Now that metabolic benefits of bariatric surgery are well recognized, bariatric success should be redefined to include the metabolic parameters [5]. It is well documented that small amounts of weight loss carry significant health benefits and perhaps individual co-morbid conditions should be measured as parameters of successful outcomes following bariatric surgery. These should importantly include type 2 diabetes, dyslipidemia and hypertension.

5.3.1 Type 2 Diabetes

Several studies have detailed the improvement in diabetes as a result of both restrictive and malabsorptive bariatric surgery. Pories published in 1995 about the effectiveness of LRYGB on the treatment of diabetes [12]. Many studies have followed substantiating the effectiveness of bariatric surgery on diabetes and hence this should be a powerful measurement of outcomes following bariatric surgery. For reporting outcomes in diabetes, Brethauer et al. recommended the following glycemic definitions for standardization [4]:

Definitions of glycemic outcomes after bariatric surgery

Outcome	*Definition*
Remission (complete)	Normal measures of glucose metabolism (HbA1c <6 %, FBG <100 mg/dL) in the absence antidiabetic medications
Remission (partial)	Sub-diabetic hyperglycemia (HbA1c 6–6.4 %, FBG 100–125 mg/dL) in the absence antidiabetic medications
Improvement	Statistically significant reduction in HbA1c and FBG not meeting criteria for remission or decrease in antidiabetic medications requirement (by discontinuing insulin or one oral agent or 1/2 reduction in dose)
Unchanged	The absence of remission or improvement as described above
Recurrence	FBG or HbA1c in the diabetic range (≥126 mg/dL and ≥6.5 %, respectively) or the need for antidiabetic medication after any period of complete or partial remission

Glycosylated hemoglobin (HbA1c), fasting blood glucose (FBG)

5.3.2 Hypertension

Whilst weight loss and bariatric surgery has been associated with benefits in hypertension, there is heterogeneity of data. Again to provide useful measurement outcomes, the following has been suggested by Brethauer et al [4].

Stage of hypertension prior to and after bariatric surgery at the defined follow-up intervals:

Prehypertension (120–140/80–89): systolic/diastolic
Stage 1 hypertension (140–159/90–99)
Stage 2 hypertension (>160/>100)

Antihypertensive medication use
Clearly define indication for medication as treatment of hypertension. Reporting medication type or class and duration of therapy is also recommended with the understanding that this may not be feasible in retrospective studies.

Definitions of blood pressure outcomes after bariatric surgery

Improvement	Decrease in dosage or number of antihypertensive medication or decrease in systolic or diastolic blood pressure on same medication (better control).
Partial Remission	Prehypertension values (120–140/80–89) off medication
Complete Remission	Normotensive (BP <120/80) off antihypertensive medication. If medication such as beta blockade is used for another indication (atrial fibrillation), this needs to be clearly described but cannot be included as complete remission due to the dual therapeutic effect of some medications

5.3.3 Dyslipidemia

The Adult Treatment Panel III (ATP III) Guidelines, 2001, of the National Heart, Lung and Blood Institute is the most widely used criteria of dyslipidemia. According to these criteria optimal values are LDL cholesterol <100 mg/dL, HDL cholesterol <40 mg/dL, total cholesterol <200 mg/dL and triglycerides <150 mg/dL. Brethauer et al. recommended ATP III Guidelines to be used for reporting dyslipidemia after bariatric surgery [4]. They suggested that outcomes be reported as below [4].

Improvement	Decrease in number or dose of lipid-lowering agents with equivalent control of dyslipidemia or improved control of lipids on equivalent medication.
Remission	Normal lipid panel (or specific component being studied) off medication

5.3.4 Other Co-morbidities

Other co-morbidities like gastroesophageal reflux, obstructive sleep apnoae etc should be reported either under a subjective or objective category based on questionnaires and/or investigations like polysomnogram, endoscopy, pH study, impedance study etc. [4].

5.4 Complication Outcomes

Since the acceptance of laparoscopic bariatric surgery, the mortality outcomes have improved significantly. Who would have thought that risk of dying from a laparoscopic bariatric procedure (0.08 %) is now about equivalent to the risk of dying from a routine laparoscopic cholecystectomy? However, all complications (major or minor), no matter the risks need to be reported as an outcome following bariatric surgery. Brethauer suggested the following way to report complications [4].

Complication	*Major*	*Minor*
Early <30 days	Early major	Early minor
Late >30 days	Late major	Late minor

Major complications include any complication that results in a prolonged hospital stay (beyond 7 days), administration of an anticoagulant, re-intervention, or re-operation. Minor complications will include everything else that is not included under major. The examples can be found in the paper.

5.5 Quality of Life Outcomes

Obesity significantly limits quality of life (QoL) and many studies have reported and attempted to validate QoL measurements for assessment following bariatric surgery. Three instruments have been extensively used: the Medical Outcome Study Short Form-36 (MOS SF-36, Rand SF-36 or SF-36), Bariatric Analysis and Reporting Outcome System (BAROS) and the Impact of Weight on Quality of Life-Lite (IWQoL-Lite).

5.6 Classification of Outcomes According to Duration of Follow-Up

One of the biggest deficiencies of the current literature on the various bariatric procedures is the lack of good long term outcomes. We should collect data and evaluate each of our procedures and document the duration of follow-up [4]:

- Short-term follow-up is defined as <3 years after intervention.
- Medium-term follow-up is defined as >3 and <5 years after intervention.
- Long-term follow-up is defined as >5 years after intervention.

Recommendations

- Weight loss is the main outcome measure in bariatric surgery and needs to include percentage of total weight loss (%TWL) in addition to changes in BMI or %EWL.
- Weight loss is insufficient as a single outcome measure and improvement in comorbidities and occurrence of complications needs to be included in the outcome parameters.
- QOL is an important outcome measure that needs to be assessed in morbidly obese patients undergoing bariatric surgery.

References

1. Reinhold RB. Critical analysis of long term weight loss following gastric bypass. Surg Gynecol Obstet. 1982;155(3):385–94.
2. MacLean LD, Rhode BM, Sampalis J, Forse RA. Results of the surgical treatment of obesity. Am J Surg. 1993;165(1):155–60; discussion 160–2.
3. Oria HE, Moorehead MK. Bariatric analysis and reporting outcome system (BAROS). Obes Surg. 1998;8(5):487–99.
4. Brethauer SA, Kim J, El Chaar M, Papasavas P, Eisenberg D, Rogers A, et al. Standardized outcomes reporting in metabolic and bariatric surgery. Obes Surg. 2015;25(4):587–606.
5. van de Laar AWJM, Acherman YIZ. Weight loss percentile charts of large representative series: a benchmark defining sufficient weight loss challenging current criteria for success of bariatric surgery. Obes Surg. 2014;24(5):727–34.
6. Busetto L, Dixon J, De Luca M, Shikora S, Pories W, Angrisani L. Bariatric surgery in class I obesity: a Position Statement from the International Federation for the Surgery of Obesity and Metabolic Disorders (IFSO). Obes Surg. 2014;24(4):487–519.
7. Chumlea WC, Baumgartner RN. Bioelectric impedance methods for the estimation of body composition. Can J Sport Sci J Can Sci Sport. 1990;15(3):172–9.
8. Van Loan MD. Bioelectrical impedance analysis to determine fat-free mass, total body water and body fat. Sports Med Auckl NZ. 1990;10(4):205–17.
9. NIH Consensus statement. Bioelectrical impedance analysis in body composition measurement. National Institutes of Health Technology Assessment Conference Statement. December 12-14, 1994. Nutr Burbank Los Angel Cty Calif. 1996;12(11–12):749–62.
10. Tyrrell VJ, Richards G, Hofman P, Gillies GF, Robinson E, Cutfield WS. Foot-to-foot bioelectrical impedance analysis: a valuable tool for the measurement of body composition in children. Int J Obes Relat Metab Disord J Int Assoc Study Obes. 2001;25(2):273–8.
11. Chumlea WC, Guo SS, Kuczmarski RJ, Flegal KM, Johnson CL, Heymsfield SB, et al. Body composition estimates from NHANES III bioelectrical impedance data. Int J Obes Relat Metab Disord J Int Assoc Study Obes. 2002;26(12):1596–609.
12. Pories WJ, Swanson MS, MacDonald KG, Long SB, Morris PG, Brown BM, et al. Who would have thought it? An operation proves to be the most effective therapy for adult-onset diabetes mellitus. Ann Surg. 1995;222(3):339–50; discussion 350–2.

Preoperative Predictors of Weight Loss After Bariatric Surgery

6

Deep Goel and Asim Shabbir

6.1 Introduction

Obesity has emerged as a major public health problem in both developed and developing countries. This is only expected to increase further into epidemic proportions in the years to come. Involvement of multiple organ systems and its strong association with comorbidity is well established. Bariatric surgery has emerged to be the most promising option for long term weight loss and resolution of co-morbidities.

Outcomes of bariatric surgery remain highly procedure and surgeon specific. A successful outcome is also highly dependent on the patient's compliance with alterations in their eating habits and levels of physical activity [1–3]. The commonest bariatric procedure in the West is the laparoscopic roux-en-y gastric bypass (LRYGB) which consistently results in the loss of 70–80 % of excess body weight. However the degree of weight loss among bariatric surgical patients post-surgery is considerably variable. Considerable effort has been made in this regard in the recent years, in order to identify specific preoperative predictive factors in these patients which may alter the degree of weight loss postoperatively thereby allowing surgeons to identify patients who are most likely to benefit from surgery, for optimal resource allocation and patient satisfaction.

The only factor which has been subjected to a meta-analysis is that of preoperative weight loss which shows a positive association with postoperative weight loss following gastric bypass surgery. Another clinical variable is baseline BMI; the higher the BMI, the lesser the patient will lose in terms of percentage of excess body

D. Goel, DNB, FRCS, FACS
Department of GI Surgery, Bariatric and Minimal Access Surgery,
BLK Hospital, Delhi, India
e-mail: goel_deep@hotmail.com

A. Shabbir, MMEd, FRCS (✉)
National University Hospital, Singapore, Singapore
e-mail: cfsasim@nus.edu.sg

P.R. Palanivelu et al. (eds.), *Bariatric Surgical Practice Guide*,
DOI 10.1007/978-981-10-2705-5_6

weight (%EWL) relative to patients with lower initial BMIs. This effect is in part an artifact of measuring weight loss in relative rather than absolute terms [4, 5].

Although the remaining data are not based on level 1 evidence other preoperatively identifiable factors which are associated with an improved outcome include Caucasian ethnicity, higher educational status, non-shift-work working patterns, female gender and divorced or single marital status. Similarly increased levels of preoperative physical activity and an absence of binge eating behavior are consistent with a favorable result whereas increased age, smoking and other socioeconomic factors have not been shown to have a significant impact. Conversely diabetes mellitus seems to have a slightly negative correlation with postoperative weight loss; however, a history of psychiatric illness has not been shown to have any significant influence.

The purpose of this chapter is to discuss the current state of evidence with regard to identification of preoperative predictive factors affecting weight loss post bariatric surgery hence assisting surgeons in patient selection.

6.2 Preoperative Weight Loss

Preoperative weight loss is postulated to help assess patient compliance and assist with patient selection. Requiring preoperative weight loss might identify patients who will comply better with the dietary restrictions after surgery. Losing weight in the weeks before surgery appears to decrease liver size, which in turn might lead to shorter operative times, lesser blood loss, lower rates of conversion from laparoscopic to open procedures, and fewer per-operative complications [6].

Because a preoperative weight loss requirement in the period immediately preceding surgery might potentially exclude some patients who would refuse to lose weight, it is critical to evaluate the evidence on whether preoperative weight loss leads to improved outcomes. Several studies have found a short-term benefit for preoperative weight loss in bariatric surgery patients as per a meta-analysis done by Masha et al. [7]. Mrad et al. found that preoperative weight loss correlated with postoperative weight loss in men but not in women. A significant short-term correlation was found at 3 months, but this effect had disappeared by 12 months [8]. Alami et al. also found significantly greater weight loss in the preoperative weight loss group at 3 months [9]. Alvarado et al. showed that an increase of 1 % in preoperative weight loss correlated with an increase of 1.8 % in the postoperative percentage excess weight loss (%EWL) at 1 year [10]. Carlin et al. found no correlation between the preoperative and postoperative %EWL at 12 months, controlling for initial BMI [11]. Alger-Mayer et al. found a positive correlation between the preoperative %EWL and post-operative %EWL at 3 years [12].

The above concept is controversial, in part because of questions of the safety of relatively rapid weight loss in an obese population before undergoing major surgery. The efficacy and justification of mandating patients to lose weight before bariatric surgery has also been challenged. The findings suggest that obese patients can lose 10 % of their excess body weight in the weeks before undergoing surgery without significant peri-operative risk. Several studies demonstrated a decreased operative time for patients who had lost weight preoperatively, although mostly this did not translate to a decreased length of stay or reduction in complication rates. Overall, it appears that preoperative weight loss results in greater total postoperative weight loss, when studies of low quality were excluded.

6.3 Preoperative BMI

Several authors have sought to determine whether or not a patient's preoperative body mass index (BMI) has any bearing on their likely outcome following surgery. The majority of those studies have concluded that while a higher preoperative BMI is associated with a greater absolute weight loss, when considered in terms of %EWL, this group tends to be worse [1, 13–17].

To date no meta-analysis of the studies specific to LRYGB has been published and consequently the significance of BMI at presentation can only be considered to be based on level 3 evidence at best. The discrepancy between absolute weight loss and %EWL has led some authors to argue that %EWL is not an appropriate measure of success in the higher initial BMI group. Percentage EWL is a relative measure that diminishes the significance of the absolute amount, i.e., kilogram of weight lost. The disparity between %EWL and absolute weight loss is also magnified by the length of post-operative follow-up. The relatively short lengths of follow-up (i.e., 12 months) of many studies may not allow sufficient time for patients with higher BMIs to shed sufficient weight to reach their weight nadir.

6.4 Ethnicity

Several studies have looked at the subject of ethnicity to see whether racial background has an influence on the degree of EWL following LRYGB. All but one of the studies that have compared Caucasians with people of Afro-Caribbean descent have found a significantly greater degree of EWL in the investigated Caucasian populations [11, 18–23]. Why these racial differences exist is not currently known. Similarly, the degree to which ethnicity can be used as a prognostic indicator is also currently unquantified but there remains a strong suggestion that certain races do experience a more favorable outcome following LRYGB than others secondary to metabolic differences.

6.5 Marital Status

Another factor which has been shown to influence EWL following LRYGB is marital status. Whether this should be viewed as a modifiable factor is open to debate but the fact that unmarried patients achieved a higher degree of EWL after LRYGB when compared with their married counterparts is still worthy of consideration [20, 24].

6.6 Binge Eating Disorder

The specific aspect of eating behavior that has attracted the most attention has been that of binge eating disorder (BED) in which a person experiences episodes of eating an objectively large amount of food in association with a subjective feeling of loss of control. A literature review in 1998 by Hsu et al. concluded that BED was associated with weight regain [25].

A recent systematic review by Mercado et al. found 2 studies reporting a positive correlation (BED being associated with greater postoperative EBWL), 4 studies reporting a negative correlation and 14 showing no difference [26]. No meta-analyses on this topic is currently available.

6.7 Physical Activity

Physical activity deserves particular attention both because the magnitude of the effect is clinically meaningful and this characteristic is potentially modifiable. The few studies that have been published have suggested that a reduced level of physical activity preoperatively is a strong predictor of decreased EWL following LRYGB [14, 24].

6.8 Out Patient Attendance

El Chaar et al. compared LRYGB patients with gastric band patients and found that while gastric band patients who had missed more than a quarter of their preoperative clinic appointments had a significantly lower postoperative %EWL than those who missed fewer than 25 %, the same was not true for those who had undergone the LRYGB [27].

6.9 Smoking

Although the precise mechanism remains unclear, the relationship between smoking cessation and weight gain is well established. Most studies till date have concentrated on the effects of smoking on postoperative morbidity and mortality. Effect of smoking on the degree of %EWL in obese patients is not well established. Those studies which have looked specifically at the effects of smoking on %EWL have found results varying from a modestly beneficial effect of smoking to a modestly detrimental effect [28–30].

6.10 Genetics

Since genotype of an individual directly determines his or her phenotype and the fact that obesity runs in families, it would be unwise to neglect its role in weight loss dynamics. A study by Gallagher et al. suggested that pairs of genetically-related patients are liable to achieve more similar degrees of %EWL following bariatric surgery compared with cohabiting but genetically unrelated couples. They concluded that heredity accounted for as much as 77 % of the variability of postoperative %EWL [31].

6.11 Diabetes

A study by Carbonell et al. looking specifically at diabetics undergoing LRYGB investigated 655 diabetic patients and suggested that patients requiring insulin, experienced significantly less postoperative %EWL at 1 year than non-diabetic patients [32]. To date no systematic review or meta-analysis looking at the predictive value of diabetes status on post-LRYGB %EWL has been published.

6.12 Conclusion

Although many factors have been implicated as being potentially predictive of the degree of %EWL that can be expected following LRYGB, only preoperative weight loss has been established on basis of level I evidence to have an effect on postoperative outcome. Role of other factors like age, sex, ethnicity, smoking, marital status, diabetes, psychiatric illness, eating behavior, genetics and preoperative BMI are only based on level III evidence and further randomized studies are needed to establish the same.

Recommendations

- Preoperative weight loss is the only factor to successfully predict postoperative weight loss after bariatric surgery
- Integrating a preoperative weight loss program would be beneficial for bariatric surgery candidates.

References

1. Melton GB, Steele KE, Schweitzer MA, Lidor AO, Magnuson TH. Suboptimal weight loss after gastric bypass surgery: correlation of demographics, comorbidities, and insurance status with outcomes. J Gastrointest Surg Off J Soc Surg Aliment Tract. 2008;12(2):250–5.
2. Ray EC, Nickels MW, Sayeed S, Sax HC. Predicting success after gastric bypass: the role of psychosocial and behavioral factors. Surgery. 2003;134(4):555–63; discussion 563–4.
3. van Hout GCM, Verschure SKM, van Heck GL. Psychosocial predictors of success following bariatric surgery. Obes Surg. 2005;15(4):552–60.
4. van de Laar A, de Caluwé L, Dillemans B. Relative outcome measures for bariatric surgery. Evidence against excess weight loss and excess body mass index loss from a series of laparoscopic Roux-en-Y gastric bypass patients. Obes Surg. 2011;21(6):763–7.

5. Bray GA, Bouchard C, Church TS, Cefalu WT, Greenway FL, Gupta AK, et al. Is it time to change the way we report and discuss weight loss? Obes Silver Spring Md. 2009;17(4):619–21.
6. Lewis MC, Phillips ML, Slavotinek JP, Kow L, Thompson CH, Toouli J. Change in liver size and fat content after treatment with Optifast very low calorie diet. Obes Surg. 2006;16(6):697–701.
7. Livhits M, Mercado C, Yermilov I, Parikh JA, Dutson E, Mehran A, et al. Preoperative predictors of weight loss following bariatric surgery: systematic review. Obes Surg. 2012;22(1):70–89.
8. Mrad BA, Stoklossa CJ, Birch DW. Does preoperative weight loss predict success following surgery for morbid obesity? Am J Surg. 2008;195(5):570–3; discussion 573–4.
9. Alami RS, Morton JM, Schuster R, Lie J, Sanchez BR, Peters A, et al. Is there a benefit to preoperative weight loss in gastric bypass patients? A prospective randomized trial. Surg Obes Relat Dis Off J Am Soc Bariatr Surg. 2007;3(2):141–5; discussion 145–6.
10. Alvarado R, Alami RS, Hsu G, Safadi BY, Sanchez BR, Morton JM, et al. The impact of preoperative weight loss in patients undergoing laparoscopic Roux-en-Y gastric bypass. Obes Surg. 2005;15(9):1282–6.
11. Carlin AM, O'Connor EA, Genaw JA, Kawar S. Preoperative weight loss is not a predictor of postoperative weight loss after laparoscopic Roux-en-Y gastric bypass. Surg Obes Relat Dis Off J Am Soc Bariatr Surg. 2008;4(4):481–5.
12. Alger-Mayer S, Polimeni JM, Malone M. Preoperative weight loss as a predictor of long-term success following Roux-en-Y gastric bypass. Obes Surg. 2008;18(7):772–5.
13. Ma Y, Pagoto SL, Olendzki BC, Hafner AR, Perugini RA, Mason R, et al. Predictors of weight status following laparoscopic gastric bypass. Obes Surg. 2006;16(9):1227–31.
14. Hatoum IJ, Stein HK, Merrifield BF, Kaplan LM. Capacity for physical activity predicts weight loss after Roux-en-Y gastric bypass. Obes Silver Spring Md. 2009;17(1):92–9.
15. Coupaye M, Sabaté JM, Castel B, Jouet P, Clérici C, Msika S, et al. Predictive factors of weight loss 1 year after laparoscopic gastric bypass in obese patients. Obes Surg. 2010;20(12):1671–7.
16. Leong B, Wilson T, Wilson EB, Snyder B. P-19: laparoscopic Roux-en-Y gastric bypass: using sBMI as a predictor of success and failure. Surg Obes Relat Dis. 2009;5(3):S30.
17. Chen EY, McCloskey MS, Doyle P, Roehrig J, Berona J, Alverdy J, et al. Body mass index as a predictor of 1-year outcome in gastric bypass surgery. Obes Surg. 2009;19(9):1240–2.
18. Anderson WA, Greene GW, Forse RA, Apovian CM, Istfan NW. Weight loss and health outcomes in African Americans and whites after gastric bypass surgery. Obes Silver Spring Md. 2007;15(6):1455–63.
19. Harvin G, DeLegge M, Garrow DA. The impact of race on weight loss after Roux-en-Y gastric bypass surgery. Obes Surg. 2008;18(1):39–42.
20. Lutfi R, Torquati A, Sekhar N, Richards WO. Predictors of success after laparoscopic gastric bypass: a multivariate analysis of socioeconomic factors. Surg Endosc. 2006;20(6):864–7.
21. Buffington CK, Marema RT. Ethnic differences in obesity and surgical weight loss between African-American and Caucasian females. Obes Surg. 2006;16(2):159–65.
22. Madan AK, Whitfield JD, Fain JN, Beech BM, Ternovits CA, Menachery S, et al. Are African-Americans as successful as Caucasians after laparoscopic gastric bypass? Obes Surg. 2007;17(4):460–4.
23. Kakade M, Stahl R, Clements R, Grams J. P-40 Impact of race on clinical outcomes after laparoscopic Roux-en-Y gastric bypass. Surg Obes Relat Dis. 2011;7(3):385–6.
24. Livhits M, Mercado C, Yermilov I, Parikh JA, Dutson E, Mehran A, et al. Behavioral factors associated with successful weight loss after gastric bypass. Am Surg. 2010;76(10):1139–42.
25. Hsu LK, Benotti PN, Dwyer J, Roberts SB, Saltzman E, Shikora S, et al. Nonsurgical factors that influence the outcome of bariatric surgery: a review. Psychosom Med. 1998;60(3):338–46.

26. Mercado C, Livhits M, Yermilov I, Parikh J, Ko CY, Gibbons MM. P-46: is binge eating disorder associated with the degree of weight loss following bariatric surgery? Surg Obes Relat Dis. 2010;6(3):S43.
27. El Chaar M, McDeavitt K, Richardson S, Gersin KS, Kuwada TS, Stefanidis D. Does patient compliance with preoperative bariatric office visits affect postoperative excess weight loss? Surg Obes Relat Dis Off J Am Soc Bariatr Surg. 2011;7(6):743–8.
28. Latner JD, Wetzler S, Goodman ER, Glinski J. Gastric bypass in a low-income, inner-city population: eating disturbances and weight loss. Obes Res. 2004;12(6):956–61.
29. Levine MD, Kalarchian MA, Courcoulas AP, Wisinski MSC, Marcus MD. History of smoking and postcessation weight gain among weight loss surgery candidates. Addict Behav. 2007;32(10):2365–71.
30. Dixon JB, Dixon ME, O'Brien PE. Pre-operative predictors of weight loss at 1-year after Lap-Band surgery. Obes Surg. 2001;11(2):200–7.
31. Gallagher R, Xing C, Varela JE, Livingston E, Puzziferri N. PL-208: genetic and environmental influence on weight loss after bariatric surgery. Surg Obes Relat Dis. 2010;6(3):S12.
32. Carbonell AM, Wolfe LG, Meador JG, Sugerman HJ, Kellum JM, Maher JW. Does diabetes affect weight loss after gastric bypass? Surg Obes Relat Dis Off J Am Soc Bariatr Surg. 2008;4(3):441–4.

Preoperative Predictors of Diabetes Remission Following Bariatric Surgery

7

Saravana Kumar and Rachel Maria Gomes

7.1 Introduction

Obesity is one of the greatest public health problems today with more than 400 million adults being obese [1]. The worldwide prevalence of type 2 diabetes mellitus (T2DM) is also rising alongside obesity with more than 300 million people suffering from T2DM of which more than 60 % of patients with T2DM are obese [2–4]. This has been commonly referred as 'diabesity'. Hence the prevention and treatment of diabesity is an important public health priority.

Bariatric surgery has now shown to play a significant role in the treatment of all components of metabolic syndrome, with more relevance pertaining to T2DM. It has been demonstrated that bariatric surgery is an effective treatment for T2DM when compared with conventional nonsurgical medical treatment in appropriately selected diabetic individuals [5, 6]. Considerable effort has been made in this regard in the recent years, in order to identify the specific preoperative variables which could serve as predicting factors of diabetes control, thereby allowing surgeons to identify patients who are most likely to benefit from surgery. The main predictors of T2DM remission are C-peptide, BMI, age, duration of diabetes, glycaemic status, insulin therapy and type of bariatric surgical procedure.

The aim of this chapter was to review the role of these factors as predictors of DM remission.

S. Kumar, MS, FMAS (✉) • R.M. Gomes, MS, FMAS
Bariatric Division, Upper Gastrointestinal Surgery and Minimal Access Surgery Unit, GEM Hospital and Research Centre, Coimbatore, India
e-mail: drsakubariatric@gmail.com; dr.gomes@rediffmail.com

P.R. Palanivelu et al. (eds.), *Bariatric Surgical Practice Guide*, DOI 10.1007/978-981-10-2705-5_7

7.2 Pre-operative Predictors of Diabetes Remission

7.2.1 C-Peptide

The ‘connecting’ peptide or C-peptide is a polypeptide released from the pancreatic beta-cells during cleavage of insulin from proinsulin and thus represents the capacity of insulin secretion, as both are secreted in equimolar amounts by the beta cells. Directly measuring insulin levels may be difficult in T2DM patients especially in those who are receiving insulin therapy. Hence measuring the C-peptide level is a valuable test to measure endogenous insulin in diabetic patients [7–9]. Obesity especially central obesity is known to be associated with insulin resistance which in turn is associated with hyperinsulinemia. Hence these patients correspondingly have higher C-peptide levels. However, with advancing T2DM beta cells are progressively destroyed, with C-peptide levels gradually becoming low.

WJ. Lee et al., in his study reported elevated baseline C-peptide >4 ng/ml in 58 % of morbidly obese patients with T2DM with a mean baseline C-peptide of 5.3 ± 3.5 ng/ml. There was a mean reduction by 64.1 % in C-peptide levels after a significant weight reduction 1 year after surgery with a T2DM remission rate of 78 % corresponding to decreasing insulin resistance and reduction in hyperinsulinemia [9]. WJ Lee et al. reported that patients with T2DM remission had higher baseline C-peptide levels than those without remission [8]. Ramos Levi et al. also reported that patients with T2DM remission had higher C-peptide levels than those without remission [10].

WJ. Lee et al. reported diabetes remission rates for those with preoperative C-peptide <3, 3–6, and >6 ng/ml to be 55.3 %, 82.0 % and 90.3 % respectively in morbidly obese T2DM [11]. Dixon et al. in a study in a Chinese population reported fasting C-peptide concentration >2.9 ng/mL to be a predictor of remission in morbidly obese T2DM [12]. In another study in Korean population Dixon et al. reported that a baseline C-peptide >2.4 ng/ml was associated with remission in morbidly obese T2DM [13]. Lakdawala et al. reported a fasting C-peptide levels more than or equal to 3 nmol/l to be a predictor of remission in morbidly obese T2DM [14]. Ramos Levi et al. reported a cutoff of C-peptide of 3.75 ng/ml for prediction of remission in morbidly obese T2DM [10]. WJ Lee et al. reported that a fasting C-peptide levels more than or equal to 3 nmol/l is the best prognostic marker of good remission after bariatric surgery even in the non-morbidly obese [15].

WJ Lee et al. reported low C-peptide levels <1 nmol/l in 1 % of morbidly obese patients with T2DM [9]. Both WJ Lee et al. and Aarts et al. reported that a preoperative fasting C-peptide less than 1 ng/l in severely obese T2DM indicated partial beta cell failure and predicted a markedly reduced chance of resolution of T2DM [16] In the study in a Korean population Dixon et al. reported that a baseline C-peptide of <2.0 ng/ml predicted a poor glycaemic response in morbidly obese T2 DM [13]. However interpretation of low C-peptide levels must be made with a corresponding level of blood glucose as fasting levels of C-peptide may be suppressed in a hyperglycaemic status [16].

7.2.2 Body Mass Index

Body mass index (BMI) has been studied extensively as a predicting variable for outcomes of T2DM following bariatric surgery. Mingrone et al. reported that the baseline BMI was unrelated to diabetes remission in morbidly obese patients [6]. Panunzi et al. also reported that the baseline BMI was unrelated to diabetes remission. They reported similar diabetes remission rates in patients with BMI of more than 35 kg/m^2 versus BMI of less than 35 kg/m^2 [17] WJ Lee et al. in a multi-institutional study found similar diabetes remission rates in patients with BMI of 30 kg/m^2 versus BMI of less than 30 kg/m^2 [11].

Some studies identified BMI as predictor of T2DM remission. Lakdawala et al. identified BMI ≥35 kg/m^2 as a predictor of long term remission [14]. Dixon et al. in a study in Korean population also identified BMI ≥35 kg/m^2 as a predictor of long term remission [12]. Robert et al. identified that at 1 year BMI less than 35 was a positive predicting factor of diabetes remission [18]. Robert et al. paradoxically demonstrated that a BMI >50 kg/m^2 was a negative predictor of T2DM remission [18].

7.2.3 Duration of T2DM

The duration of T2DM reflects the natural course of the disease of progressive deterioration of beta cell function. Hence more the duration of disease, the lower the residual islet cell amount is likely to be.

WJ Lee et al. reported that less than 4 years of duration of DM will have a better outcome than those with more than 8 years (only 4 % remission rate). Hence this was added as a component in his scoring system [8, 11, 21]. Lakdawala et al. reported patients with less than 5 years duration of DM had remission rate is nearing 100 % whereas those with 5–15 years the remission rate varied between 60 and 75 % [14]. Similarly, Dixon et al. also reported that longer the duration of DM, the remission rates were lower [12, 22]. Rosenthal et al. noted that the T2DM remission rate was very low in patients who had a duration of T2DM of greater than 5 years and received sleeve gastrectomies [23]. A multi-institutional study by Lee et al. showed that the duration of T2DM was the most important predictor of T2DM remission after bariatric surgery [11]. In a study by Robert et al., T2DM less than 4 years duration was reported as a positive predictor factor for remission at 1 year after bariatric surgery [18]. Blackstone et al. in T2DM after RYGB study also supported the shorter duration of T2DM less than 4 years as a positive predictive factor [24]. Yan et al. identified that patients with a complete remission had a significantly shorter history of diabetes [25].

7.2.4 Age of the Patient

Age reflects the general reserve of beta-cell function which gradually declines with increasing age. Hamza et al. reported younger age to be an independent predictor of T2DM remission. They also reported that each additional 12 years of age reduced the chance of T2DM remission by 20 % [26]. WJ Lee et al. had reported that patients less than 40 years of age showed better remission rate than patients over 40 years of age which later became a part of his scoring index [9, 21]. Lakdawala et al. reported better remission rates in younger patients, with patients over 60 years associated with significantly poor outcomes [14].

7.2.5 Glycemic Status

HbA1c levels indicate glycaemic control, with higher HbA1c levels indicating poor glycaemic control. High HbA1c with poor glycaemic control may be related to either higher insulin resistance or lower beta cell function. It has been noted from various studies that patients with better glycemic control (HbA1C <7) have better remission of DM [20, 24, 27–29]. Patients who require only OHA to have a good glycemic control have reported higher remission rates than those requiring insulin, the latter indicating poor beta cell reserve. WJ Lee in his analyses, found that the patients who did not receive insulin therapy are more likely to have T2DM remission after surgery [21]. Robert et al., Arterburn et al. and Jurowich et al. also identified that insulin therapy as a preoperative predictive factor of diabetes remission [18, 27, 28].

7.2.6 Type of Procedure

Depending on the surgical procedure, the DM remission rate can range from 45 to 97 % of patients. Panunzi et al. in a meta-analysis reported diabetes remission of 89 % after bilio-pancreatic diversion, 77 % after Roux-en-Y bypass, 62 % after gastric banding, and 60 % after sleeve gastrectomy [17]. Another metanalysis by Buchwald et al. reported similar results [30]. This difference in T2DM may be related to a difference in physiologic mechanisms. However comparing the outcomes of T2DM with relation to procedures is difficult as disease severity varies within each surgical subgroup. WJ Lee et al. identified that in patients with low C-peptide levels outcomes after gastric bypass is significantly better compared to a restrictive procedure [8].

Several studies have reported that T2DM remission is more related to the percentage of weight loss rather than the baseline weight implicating that procedures with better weight loss lead to higher remission rates [12, 19–21].

Conclusions

Remission of diabetes is dependent on many factors. Elderly patients, duration of T2DM >4–5 years, poor glycaemic control and need for insulin therapy all corresponding to low beta cell function and are associated with lower rates of remission of T2DM. Beta cell function is an important factor in predicting diabetes remission. Beta cell function can be estimated by measuring C peptide levels to give a more accurate idea of residual beta cell function. Fasting C-peptide levels more than >3–4 ng/ml is a predictor of T2DM remission and levels less than 1 ng/ml predicted a markedly reduced chance of resolution. Relationship of T2 DM remission and BMI are conflicting but higher BMI may be a predictor of T2DM remission. Diabetes resolution was better after bilio-pancreatic diversion followed by roux-en-Y bypass, then sleeve gastrectomy and gastric banding which may be related to both physiological mechanisms and degree of weight loss. T2DM remission is more related to the percentage of weight loss rather than the baseline weight.

Recommendations

- Severity of type 2 diabetes mellitus predicts remission post-bariatric surgery.
- Clinical factors reflecting the severity of diabetes mellitus include age, BMI, duration of T2DM, glycaemic control, need for insulin therapy and residual beta cell function.
- Higher the malabsorption better the weight loss and higher the remission of diabetes.

References

1. Raffaelli M, Sessa L, Mingrone G, Bellantone R. Assessing the obese diabetic patient for bariatric surgery: which candidate do I choose? Diabetes Metab Syndr Obes Targets Ther. 2015;8:255–62.
2. Colditz GA, Willett WC, Rotnitzky A, Manson JE. Weight gain as a risk factor for clinical diabetes mellitus in women. Ann Intern Med. 1995;122(7):481–6.
3. Kramer H, Cao G, Dugas L, Luke A, Cooper R, Durazo-Arvizu R. Increasing BMI and waist circumference and prevalence of obesity among adults with Type 2 diabetes: the National Health and Nutrition Examination Surveys. J Diabetes Complications. 2010;24(6):368–74.
4. Wong K, Glovaci D, Malik S, Franklin SS, Wygant G, Iloeje U, et al. Comparison of demographic factors and cardiovascular risk factor control among U.S. adults with type 2 diabetes by insulin treatment classification. J Diabetes Complications. 2012;26(3):169–74.
5. Schauer PR, Bhatt DL, Kashyap SR. Bariatric surgery versus intensive medical therapy for diabetes. N Engl J Med. 2014;371(7):682.
6. Mingrone G, Panunzi S, De Gaetano A, Guidone C, Iaconelli A, Leccesi L, et al. Bariatric surgery versus conventional medical therapy for type 2 diabetes. N Engl J Med. 2012;366(17):1577–85.
7. Lee W-J, Almulaifi A, Tsou JJ, Ser K-H, Lee Y-C, Chen S-C. Laparoscopic sleeve gastrectomy for type 2 diabetes mellitus: predicting the success by ABCD score. Surg Obes Relat Dis Off J Am Soc Bariatr Surg. 2015;11(5):991–6.
8. Lee W-J, Chong K, Chen J-C, Ser K-H, Lee Y-C, Tsou J-J, et al. Predictors of diabetes remission after bariatric surgery in Asia. Asian J Surg Asian Surg Assoc. 2012;35(2):67–73.
9. Lee W-J, Chong K, Ser K-H, Chen J-C, Lee Y-C, Chen S-C, et al. C-peptide predicts the remission of type 2 diabetes after bariatric surgery. Obes Surg. 2012;22(2):293–8.
10. Ramos-Leví AM, Matía P, Cabrerizo L, Barabash A, Torrejón MJ, Sánchez-Pernaute A, et al. C-peptide levels predict type 2 diabetes remission after bariatric surgery. Nutr Hosp. 2013;28(5):1599–603.

11. Lee W-J, Hur KY, Lakadawala M, Kasama K, Wong SKH, Lee Y-C. Gastrointestinal metabolic surgery for the treatment of diabetic patients: a multi-institutional international study. J Gastrointest Surg Off J Soc Surg Aliment Tract. 2012;16(1):45–51; discussion 51–2.
12. Dixon JB, Chuang L-M, Chong K, Chen S-C, Lambert GW, Straznicky NE, et al. Predicting the glycemic response to gastric bypass surgery in patients with type 2 diabetes. Diabetes Care. 2013;36(1):20–6.
13. Dixon JB, Hur K-Y, Lee W-J, Kim M-J, Chong K, Chen S-C, et al. Gastric bypass in Type 2 diabetes with BMI < 30: weight and weight loss have a major influence on outcomes. Diabet Med J Br Diabet Assoc. 2013;30(4):e127–34.
14. Bhasker AG, Remedios C, Batra P, Sood A, Shaikh S, Lakdawala M. Predictors of remission of T2DM and metabolic effects after laparoscopic Roux-en-y gastric bypass in obese Indian diabetics-a 5-year study. Obes Surg. 2015;25(7):1191–7.
15. Lee W-J, Ser K-H, Chong K, Lee Y-C, Chen S-C, Tsou J-J, et al. Laparoscopic sleeve gastrectomy for diabetes treatment in nonmorbidly obese patients: efficacy and change of insulin secretion. Surgery. 2010;147(5):664–9.
16. Aarts EO, Janssen J, Janssen IMC, Berends FJ, Telting D, de Boer H. Preoperative fasting plasma C-peptide level may help to predict diabetes outcome after gastric bypass surgery. Obes Surg. 2013;23(7):867–73.
17. Panunzi S, De Gaetano A, Carnicelli A, Mingrone G. Predictors of remission of diabetes mellitus in severely obese individuals undergoing bariatric surgery: do BMI or procedure choice matter? A meta-analysis. Ann Surg. 2015;261(3):459–67.
18. Robert M, Ferrand-Gaillard C, Disse E, Espalieu P, Simon C, Laville M, et al. Predictive factors of type 2 diabetes remission 1 year after bariatric surgery: impact of surgical techniques. Obes Surg. 2013;23(6):770–5.
19. Sugerman HJ, Wolfe LG, Sica DA, Clore JN. Diabetes and hypertension in severe obesity and effects of gastric bypass-induced weight loss. Ann Surg. 2003;237(6):751–6; discussion 757–8.
20. Jiménez A, Casamitjana R, Flores L, Viaplana J, Corcelles R, Lacy A, et al. Long-term effects of sleeve gastrectomy and Roux-en-Y gastric bypass surgery on type 2 diabetes mellitus in morbidly obese subjects. Ann Surg. 2012;256(6):1023–9.
21. Lee MH, Lee W-J, Chong K, Chen J-C, Ser K-H, Lee Y-C, et al. Predictors of long-term diabetes remission after metabolic surgery. J Gastrointest Surg Off J Soc Surg Aliment Tract. 2015;19(6):1015–21.
22. Dixon JB, O'Brien PE. Health outcomes of severely obese type 2 diabetic subjects 1 year after laparoscopic adjustable gastric banding. Diabetes Care. 2002;25(2):358–63.
23. Rosenthal R, Li X, Samuel S, Martinez P, Zheng C. Effect of sleeve gastrectomy on patients with diabetes mellitus. Surg Obes Relat Dis Off J Am Soc Bariatr Surg. 2009;5(4):429–34.
24. Blackstone R, Bunt JC, Cortés MC, Sugerman HJ. Type 2 diabetes after gastric bypass: remission in five models using HbA1c, fasting blood glucose, and medication status. Surg Obes Relat Dis Off J Am Soc Bariatr Surg. 2012;8(5):548–55.
25. Yan H, Tang L, Chen T, Kral JG, Jiang L, Li Y, et al. Defining and predicting complete remission of type 2 diabetes: a short-term efficacy study of open gastric bypass. Obes Facts. 2013;6(2):176–84.
26. Hamza N, Abbas MH, Darwish A, Shafeek Z, New J, Ammori BJ. Predictors of remission of type 2 diabetes mellitus after laparoscopic gastric banding and bypass. Surg Obes Relat Dis Off J Am Soc Bariatr Surg. 2011;7(6):691–6.
27. Arterburn DE, Bogart A, Sherwood NE, Sidney S, Coleman KJ, Haneuse S, et al. A multisite study of long-term remission and relapse of type 2 diabetes mellitus following gastric bypass. Obes Surg. 2013;23(1):93–102.

28. Jurowich C, Thalheimer A, Hartmann D, Bender G, Seyfried F, Germer CT, et al. Improvement of type 2 diabetes mellitus (T2DM) after bariatric surgery – who fails in the early postoperative course? Obes Surg. 2012;22(10):1521–6.
29. Schauer PR, Burguera B, Ikramuddin S, Cottam D, Gourash W, Hamad G, et al. Effect of laparoscopic Roux-En Y gastric bypass on type 2 diabetes mellitus. Ann Surg. 2003;238(4):467–84; discussion 84–5.
30. Buchwald H, Estok R, Fahrbach K, Banel D, Jensen MD, Pories WJ, et al. Weight and type 2 diabetes after bariatric surgery: systematic review and meta-analysis. Am J Med. 2009;122(3):248–56.e5.

Part III

Technical Considerations

8 Standardization of Technique in Sleeve Gastrectomy

Jayshree Todkar and Rachel Maria Gomes

8.1 Introduction

Laparoscopic sleeve gastrectomy (LSG) is a restrictive bariatric procedure without a diverting malabsorptive component. It involves resection of a large part of the body and the fundus of the stomach along the greater curvature to provide increased satiety and decreased appetite. The LSG has been seen over time to be an effective bariatric surgery operation and a sensible option in high risk patients [1]. It has thus evolved to be the most popular bariatric stand-alone operation in India [2].

LSG for weight loss was first described by Marceau in 1993 as a component of the bilio-pancreatic diversion with duodenal switch (BPD/DS) [3]. Here the distal gastrectomy of Scopinaro's BPD/DS was modified into a vertical gastrectomy or a sleeve gastrectomy. LSG was subsequently performed as a component of single staged BPD/DS and as the initial stage of a two-staged approach for super obese patients who were considered a high risk group for a combined procedure [4]. Regan et al. in 2003 also described it as the initial stage of a two-staged laparoscopic roux-en-Y gastric bypass (LRYGB), consisting of LSG followed by LRYGB in superobese patients [5]. Over time in addition to the safety profile of LSG in super obese patients, the effectiveness of LSG in isolation was identified in regards to

J. Todkar, MS, Dip. Laparoscopic Surg, FBMS
Department of Bariatric Surgery, Ruby Hall Clinic,
Poona Hospital, Apollo Spectra Hospital, Pune, India
Dr LH Hiranandani Hospital, Mumbai, India
e-mail: jayatodkar@gmail.com

R.M. Gomes, MS, FMAS (✉)
Bariatric Division, Upper Gastrointestinal Surgery and Minimal Access Surgery Unit,
GEM Hospital and Research Centre, Coimbatore, India
e-mail: dr.gomes@rediffmail.com

P.R. Palanivelu et al. (eds.), *Bariatric Surgical Practice Guide*,
DOI 10.1007/978-981-10-2705-5_8

percentage of excess weight loss (%EWL) and resolution of obesity comorbid conditions. LSG has now evolved to be a standard bariatric stand-alone operation.

Besides safety profile and effectiveness LSG has been a popular surgical approach among the bariatric community due to its perceived simplicity of surgical technique. Its prominent advantages are lack of an intestinal bypass (thus avoiding an anastomosis and diversion malabsorption), shorter operating times and no implantation of a foreign body. The wide variation in technique used by different bariatric surgeons has however been a part of evolution of this procedure with many showing to have an effect on eventual mid-term and long-term outcomes. The aim of this chapter was to summarize the existing evidence on LSG technique.

8.2 Size of the Bougie

A bougie is routinely used to size a LSG during stapler transection. The final volume of the sleeve will depend upon both the size of the bougie, the tightness of application of the stapler in relation to the bougie and also the use of imbricating sutures. No consensus exists as to what size of bougie is most effective. Though the aim would be to reduce the gastric volume as much as possible this has to be balanced with safety, as it is known from existing literature that more tighter the sleeve, the chances of leak could be higher, possibly because of higher intragastric pressures. Gagner et al. describe an inverse relation between the size of the bougie and the rate of leaks and advocate the use of catheters between 50 and 60 Fr [6]. However as 1 Fr is equivalent to 0.33 mm, 32 Fr bougies have a 1.1-cm diameter, 36 Fr bougies have a 1.2 cm diameter, and 40 Fr bougies have 1.3 cm diameter and so on thus making the differences between sizes minimal. Most authors reporting more than 50 % EWL after 1 year utilized different bougie sizes ranging from 32 to 48 Fr, whereas studies reporting EWL less than 50 % after 1 year comprised a bougie size ranging from 46 to 60 Fr [5, 7–11]. Weiner et al. compared three groups of patients (one in which no bougie is introduced to calibrate, one using 44 Fr catheters, and another using 32 Fr catheters) and concluded no differences in short-term results but, after 2 years, the results in favor of the more restrictive groups [12]. However in a systematic review and meta-analysis of 9991 cases Parikh et al. retrospectively compared results among patients that utilized 40 and 60 Fr catheters, with no differences between groups after 6 and 12 months. However they identified that utilizing a bougie ≥40 Fr may decrease leak without impacting %EWL up to 3 years [13]. In the International Sleeve Gastrectomy Expert Panel Consensus Statement majority voted size 32–36 Fr (translating to a diameter of 1.1–1.2 cm) as ideal. In India there exists a standard available bougie size of 38 Fr (12.7 mm, 38 Fr, Gastric Calibration Tube, Ethicon Endo-Surgery) which is most commonly used by most surgeons. Although some studies have suggested that bougie size impacts weightloss, in general most studies have shown variable results with regards to bougie size and weight loss outcomes. Hence it can be concluded that surgeons do not require to be too restrictive and a size of around 40F could probably be ideal.

8.3 Beginning of the Distal Section of the Stomach

Another important step to be considered in LSG is the length of antrum required to be preserved to maintain normal gastric emptying and understanding the effect of this on mid-term and long-term outcomes, as increased preservation may theoretically decrease the extent of restriction. Most authors in initial studies had performed the resection at 6–7 cm from the pylorus in order to preserve the entire gastric antrum to promote proper gastric emptying. Later surgeons moved closer to the pylorus, about 3–4 cm from the pylorus resulting in preservation of part of the antrum still allowing for good gastric emptying but increasing the restriction of the procedure. Mognol et al. and Baltasar et al. then advocated radical antral resection with a transection beginning about 2 cm from the pylorus to improve restriction, especially when it is performed as a standalone procedure. But the concern of failure of stomach evacuation after radical excision of the antrum existed. However gastric emptying studies have actually shown an increase in gastric emptying post-operatively even with radical resection of the antrum during LSG [14]. Complications such as failure of stomach evacuation were not observed suggesting that even more radical resection of the pyloric antrum with increased restriction is possible. In fact increased gastric emptying may actually be more beneficial to eventual weight loss. Sánchez-Santos et al., in the results of the Spanish National Registry, reported that groups who begin gastrectomy closest to the pylorus obtain better weight-loss results in the follow-up [15]. However in the large metanalysis by Parikh et al. comparison of <5 cm versus >5 cm showed no difference in leak rate or weight loss [13]. As per experts opinion in the International Sleeve Gastrectomy Expert Panel Consensus Statement majority voted that surgeons would prefer beginning the distal section 2–6 cm from the pylorus [16]. Thus as increasing data is supporting the beginning of the distal section closer to the pylorus it can be concluded that a distal section < or equal to 5 cm from the pylorus is ideal.

8.4 Staplers

Studies performed by measurement of tissue thickness of human stomach on excised gastric specimens from obese patients show that stomach thickness varies from thinnest at the proximal end near the esophageal junction to thickest near the antrum [17]. Due to this variation in stomach thickness, laparoscopic linear cutting staplers should be tailored accordingly. As per experts opinion in the International Sleeve Gastrectomy Expert Panel Consensus Statement majority voted that nothing less than a blue load (closed staple height 1.5 mm) should be used on any part of a LSG. Some dissenters voted against because they recommended that nothing less than a green load (closed staple height 2.0 mm) should be used on any part of a LSG. It was voted that when using buttressing materials, anything lesser than green load should be avoided. When resecting the antrum, it is advisable not to use a stapler lesser than a green load (closed staple height 2.0 mm). When performing revision surgery, firings should be green or larger.

In routine practice staple loads could be blue, gold, green, or black for the Ethicon Echelon™ stapler or blue, green for the Covidien Endo GIA™ stapler or tan, purple, or black for the Covidien Endo GIA Tristaple™ load. The surgeon starts with the thickest load at the antrum and then chooses subsequent staple loads based on how the tissues feel. Interestingly a recent study showed that this subjective assessment has a high chance of choosing incorrect staple heights but implications of this in clinical practice is not known [18]. Considering the fact that the existing staplers have provided reasonably good outcomes and there presently exists no technology for intraoperative measurement of tissue thickness to guide the choice of stapler load, choice should be made according the anatomical location and subjective assessment of tissue thickness.

8.5 Proximal Section of the Stomach

The distal esophagus and esophagogastric junction are supplied on the right and anterior side by branches of the left gastric artery and left inferior phrenic artery and on the posterior and left side by fundic branches of the splenic artery, the posterior gastric artery and the phrenic branches [19]. A LSG requires complete dissection of the fundus by division of the short gastric vessels, of the posterior gastric artery, and of the phrenic branches. Thus a "critical area" of vascularization may occur laterally, just at the esophago-gastric junction at the angle of His [19]. Hence one needs to take utmost caution at this region as undue ischaemia can increase the chance of leak. Also it is recommended that the proximal section (last section) is performed 1–2 cm away from the gastroesophageal junction [19].

It is also important to completely mobilize the fundus laterally and posteriorly before transection, removing the fundus completely, preventing the possibility of dilatation and subsequent weight regain as this is the most distensible portion of the stomach

8.6 Suture Reinforcement

Many different reinforcement options have been used after LSG. Dapri et al. showed, through a prospective RCT, with three treatment arms (non-reinforced, suture reinforced, and stapler-load buttressing) a difference in intraoperative blood loss but no difference for leak rate after staple-line reinforcement. Operative times were increased with the use of oversuturing. Bleeding was the least with the use of staple load buttressing [20]. Albanopoulos et al. through a prospective RCT, with two treatment arms (suture reinforced and stapler-load buttressing) demonstrated no significant difference in terms of bleeding and postoperative leak between the two techniques [21]. Musella et al. through a prospective RCT, with two treatment arms (non-reinforced and suture reinforced) showed no difference in the rate of leak or bleeding but did show a higher rate of stenosis with staple-line reinforcement [22]. In the large metanalysis by Parikh et al. buttressing did not affect leak rate [13]. Similarly, in a systemic review of 4881 patients undergoing sleeve gastrectomy,

Knapps et al. found no significant differences in leak rates, mortality, and overall morbidity between reinforced and unreinforced patients [23]. In another metanalysis by Chen et al. no significant differences in leak rates, mortality, and overall morbidity were observed between reinforced and unreinforced patients [24]. A recent meta-analysis by Choi et al. analyzed the outcomes for 1345 patients and found that staple line reinforcement with a buttress significantly reduced the incidence of bleeding, leakage, and overall complications. Oversewing did not demonstrate such advantage and, in fact, was found to increase the bleeding risk [25]. A recent systematic review by Michel Gagner of 88 studies including 8920 patients found leak rates and complication rates of 1.1 and 5.5 % with absorbable polymer membrane 2.0 and 6.3 % with oversewing, 2.6 and 8.9 % with no reinforcement, and 3.3 and 7.8 % with nonabsorbable bovine pericardial strips, respectively. They concluded that leak rate in LSG was significantly lower using APM staple-line reinforcement than oversewing, BPS reinforcement, or no reinforcement [26]. In the metanalysis by Shikora et al., in sleeves and bypasses, suture oversewing was better than no reinforcement but not as effective as bovine pericardium for leak (2.45 %) and bleed (2.69 %) rates [27].

In conclusion, many different reinforcement options have and are being used. Staple line buttressing has been shown in several publications to decrease bleeding and possibly even reduce leak rates. Oversewing may be better than no reinforcement at all. Since the leak rate after LSG is low, evidence generation is difficult as powering a study sufficiently to result in statistically significant differences would require large numbers of patients and is very difficult to perform. Without large long term data, it is very difficult to suggest routine staple reinforcement. In a the survey of expert sleeve gastrectomy surgeons for the International Sleeve Gastrectomy Expert Panel Consensus Statement 100 % of participants agreed that reinforcement reduced bleeding but consensus was not achieved on leaks. In this statement, Rosenthal et al. reported data that showed that 63 % suture-reinforced the staple line and only 21 % used a buttressing material which may have been related to the "high" cost of buttressing. Even for those using oversewing, suture material (absorbable vs. nonabsorbable) and the sewing technique (baseball stitch, simple oversewing, locking, imbricating, etc.) is variable. While some surgeons oversew the entire staple line, others perform only at selected regions of the staple line. Hence, based on current literature no one technique can be recommended and this can be based on individual surgeon experience and preference.

8.7 Banding the Sleeve

The concept of using a non-adjustable band/ring was first used for LRYGB as reported by Fobi et al. [28]. This was based on the concept of preventing dilatation of the gastric pouch in the long term and hence subsequent weight regain. The same principle has also been attempted with LSG as well. The first study of banded laparoscopic sleeve gastrectomy (BLSG) studied 27 patients who underwent a LSG followed by placement of a band of biological tissue (AlloDerm) at 6 cm from the gastroesophageal junction. These patients were compared to 54 patients with a LRYGB matched for sex, age, and initial body mass index. All 27 patients had improvement or resolution of their diabetes, hypertension, hyperlipidemia, and sleep apnea after BLSG similar to the control LRYGB group. There were no deaths, but one had a pulmonary embolus and another had a leak. Symptoms of gastroesophageal reflux disease generally improved. This was the first study to document the feasibility and possible benefits of BLSG [29]. In another retrospective study, 25 patients who underwent BLSG using a MiniMizer® ring were selected for matched-pair analysis. Ring implantation did not increase the duration of surgery or early surgical complications. At 12 months vomiting was significantly increased in the BLSG patients. At 12 months follow-up, excess weight loss and new onset reflux was equal in both groups but the incidence of postoperative vomiting was significantly raised when patients started to increase eating volume [30]. With only limited data available, presently no recommendations can be made with regard to the use of band over a sleeve.

Recommendations

- A bougie size of around 40F is ideal in constructing a sleeve gastrectomy
- The first stapler firing in sleeve gastrectomy needs to be less than or at 5 cm from the pylorus.
- Choice of stapler load should be made according the anatomical location and subjective assessment of tissue thickness.
- Complete mobilization and resection of the fundus is to be performed.
- The last stapler firing should be carefully performed avoiding the gastroesophageal junction.
- Staple line buttressing/reinforcement reduces bleeding
- No recommendations can be made with regard to the use of band over a sleeve.

References

1. Todkar JS, Shah SS, Shah PS, Gangwani J. Long-term effects of laparoscopic sleeve gastrectomy in morbidly obese subjects with type 2 diabetes mellitus. Surg Obes Relat Dis. 2010;6(2):142–5.
2. Eisenberg D, Bellatorre A, Bellatorre N. Sleeve gastrectomy as a stand-alone bariatric operation for severe, morbid, and super obesity. JSLS. 2013;17(1):63–7.
3. Marceau P, Biron S, Bourque RA, Potvin M, Hould FS, Simard S. Biliopancreatic diversion with a new type of gastrectomy. Obes Surg. 1993;3(1):29–35.
4. Ren CJ, Patterson E, Gagner M. Early results of laparoscopic biliopancreatic diversion with duodenal switch: a case series of 40 consecutive patients. Obes Surg. 2000;10(6):514–23; discussion 524.
5. Regan JP, Inabnet WB, Gagner M, Pomp A. Early experience with two-stage laparoscopic Roux-en-Y gastric bypass as an alternative in the super-super obese patient. Obes Surg. 2003;13(6):861–4.

6. Gagner M. Leaks after sleeve gastrectomy are associated with smaller bougies: prevention and treatment strategies. Surg Laparosc Endosc Percutan Tech. 2010;20(3):166–9.
7. Moon Han S, Kim WW, Oh JH. Results of laparoscopic sleeve gastrectomy (LSG) at 1 year in morbidly obese Korean patients. Obes Surg. 2005;15(10):1469–75.
8. Mognol P, Chosidow D, Marmuse J-P. Laparoscopic sleeve gastrectomy as an initial bariatric operation for high-risk patients: initial results in 10 patients. Obes Surg. 2005;15(7):1030–3.
9. Langer FB, Bohdjalian A, Felberbauer FX, Fleischmann E, Reza Hoda MA, Ludvik B, et al. Does gastric dilatation limit the success of sleeve gastrectomy as a sole operation for morbid obesity? Obes Surg. 2006;16(2):166–71.
10. Baltasar A, Serra C, Pérez N, Bou R, Bengochea M, Ferri L. Laparoscopic sleeve gastrectomy: a multi-purpose bariatric operation. Obes Surg. 2005;15(8):1124–8.
11. Himpens J, Dapri G, Cadière GB. A prospective randomized study between laparoscopic gastric banding and laparoscopic isolated sleeve gastrectomy: results after 1 and 3 years. Obes Surg. 2006;16(11):1450–6.
12. Weiner RA, Weiner S, Pomhoff I, Jacobi C, Makarewicz W, Weigand G. Laparoscopic sleeve gastrectomy – influence of sleeve size and resected gastric volume. Obes Surg. 2007;17(10):1297–305.
13. Parikh M, Issa R, McCrillis A, Saunders JK, Ude-Welcome A, Gagner M. Surgical strategies that may decrease leak after laparoscopic sleeve gastrectomy: a systematic review and meta-analysis of 9991 cases. Ann Surg. 2013;257(2):231–7.
14. Michalsky D, Dvorak P, Belacek J, Kasalicky M. Radical resection of the pyloric antrum and its effect on gastric emptying after sleeve gastrectomy. Obes Surg. 2013;23(4):567–73.
15. Sánchez-Santos R, Masdevall C, Baltasar A, Martínez-Blázquez C, Martínez-Blázquez C, García Ruiz de Gordejuela A, Ponsi E, et al. Short- and mid-term outcomes of sleeve gastrectomy for morbid obesity: the experience of the Spanish National Registry. Obes Surg. 2009;19(9):1203–10.
16. Rosenthal RJ, International Sleeve Gastrectomy Expert Panel, Diaz AA, Arvidsson D, Baker RS, Basso N, et al. International sleeve gastrectomy expert panel consensus statement: best practice guidelines based on experience of >12,000 cases. Surg Obes Relat Dis. 2012;8(1):8–19.
17. Elariny H, González H, Wang B. Tissue thickness of human stomach measured on excised gastric specimens from obese patients. Surg Technol Int. 2005;14:119–24.
18. Huang R, Gagner M. A thickness calibration device is needed to determine staple height and avoid leaks in laparoscopic sleeve gastrectomy. Obes Surg. 2015;25(12):2360–7.
19. Basso N, Casella G, Rizzello M, Abbatini F, Soricelli E, Alessandri G, et al. Laparoscopic sleeve gastrectomy as first stage or definitive intent in 300 consecutive cases. Surg Endosc. 2011;25(2):444–9.
20. Dapri G, Cadière GB, Himpens J. Reinforcing the staple line during laparoscopic sleeve gastrectomy: prospective randomized clinical study comparing three different techniques. Obes Surg. 2010;20(4):462–7.
21. Albanopoulos K, Alevizos L, Flessas J, Menenakos E, Stamou KM, Papailiou J, et al. Reinforcing the staple line during laparoscopic sleeve gastrectomy: prospective randomized clinical study comparing two different techniques. Preliminary results. Obes Surg. 2012;22(1):42–6.
22. Musella M, Milone M, Bellini M, Leongito M, Guarino R, Milone F. Laparoscopic sleeve gastrectomy. Do we need to oversew the staple line? Ann Ital Chir. 2011;82(4):273–7.
23. Knapps J, Ghanem M, Clements J, Merchant AM. A systematic review of staple-line reinforcement in laparoscopic sleeve gastrectomy. JSLS. 2013;17(3):390–9.
24. Chen B, Kiriakopoulos A, Tsakayannis D, Wachtel MS, Linos D, Frezza EE. Reinforcement does not necessarily reduce the rate of staple line leaks after sleeve gastrectomy. A review of the literature and clinical experiences. Obes Surg. 2009;19(2):166–72.
25. Choi YY, Bae J, Hur KY, Choi D, Kim YJ. Reinforcing the staple line during laparoscopic sleeve gastrectomy: does it have advantages? A meta-analysis. Obes Surg. 2012;22(8):1206–13.

26. Gagner M, Buchwald JN. Comparison of laparoscopic sleeve gastrectomy leak rates in four staple-line reinforcement options: a systematic review. Surg Obes Relat Dis. 2014;10(4):713–23.
27. Shikora SA, Mahoney CB. Clinical benefit of gastric staple line reinforcement (SLR) in gastrointestinal surgery: a meta-analysis. Obes Surg. 2015;25(7):1133–41.
28. Fobi M. Why the operation I prefer is silastic ring vertical gastric bypass. Obes Surg. 1991;1(4):423–6.
29. Alexander JW, Martin Hawver LR, Goodman HR. Banded sleeve gastrectomy – initial experience. Obes Surg. 2009;19(11):1591–6.
30. Karcz WK, Karcz-Socha I, Marjanovic G, Kuesters S, Goos M, Hopt UT, et al. To band or not to band – early results of banded sleeve gastrectomy. Obes Surg. 2014;24(4):660–5.

Technical Considerations of Laparoscopic Gastric Plication with or Without a Band

9

Chih-Kun Huang, Abhishek Katakwar, Jasmeet Singh Ahluwalia, Vijayraj Gohil, Chia-Chia Liu, and Ming-Che Hsin

9.1 Introduction

Successful weight loss and resolution of comorbidities, coupled with improved minimally invasive procedures, has accounted for the recent rise in the number of bariatric surgeries worldwide [1]. Laparoscopic adjustable gastric banding (LAGB) qualifies as a safe and reversible procedure with a percentage of excess weight loss of %EWL of 50% at the end of 3 years. However, if patients do not have good compliance and there is a diet modification leading to intake of calorie-dense liquids, only 40–60% of these patients are able to maintain acceptable long-term weight loss [2–6]. Other, band complications such as erosion, infection, and slippage are believed to be associated with frequent adjustments, though adjustments are the most important factor affecting weight loss and unfavorable long-term outcomes [2]. The last decade has seen rise in the popularity of laparoscopic sleeve gastrectomy (LSG) and has shown promise in mid-term results [7]. However, this

C.-K. Huang, MD (✉) • C.-C. Liu • M.-C. Hsin, MD
Body Science & Metabolic Disorders International (B.M.I) Medical Center, China Medical University Hospital, Taichung, Taiwan
e-mail: dr.ckhuang@hotmail.com; lccamyliu@gmail.com; matthsin@gmail.com

A. Katakwar, MS
Bariatric and Metabolic Surgery Centre, Asian Institute of Gastroenterology, Somajiguda, Hyderabad, Telangana, India
e-mail: abhishekkatakwar@gmail.com

J.S. Ahluwalia, MS
Global Hospital, Jalandhar, Punjab, India
e-mail: docjasmeet@gmail.com

V. Gohil, MS
Asia-Prio Bariatric and Metabolic Surgery Center, Oasis International Hospital, Chaoyang District, Beijing, China
e-mail: drvijayrajgohil@gmail.com

P.R. Palanivelu et al. (eds.), *Bariatric Surgical Practice Guide*,
DOI 10.1007/978-981-10-2705-5_9

procedure has the longest staple line among all bariatric procedures which gives rise to the concerns of staple line leak, bleeding and stricture. Furthermore, post-operative decrease in lower esophageal sphincter pressure has been observed [8]. Another gold stand procedure is roux-en-Y gastric bypass which carries the paradox of excellent weight loss but long-term vitamin deficiency [9, 10].

Talebpour and Amoli introduced the concept of plication of the greater curvature without cutting the stomach and published their 12-year results with acceptable outcomes [11]. Specifically, gastric plication does not involve gastric resection, intestinal bypass, or placement of a foreign body, and this could potentially provide a lower risk alternative that will appeal to patients and referring physicians. The rationale for this procedure addresses issues that might limit the acceptance of other bariatric procedures.

LAGB can be combined with plication. Referred to as the laparoscopic adjustable gastric banded plication (LAGBP); invented by Chih-Kun Huang, it has been recently reported as a novel bariatric procedure with good 4-year results [12]. Here in, we describe laparoscopic gastric plication (LGP) as a standalone surgical technique as well as LAGBP.

9.2 Laparoscopic Gastric Plication

The operation involves mobilizing the greater curvature of the stomach, similar to the dissection for sleeve gastrectomy, and infolding or imbricating the stomach to achieve gastric restriction. Increasing number of LGP procedures are being performed worldwide, and this operation is being marketed as a new option for surgical weight loss by some practices.

In 2011, American Society for Metabolic and Bariatric Surgery issued recommendations regarding gastric plication for the treatment of obesity [13]:

1. Gastric plication procedures should be considered investigational at present. This procedure should be performed under a study protocol with third-party oversight (local or regional ethics committee, institutional review board, data monitoring and safety board, or equivalent authority) to ensure continuous evaluation of patient safety and to review adverse events and outcomes.
2. Reporting of short- and long-term safety and efficacy outcomes in the medical literature is strongly encouraged. Data for these procedures should also be reported to a program's center of excellence database.

9.2.1 Surgical Technique

All patients should receive prophylaxis against deep vein thrombosis and antibiotics as per the policy of the hospital before starting the procedure. A bariatric operating table providing at least 45° of reverse Trendelenburg position is preferable.

Room Setup: Patient lies supine on the table with arms extended. Patient must be fastened to the table to prevent slippage during change of posture. Adequate padding must be ensured. Surgeon stands on the right side, camera-surgeon and first assistant on the left side of the patient.

Port placement: Four or five ports are used. Pneumo-peritoneum is created using veress needle. Surgeon's left hand port in right upper quadrant (5 mm) and right hand at supraumbilicus (15 mm). 5 mm assistant port is in left upper quadrant.

Liver retraction: The left lobe of liver could be retracted by Nathanson liver retractor or elevated using T-shaped liver suspension technique [14].

Mobilisation of greater curvature: The junction of right and left gastro-epiploic vessels is seen and greater omentum is divided close to the stomach above this point till left crus of diaphragm is clearly seen. Below this point, the omentum is divided distally but preserving right gastro-epiploic vessels thereby maintaining arterial supply and venous drainage of plicated stomach. This helps in decreasing edema of the stomach wall. Dissection is carried out distally till 3 cm from the pylorus.

Gastric plication formula: Stomach is measured transversely at the level of 6 cm below gastroesophageal junction ("x" cm) and plication formula is applied to determine the amount of plication ($y=(x+1)/2$). Stomach is marked from lesser curvature side "y" cm away.

Plication: It is started from 0.5 cm from esophago-cardiac junction and progresses till 3 cm from pylorus. The greater curvature is inverted interruptedly using non-absorbable sutures (2–0 Ethibond Excel Ethicon, St. Stevens-Woluwe, Belgium) at every 2 cm and is then reinforced with a continuous seromuscular suture (polypropylene 2–0). Continuous second layer is important in preventing herniation of inverted stomach out of the first layer.

9.2.2 Postoperative Management

Cefazolin (1 g every 8 h), Pantoprazole (40 mg every 24 h), and Dexamethasone (5 mg every 8 h) are intravenously administered to the patients for 1–2 days postoperatively. Moreover, we add serotonin receptor antagonist, Navoban (Sandoz Pharma Ltd, Basel, Switzerland), to alleviate obvious nausea and/or vomiting in the immediate postoperative period. Patients are given oral sips of water 4–6 h after the surgery. Patients are discharged if there is no vomiting and they are able to drink enough liquids. Oral PPIs are given for 1–3 months following surgery. Liquid diet is prescribed for the first week followed by pureed diet for the second week. This is followed by semi-solid diet for another 2 weeks after which solid food is introduced in a stepwise fashion. During the first year, all patients are prescribed multivitamins and iron supplements. Follow-up visits are scheduled every 3 months. Full evaluation of patient including upper gastrointestinal endoscopy is performed after 1 year for surveillance and yearly thereafter.

9.2.3 Results

LGP appears to be an effective operation for the treatment of morbid obesity. In the systemic review of 521 patients of prospective studies, the rate of reported complications reached 15.1 % and reoperation rate was 3 % [15]. Minor complications were at a rate of 10.7 %, with nausea, vomiting, and sialorrhea being the most common in 5.7 %, intraoperative bleeding which was managed without the need for conversion or transfusions in 1.7 %, and dysphagia or obstruction which was successfully managed conservatively in 2.6 %. Major complications presented at a rate of 4.4 %. Major complications that required reoperation were at a rate of 3 %, the most common causes being gastric obstruction (due to fold prolapse, fold edema, adhesions, or accumulation of fluid within the gastric fold) in 1.5 %, leaks due to suture line disruption and herniation in 0.7 %, and gastric fistula in 0.1 %. No worsening of GERD symptoms or new GERD onset was reported.

Another systematic review yielded 14 studies encompassing 1450 LGP procedures. The mean preoperative body mass index (BMI) ranged from 31.2 to 44.5 kg/m^2, and 80.8 % of the patients were female. Operative time ranged from 50 to 117.9 min (average 79.2 min). Hospital stay varied from 0.75 to 5 days (average 2.4 days). The percentage of excessive weight loss (% EWL) for LGP varied from 31.8 to 74.4 % with follow-up from 6 to 24 months. No mortality was reported in these studies and the rate of major complications requiring reoperation ranged from 0 to 15.4 % (average 3.7 %) [16].

All studies show a % EWL in the range of 50 % on 6 months and 60 % on 12 months. Studies with longer follow-up periods indicate a durable result for up to 36 months. Complication rates appears to be low. However, the long-term results show a trend towards weight gain after 1 year of plication due to dilatation of the plicated stomach [17–19].

9.3 Laparoscopic Adjustable Gastric Band Plication

We previously reported a case wherein augmented weight loss was achieved after LAGB by gastric plication. This effectiveness in weight loss demonstrated by combining both procedures led to the invention of LAGBP [20]. So, in 2009 we introduced this new procedure to overcome the concerns raised by LSG, LAGB and plication and named it as laparoscopic adjustable gastric banded plication (LAGBP) [21]. By maintaining the gastrointestinal continuity and being a relatively reversible procedure, laparoscopic adjustable gastric banded plication (LAGBP) compensates the lacunae of current surgical options [22, 23]. LAGBP can achieve moderate weight loss from the initial greater curvature plication and further weight loss could be augmented and maintained by adjusting the band during long-term follow-up. Moreover, LAGBP has been reported a comparable weight loss effect with sleeve gastrectomy and can achieve 54.9 to 56.3 % and 65.8 to 66.9 % EWL at 12 and 24 post-operative months, respectively [24]. Several authors have reported variations in their technique, bougie size and suture material used to perform isolated plication [19, 25]. Our initial technique of placing the band first and then plicating the stomach resulted in higher incidence of gastric fundus herniation compared to that reported in a systematic review [26]. After our first 65 cases, since March 2012, we have modified our surgical techniques to avert the serious complications like gastric fundal herniation. Firstly, we switched from "banding-first" method to "plication-first" technique to facilitate complete fundus plication. Secondly, every individual's stomach is different in size; stomach should be plicated based on the gastric plication formula (GPF) to ensure adequate plication. Third, devascularization of all greater curvature vessels impaired venous return of stomach and causing more edema after surgery. By preserving the right gastroepiploic vessels, we improved postoperative vomiting and gastric fundal herniation [27]. Fourth, we replaced the second layer plication from 2-O Ethibond Excel to continuous 2-O Prolene sutures (Ethicon, Somerville, NJ, USA), to tighten the outer layer of greater curvature plication. This technique has become our standard and the same is described later in technique.

9.3.1 Indications

- As for other bariatric procedures, BMI >40 or BMI >35 with co-morbidity is an indication for surgery [28].
- This BMI limit may be reduced by 3 for Asian population as per Asia Pacific surgical criteria; BMI >37 or BMI >32 with co-morbidity [29] Thorough preoperative evaluation should be done as for any other bariatric procedure as per protocols of the institution.

9.3.2 Contraindication

- Large hiatus hernia or severe gastro-esophageal reflux is a relative contra- indication.
- Patients who cannot follow-up in the clinic for weight loss monitoring and band adjustments must not be offered this procedure.
- Patients allergic to silicon.

9.3.3 Surgical Technique

After the plication is done (same technique described as above), we placed an adjustable gastric band.

Adjustable gastric band: Band is then placed using pars flaccida technique with minimal dissection and is locked in proper position. The band is checked for proper functioning after its placement. Band need not be fixed to the stomach. The reservoir port is placed over anterior rectus sheath near the umbilicus.

9.3.4 Post-operative Course

We use the same care process as plication surgery. After discharge, patient is scheduled in clinic 1 week following surgery and thereafter at 1, 3, 6, 9, 12 months. Following which a 6 monthly follow-up is done. Adjustment of the gastric band is started mostly from the third month depending on patient's satiety, amount of food intake, and weight loss. Full evaluation of patient including upper GI endoscopy is performed after 1 year for surveillance and yearly thereafter.

9.4 Complications

1. Nausea/vomiting: This can be usually managed with anti-emetics, prokinetics, antacids and adequate hydration. A recent systematic review reported that 8 % of patients who underwent gastric plication developed nausea and vomiting [15]. The feeling of postoperative gastric fullness or gastric spasm was the possible reason, which would subside after adaptation [11]. Most cases resolved within a week with PPI's, anti-emetics, and anti-inflammatory drugs without requiring admission.
2. Acute gastric obstruction: A too tight plication can result in acute gastric obstruction and will require emergent release of plication sutures. This condition settles promptly after the reversal of plication.
3. Herniation of plicated stomach: Gastric fold herniation (GFH) is a devastating complication after greater curvature plication with an incidence varying from 0.1 to 7.6 % [17, 19, 26]. It is defined as the herniation of gastric tissue through the plicated stomach sutures. Patients who present with intractable abdominal pain or vomiting following LAGBP require urgent radiological studies, such as upright plain films or abdominal CT, to exclude the possible existence of GFH. In the upright abdominal plain film, GFH can be diagnosed by the presence of a gastric bubble. An abdominal CT is the most sensitive study, which will typically demonstrate bulging of the herniated segment from the plicated stomach. GFHs usually warrants urgent reoperation once diagnosed. If left untreated, the congested stomach would eventually progress to full thickness ischemia, necrosis, and even perforation. The surgical options would be deplication of the sutures, resection of the herniated segment, and removal of the adjustable gastric band or re-plication. We postulated that the incidence of GFH was multifactorial, resulting from early and late. Early GFH, which occurred within a week, could be attributed to technical issues such as edematous stomach, inappropriate suture material, widely placed plication sutures, and forceful vomiting. Late causes could be due to disruption of the suture line as seen in chronic vomiting and raised intragastric pressure [11].
4. Gastric perforation: This is a rare but serious complication of LAGBP. A high degree of clinical suspicion is important. Pain, tachycardia and high leukocyte count should raise the surgeon's alarm. Computed tomography of abdomen or contrast study may be performed but in the end, clinical judgment must prevail.

Laparoscopic exploration should be performed earlier, band removed and plication must be released. Perforation can usually be repaired primarily. However, wedge resection or sleeve gastrectomy may be required for the ischemic part.
5. Band erosion or infection: As with LAGB, band may get infected and usually needs removal.
6. Band slippage: It can present with persistent vomiting and severe GERD. X-ray can detect the loss of 45° angle between band and horizontal line. Mostly it needs removal of band which can be replaced 3 months later.

Conclusion

Laparoscopic plication and adjustable gastric banded plication are new and effective procedures for weight loss. The short term and long term results have been comparable to other procedures like sleeve gastrectomy. Although still considered investigational, it can be selectively performed especially for patients who do not prefer stapling of the stomach.

Recommendation

- Laparoscopic plication and adjustable gastric banded plication can be selectively performed especially for patients who do not prefer stapling of the stomach.

References

1. Angrisani L, Santonicola A, Iovino P, Formisano G, Buchwald H, Scopinaro N. Bariatric surgery worldwide 2013. Obes Surg. 2015;25(10):1822–32.
2. Nguyen NT, Slone JA, Nguyen X-MT, Hartman JS, Hoyt DB. A prospective randomized trial of laparoscopic gastric bypass versus laparoscopic adjustable gastric banding for the treatment of morbid obesity: outcomes, quality of life, and costs. Ann Surg. 2009;250(4):631–41.
3. Suter M, Calmes JM, Paroz A, Giusti V. A 10-year experience with laparoscopic gastric banding for morbid obesity: high long-term complication and failure rates. Obes Surg. 2006;16(7):829–35.
4. Wölnerhanssen BK, Peters T, Kern B, Schötzau A, Ackermann C, von Flüe M, et al. Predictors of outcome in treatment of morbid obesity by laparoscopic adjustable gastric banding: results of a prospective study of 380 patients. Surg Obes Relat Dis. 2008;4(4):500–6.
5. O'Brien PE, McPhail T, Chaston TB, Dixon JB. Systematic review of medium-term weight loss after bariatric operations. Obes Surg. 2006;16(8):1032–40.
6. O'Brien PE, MacDonald L, Anderson M, Brennan L, Brown WA. Long-term outcomes after bariatric surgery: fifteen-year follow-up of adjustable gastric banding and a systematic review of the bariatric surgical literature. Ann Surg. 2013;257(1):87–94.
7. ASMBS Clinical Issues Committee. Updated position statement on sleeve gastrectomy as a bariatric procedure. Surg Obes Relat Dis. 2012;8(3):e21–6.
8. Braghetto I, Lanzarini E, Korn O, Valladares H, Molina JC, Henriquez A. Manometric changes of the lower esophageal sphincter after sleeve gastrectomy in obese patients. Obes Surg. 2010;20(3):357–62.
9. Gong K, Gagner M, Pomp A, Almahmeed T, Bardaro SJ. Micronutrient deficiencies after laparoscopic gastric bypass: recommendations. Obes Surg. 2008;18(9):1062–6.

10. Damms-Machado A, Friedrich A, Kramer KM, Stingel K, Meile T, Küper MA, et al. Pre- and postoperative nutritional deficiencies in obese patients undergoing laparoscopic sleeve gastrectomy. Obes Surg. 2012;22(6):881–9.
11. Talebpour M, Motamedi SMK, Talebpour A, Vahidi H. Twelve year experience of laparoscopic gastric plication in morbid obesity: development of the technique and patient outcomes. Ann Surg Innov Res. 2012;6(1):7.
12. Ahluwalia JS, Kuo H-C, Chang P-C, Sun P-L, Hung K-C, Huang C-K. Standardized technique of laparoscopic adjustable gastric banded plication with 4-year results. Obes Surg. 2015;25(9):1756–7.
13. Clinical Issues Committee. ASMBS policy statement on gastric plication. Surg Obes Relat Dis. 2011;7(3):262.
14. Zachariah SK, Tai C-M, Chang P-C, Se AO, Huang C-K. The "T-suspension tape" for liver and gallbladder retraction in bariatric surgery: feasibility, technique, and initial experience. J Laparoendosc Adv Surg Tech A. 2013;23(4):311–5.
15. Kourkoulos M, Giorgakis E, Kokkinos C, Mavromatis T, Griniatsos J, Nikiteas N, et al. Laparoscopic gastric plication for the treatment of morbid obesity: a review. Minim Invasive Surg. 2012;2012:696348.
16. Ji Y, Wang Y, Zhu J, Shen D. A systematic review of gastric plication for the treatment of obesity. Surg Obes Relat Dis. 2014;10(6):1226–32.
17. Skrekas G, Antiochos K, Stafyla VK. Laparoscopic gastric greater curvature plication: results and complications in a series of 135 patients. Obes Surg. 2011;21(11):1657–63.
18. Talebpour M, Amoli BS. Laparoscopic total gastric vertical plication in morbid obesity. J Laparoendosc Adv Surg Tech A. 2007;17(6):793–8.
19. Ramos A, Galvao Neto M, Galvao M, Evangelista LF, Campos JM, Ferraz A. Laparoscopic greater curvature plication: initial results of an alternative restrictive bariatric procedure. Obes Surg. 2010;20(7):913–8.
20. Huang C-K, Asim S, Lo C-H. Augmenting weight loss after laparoscopic adjustable gastric banding by laparoscopic gastric plication. Surg Obes Relat Dis. 2011;7(2):235–6.
21. Huang C-K, Lo C-H, Shabbir A, Tai C-M. Novel bariatric technology: laparoscopic adjustable gastric banded plication: technique and preliminary results. Surg Obes Relat Dis. 2012;8(1):41–5.
22. Goel R, Chang P-C, Huang C-K. Reversal of gastric plication after laparoscopic adjustable gastric banded plication. Surg Obes Relat Dis. 2013;9(1):e14–5.
23. Pattanshetti S, Tai C-M, Yen Y-C, Lin H-Y, Chi S-C, Huang C-K. Laparoscopic adjustable gastric banded plication: evolution of procedure and 2-year results. Obes Surg. 2013;23(11):1934–8.
24. Mui WL-M, Lee DW-H, Lam KK-Y, Tsung BYS. Laparoscopic greater curve plication in Asia: initial experience. Obes Surg. 2013;23(2):179–83.
25. Brethauer SA, Harris JL, Kroh M, Schauer PR. Laparoscopic gastric plication for treatment of severe obesity. Surg Obes Relat Dis. 2011;7(1):15–22.
26. Abdelbaki TN, Huang C-K, Ramos A, Neto MG, Talebpour M, Saber AA. Gastric plication for morbid obesity: a systematic review. Obes Surg. 2012;22(10):1633–9.
27. Malapan K, Ghinagow A, Vij A, Chang P-C, Hsin M-C, Huang C-K. Laparoscopic adjustable gastric banded plication (Lagbp): standardization of surgical technique and analysis of surgical outcomes. Obes Surg. 2016;26(1):85–90.
28. NIH conference. Gastrointestinal surgery for severe obesity. Consensus development conference panel. Ann Intern Med. 1991;115(12):956–61.
29. Lee W-J, Wang W. Bariatric surgery: Asia-Pacific perspective. Obes Surg. 2005;15(6):751–7.

Standardization of Technique in Roux-en-Y Gastric Bypass

10

Randeep Wadhawan

10.1 Introduction

The laparoscopic roux-en-Y gastric bypass (LRYGB) is widely considered as the gold standard in bariatric surgery; achieving superior weight-loss with acceptable complication rates [1]. It has generally been considered as a reference bariatric surgical procedure when comparing the outcomes of a new procedure. LRYGB is also a metabolic procedure as it results in significant improvements of diabetes mellitus, hypertension, dyslipidemia and sleep apnea, along with a subsequent reduction in overall mortality. Though the technique is now well defined, controversies continue to exist at certain aspects of the configuration [2].

Literature suggests that surgeons worldwide have used different techniques with respect to pouch creation, stoma diameter, limb lengths, defect closure and use of a band. Though their approaches have been different, most have been able to produce excellent results in terms of achievement of excess weight loss and remission of co-morbidities. This article analyses the different techniques, to highlight the differences among them and to lay forward the recommendations based on evidence.

10.2 Pouch Creation

The restrictive effect of LRYGB is obtained by creating a small gastric pouch along the lesser curvature with a narrow gastrojejunostomy. It is further accentuated through bypassing the stomach, duodenum, and various lengths of the proximal jejunum, as well as dumping, stasis, and changes of gastrointestinal hormones such as ghrelin. Roberts et al. have suggested that it is actually pouch volume more than stoma diameter that truly impacts satiety and affects weight loss [2].

R. Wadhawan, MS, FIAGES, FMAS, FAIS, FICS
Department of Minimal Access, Bariatric and GI Surgery Fortis Hospital, New Delhi, India
e-mail: randeepwadhawan@yahoo.com

P.R. Palanivelu et al. (eds.), *Bariatric Surgical Practice Guide*,
DOI 10.1007/978-981-10-2705-5_10

In LRYGB, the pouch formation is the most demanding part of the operation. The laparoscopic perigastric dissection technique, especially in super obese or male patients with a big amount of local fatty tissue, may be very demanding and comes along with a higher intraoperative complication rate due to bleeding or disorientation. Preservation of vagus nerve is essential during pouch formation to reduce postoperative dumping syndrome [3].

Kelvin Higa has suggested that the first firing during the creation of pouch should begin no more than 5 cm distal to OG junction [4]. He has also suggested dissection of hiatus routinely and repair of the hiatal hernia along with removing the fat pad overlying the angle of His, which according to him will allow more precise and consistent pouch creation with better long term performance and lower complications. Radwin Kassir et al. have suggested the transverse firing of the first stapler to be at 6 cm distal to the cardia or 2 cm proximal to the incisura for an ideal pouch size [5]. Gastric pouch anatomy plays a significant role in weight loss in addition to volume. Capella at al demonstrated that long narrow pouches have less tendency to enlarge and should delay the transit more than wider pouches and produce better weight loss [6]. Hence, an ideal pouch is a small narrow pouch based on the lesser curvature.

10.3 Stoma

Since the introduction of the laparoscopic technique in 1994, a variety of surgical techniques to construct the gastrojujenal (GJ) anastomosis have been developed, with no consensus on one ideal technique. Three types of anastomosis are commonly performed: hand-sewn anastomosis (HSA), linear-stapled anastomosis (LSA), and circular-stapled anastomosis (CSA). Literature has been conflicting regarding the superiority of a particular technique, in reducing the early complications [7–9]. In the USA, the percentage of surgeons using the circular stapler, linear stapler and hand sewing for GJ is 43, 41 and 21 % and the selection of a particular anastomotic technique is usually based on the surgeon's preference [10].

Anastomotic leak and stricture formation are the well known complications of GJ. Various studies have yielded different rates of stricture from 3 to 8 % with HSA, 0 to 6 % with LSA, and 5 to 31 % with CSA. Many series have shown that the use of a 21-mm circular stapler is associated with higher rates of stricture, and most surgeons prefer the use of 25-mm circular staplers to avoid this complication [8, 11–22]. Nguyen et al. and Cottan et al. found no significant difference in weight loss while using either 21 or 25 mm circular stapler [13, 23].

Studies have shown comparable outcomes in terms of weight loss when using either linear or circular stapler in GJ [9, 12, 24, 25]. A meta-analysis by Giordano et al. including eight studies comparing CSA and LSA found a statistically significant benefit for the LSA group with a reduced risk of developing a GJA stricture, reduced risk for wound infections and a significant shorter operative time, while no significant differences in the risk of leakage and weight loss at 1-year follow-up [7, 9, 12, 25]. Another meta-analysis by Penna et al. confirmed these results [26]. The anastomotic leak rate for circular stapler is about 0–6.6 %, while for linear stapler it is 0–5.1 % [8]. The issues of GJ leaks and stricture have been discussed in detail later in under Chap. 26 and 27.

There is currently no consensus on the technique of choice, as most of the series published, conclude that all three techniques are safe for performing GJ anastomosis in LRYGB and there are no significant differences regarding the complications. However, these studies are limited by the fact that most centers specialized in bariatric surgery use just one type of GJ anastomosis. Moreover, the studies comparing different GJ anastomotic techniques are retrospective, with a disparate number of patients in each group and, in most cases, limited follow-up. Extrapolating this data, an ideal stoma diameter would be 25 mm irrespective of the technique used.

10.4 Limb Length

The mechanism by which LRYGB induces weight loss includes a restrictive and a malabsorptive component. The small gastric pouch restricts the amount of food that can be ingested, and the bypass of a segment of duodenum and small bowel provides a degree of malabsorption. The degree of malabsorption can be modified by altering the length of these limbs. Though most surgeons use a body mass index (BMI) cut off to vary the length of their limbs, variability exists amongst surgeons even for similar patient BMIs [27].

Brolin et al. in a randomised controlled study randomized superobese patients (n = 45) to a 75 cm alimentary limb (biliopancreatic limb = 15 cm) versus a 150 cm alimentary limb (biliopancreatic limb = 30 cm) LRYGB. They concluded that a longer limb resulted in significantly greater weight loss than conventional LRYGB but did not cause additional metabolic sequelae or diarrhea [28].

Choban et al. in a randomised controlled study randomized patients with a BMI ≤50 (n = 69) to a 75 cm versus a 150 cm alimentary limb and those with a BMI ≥50 to a 150 cm versus a 250 cm alimentary limb (biliopancreatic limb = 30 cm in all) LRYGB. They concluded that there was no benefit to longer Roux limb lengths for patients with BMI <50 but in superobese patients longer alimentary limb-lengths may be associated with a higher percent of patients achieving >50 % EWL. Thus superobese might benefit from Roux limbs of atleast 150 cm [29].

Inabnet et al. in a randomised controlled study randomized patients with a BMI ≤50 (n = 48) to an either a short limb (biliopancreatic limb = 50 cm, alimentary limb = 100 cm) or long limb (biliopancreatic limb = 100 cm, alimentary limb = 150 cm) LRYGB. They observed no weight loss or nutritional differences between the two groups up to 1 year postoperatively but noted a higher incidence of internal hernias in the longer-limb group. They concluded that increasing the Roux limb length in non-superobese patients did not improve weight loss and may increase the incidence of internal hernias. The main limitation of this study was its short follow-up and its small sample size [30].

The study by Christou et al. reported the longest follow-up to date (10 years) and did not demonstrate a benefit to longer Roux limbs independent of BMI in the long term [31].

Interestingly, a recently published study by Savassi-Rocha et al., based on the total length of the small intestine which is between 400 and 900 cm, concluded that constructing longer Roux limbs in the range of 150 cm is unlikely to lead to better weight loss in the majority of patients when the common channel length is not considered [32]. A few publications considered the length of the common channel during the creation of the gastric bypass. Nelson et al. reported results of a postoperative survey on mostly superobese patients that received a distal bypass with a 100-cm common channel, with follow-up of 4 years, 82 % patients losing >50 % of their excess weight [33]. Furthermore, resolution of diabetes reached 94 %, hypertension 65 %, sleep apnea 48 %, and patient satisfaction with the surgery was 90 %. Nevertheless, many patients experienced mild food intolerance and occasional loose stools (71–82 %) with 4 % of patients requiring reoperation with proximal relocation of the Roux limb for symptom resolution. The study by Brolin et al. found that distal RYGB (75 cm common channel) was more effective than a 150-cm Roux but at the expense of higher malabsorptive complications and a small but real incidence of reoperation for reversal [34].

Higa in his data has reported that varying the biliopancreatic limb up to 100 cm has failed to show a difference in excess weight loss in the long term [4].

In conclusion, the currently available literature supports the notion that a longer Roux limb (at least 150 cm) may be associated with a very modest weight loss advantage in the short term in superobese patients but has no significant impact on patients with BMI ≤50. Nevertheless, there is convincing evidence that the degree of malabsorption after RYGB is influenced mainly by the length of the common channel rather than the lengths of the Roux or biliopancreatic limbs as constructed currently by the majority of bariatric surgeons.

10.5 Defect Closure

Internal hernias (IH) are a known potential complication of LRYGB. The incidence of IH has been reported to range from 3 to 4.5 % after LRYGB [35, 36]. The incidence of internal hernias with LRYGB is more when compared to open surgery due to decreased adhesion formation during laparoscopic surgery. Management of internal hernias have been discussed in detail later in the chapter 24 on internal hernias.

Three anatomical spaces have been described as the possible sites for the internal hernias caused by this surgery:

1. The mesocolic space. This is created when the alimentary limb is taken retrocolic through the transverse mesocolon for the GJ.
2. The Petersen space. This is created between the alimentary limb and the mesocolon, when the alimentary limb is taken antecolic for the GJ.
3. The intermesenteric space behind the jejunojejunal anastomosis.

The location of internal hernias has been documented with transverse mesocolon hernias commonest followed by entero-enterostomy and then Peterson's space hernias.

Routine closure of all potential defects with non-absorbable sutures is generally preferred [37]. While these are all laudable measures, more significant technical changes such as antecolic versus retrocolic may produce more significant reduction in the incidence of IH [38]. Champion and Williams mention that there was no reduction in IH after closing the mesentery in a retrocolic technique, while there was a significant reduction when using the antecolic technique, even without closure [39]. Higa et al. did refer to a large reduction in numbers after closing the mesentery in the retrocolic technique employing nonabsorbable sutures, although there was still a 3 % rate even after the closures [40]. Miyashiro et al., in results shared by Carmody et al., mention the complete absence of IH after using the retrocolic technique with the closure of the mesentery, pointing out that out of the 1.3 % of patients with intestinal obstruction, none were caused by IH [41, 42]. A large series of 1,400 patients undergoing LRYGB with an antecolic GJ without closure of any potential hernia defects reported an extremely low incidence of internal hernias [43].

Christopher W et al. published no IH in their technique without closure of the defects which included an antecolic ante-gastric gastrojejunostomy (GJ), division of the greater omentum, a long jejunojejunostomy (JJ) performed with three staple-lines, a short (<4 cm) division of the small bowel mesentery, and placement of the JJ above the colon in the left upper quadrant. Mazen R. Al-Mansouret al noted an IH incidence of 6.2 % in their study while the literature reports a 0–6.9 %. Incidence of IH changed after a routine closure of Petersen's space defect reducing the percentage of patients with Petersen hernias from 83.9 to 33.3 %, therefore submitting that closure of Petersen's space defect has the potential to reduce the incidence of IH after RYGB.

Hence it's preferred to close all potential defects using non-absorbable sutures, although the outcomes of closure of Petersens defect still remain controversial.

10.6 Band

Stomal dilatation has been long recognized as one of the causes of weight regain after LRYGB. Interventions to reduce the size of the gastric pouch or stoma may help reinitiate weight loss [44]. These findings have led some surgeons to believe that placement of a band proximal to gastrojejunostomy at the time of the primary operation will reduce dilatation of gastric pouch, stoma and small bowel, thus resulting in superior long-term weight loss outcomes. Linner's concept of preventing weight regain by reinforcing the stoma against dilating was reintroduced in 1989 by Fobi et al. by placing the band around the gastric pouch, as used in the vertical banded gastroplasty and silastic ring vertical gastroplasty [45]. This modified gastric bypass appears to provide more weight loss that is maintained over a longer period of time [46]. Fobi et al. found that >90.0 % of patients lost and, more importantly, maintained ≥50.0% EWL at ≥5 years [47].

The randomised controlled trial by Bessler et al. of banded and non-banded bypass in super-obese patients showed a statistically significant superior weight loss at 36 months in the banded group compared to the non-banded group [46]. Heneghan et al. found statistically superior weight loss in banded bypass patients at 24 months compared to the nonbanded bypass group in their matched cohort study. On subgroup analysis, they found a significant weight loss difference in those with BMI >50 but not in those with BMI <50 [48]. Awad et al. confirmed significantly better weight loss with banded bypass in their long-term retrospective comparison of banded and non-banded bypass [49].

Band erosion is a known complication of banded bypass. Fobi and colleagues saw erosion in 1.63 % patients. Awad et al. found over a 10-year period that polyurethane does not erode [49]. In their PTFE group, they had three erosions and authors hence switched over to a polyurethane band subsequently. Heneghan et al. had a low erosion rate of 1.5 % [48]. They recommended that band should be placed at least 2 cm above the gastroenterostomy. Size of the band has a definite correlation towards food intolerance. In randomised study by Bessler et al. with the use of 5.5 cm ring size, they found that banded patients were more likely to experience food intolerance [46].

Currently, there is no consensus of opinion on whether the ring size should be tailored to the patient [48]. Some authors have tried using different ring sizes in different age groups; 6.0 cm for those <50 years and 6.5 cm for >50 years but then moved to 6.5 cm for all patients. Moreover, the same authors did not find any significant difference in weight loss at 2 and 5 years in their patients who had a 5.5-, 6.0-, or 6.5-cm silastic ring [50].

10.7 Leak Test

Giovanni Quartararo et al. in a systematic review of literature evaluated 22 studies encompassing a total of 19,389 patients [51]. All of the studies except for six reported a routine intraoperative test (blue-methylene or pneumatic test) to detect a possible leakage in the gastrointestinal anastomosis. Sixteen studies reported the use of routine upper gastrointestinal series (UGIS) and in three studies UGIS was performed selectively based on clinical signs. In the last decade, the use of UGIS has been debated due to its lack of sensitivity, low positive predictive value, and cost-effectiveness. The majority of studies found gastrografin to be the main contrast used for UGIS after RYGB. Lee et al. propose the use of selective UGIS based on the combination of clinical signs and positive amylase in drainages in order to improve the detection rate of the procedure. Many authors suggest the effectiveness of CT scans with oral gastrografin administration when the suspect of an anastomotic leakage is high and its efficacy has been demonstrated in many studies conducted. Arguments in favour of routine use of postoperative UGIS in LRYGB patients seem to highlight the necessity of a useful "instrument" during the surgeons learning curve to evaluate both the technical aspects and the legal medical value before patient discharge or in cases of unsatisfactory weight loss.

Recommendations

- An ideal pouch is a short narrow pouch beginning 5–6 cm distal to the OG junction created along the lesser curvature. Restrictive action of LRYGB is primarily dependent on pouch volume and stoma size.
- A stoma size of 25 mm is appropriate irrespective of the technique of anastomosis.
- Antecolic construction of the gastro-jejunostomy is the preferred approach
- The standard LRYGB is based on the length of the alimentary limb. The biliopancreatic limb is to be kept short.
- The alimentary limb can be kept at 75 cm for patients with BMI <50 BMI. In superobese patients >50 BMI the alimentary limb can be kept at 150 cm.
- All potential defects during LRYGB should be closed to decrease the possibility of internal hernias although the outcomes of closure of Petersons defect are controversial. The choice of suture material should be nonabsorbable.
- Banded LRYGB patients will have better weight loss in the long term than the non banded LRYGB patients particularly in the superobese.

References

1. Kassir R, Breton C, Lointier P, Blanc P. Laparoscopic Roux-en-Y gastric bypass with hand-sewn gastrojejunostomy using an absorbable bidirectional monofilament barbed suture: review of the literature and illustrative case video. Surg Obes Relat Dis. 2014;10(3):560–1.
2. Roberts K, Duffy A, Kaufman J, Burrell M, Dziura J, Bell R. Size matters: gastric pouch size correlates with weight loss after laparoscopic Roux-en-Y gastric bypass. Surg Endosc. 2007;21(8):1397–402.
3. Frantzides CT, Carlson MA, Shostrom VK, Roberts J, Stavropoulos G, Ayiomamitis G, et al. A survey of dumping symptomatology after gastric bypass with or without lesser omental transection. Obes Surg. 2011;21(2):186–93.
4. Higa K, Ho T, Tercero F, Yunus T, Boone KB. Laparoscopic Roux-en-Y gastric bypass: 10-year follow-up. Surg Obes Relat Dis. 2011;7(4):516–25.
5. Kassir R, Lointier P, Tiffet O, Breton C, Blanc P. Laparoscopic Roux-en-Y gastric bypass: creation of the neogastric pouch. Obes Surg. 2015;25(1):131–2.
6. Capella RF, Iannace VA, Capella JF. An analysis of gastric pouch anatomy in bariatric surgery. Obes Surg. 2008;18(7):782–90.
7. Bendewald FP, Choi JN, Blythe LS, Selzer DJ, Ditslear JH, Mattar SG. Comparison of hand-sewn, linear-stapled, and circular-stapled gastrojejunostomy in laparoscopic Roux-en-Y gastric bypass. Obes Surg. 2011;21(11):1671–5.
8. Gonzalez R, Lin E, Venkatesh KR, Bowers SP, Smith CD. Gastrojejunostomy during laparoscopic gastric bypass: analysis of 3 techniques. Arch Surg. 2003;138(2):181–4.
9. Abdel-Galil E, Sabry AA. Laparoscopic Roux-en-Y gastric bypass – evaluation of three different techniques. Obes Surg. 2002;12(5):639–42.
10. Madan AK, Harper JL, Tichansky DS. Techniques of laparoscopic gastric bypass: on-line survey of American Society for Bariatric Surgery practicing surgeons. Surg Obes Relat Dis. 2008;4(2):166–72; discussion 172–3.

11. Rondan A, Nijhawan S, Majid S, Martinez T, Wittgrove AC. Low anastomotic stricture rate after Roux-en-Y gastric bypass using a 21-mm circular stapling device. Obes Surg. 2012;22(9):1491–5.
12. Leyba JL, Llopis SN, Isaac J, Aulestia SN, Bravo C, Obregon F. Laparoscopic gastric bypass for morbid obesity-a randomized controlled trial comparing two gastrojejunal anastomosis techniques. JSLS. 2008;12(4):385–8.
13. Nguyen NT, Stevens CM, Wolfe BM. Incidence and outcome of anastomotic stricture after laparoscopic gastric bypass. J Gastrointest Surg. 2003;7(8):997–1003; discussion 1003.
14. Alasfar F, Sabnis AA, Liu RC, Chand B. Stricture rate after laparoscopic Roux-en-Y gastric bypass with a 21-mm circular stapler: the Cleveland clinic experience. Med Princ Pract. 2009;18(5):364–7.
15. Gould JC, Garren M, Boll V, Starling J. The impact of circular stapler diameter on the incidence of gastrojejunostomy stenosis and weight loss following laparoscopic Roux-en-Y gastric bypass. Surg Endosc. 2006;20(7):1017–20.
16. Dolce CJ, Dunnican WJ, Kushnir L, Bendana E, Ata A, Singh TP. Gastrojejunal strictures after Roux-en-Y gastric bypass with a 21-MM circular stapler. JSLS. 2009;13(3):306–11.
17. Blackstone RP, Rivera LA. Predicting stricture in morbidly obese patients undergoing laparoscopic Roux-en-Y gastric bypass: a logistic regression analysis. J Gastrointest Surg. 2007;11(4):403–9.
18. Da Costa M, Mata A, Espinós J, Vila V, Roca JM, Turró J, et al. Endoscopic dilation of gastrojejunal anastomotic strictures after laparoscopic gastric bypass. Predictors of initial failure. Obes Surg. 2011;21(1):36–41.
19. Ukleja A, Afonso BB, Pimentel R, Szomstein S, Rosenthal R. Outcome of endoscopic balloon dilation of strictures after laparoscopic gastric bypass. Surg Endosc. 2008;22(8):1746–50.
20. Ruiz-de-Adana JC, López-Herrero J, Hernández-Matías A, Colao-Garcia L, Muros-Bayo J-M, Bertomeu-Garcia A, et al. Laparoscopic hand-sewn gastrojejunal anastomoses. Obes Surg. 2008;18(9):1074–6.
21. Takata MC, Ciovica R, Cello JP, Posselt AM, Rogers SJ, Campos GM. Predictors, treatment, and outcomes of gastrojejunostomy stricture after gastric bypass for morbid obesity. Obes Surg. 2007;17(7):878–84.
22. Fisher BL, Atkinson JD, Cottam D. Incidence of gastroenterostomy stenosis in laparoscopic Roux-en-Y gastric bypass using 21- or 25-mm circular stapler: a randomized prospective blinded study. Surg Obes Relat Dis. 2007;3(2):176–9.
23. Cottam DR, Fisher B, Sridhar V, Atkinson J, Dallal R. The effect of stoma size on weight loss after laparoscopic gastric bypass surgery: results of a blinded randomized controlled trial. Obes Surg. 2009;19(1):13–7.
24. Giordano S, Tolonen P, Victorzon M. Comparision of linear versus circular stapling techniques in laparoscopic gastric bypass surgery – a pilot study. Scand J Surg. 2010;99(3):127–31.
25. Bohdjalian A, Langer FB, Kranner A, Shakeri-Leidenmühler S, Zacherl J, Prager G. Circular- vs. linear-stapled gastrojejunostomy in laparoscopic Roux-en-Y gastric bypass. Obes Surg. 2010;20(4):440–6.
26. Penna M, Markar SR, Venkat-Raman V, Karthikesalingam A, Hashemi M. Linear-stapled versus circular-stapled laparoscopic gastrojejunal anastomosis in morbid obesity: meta-analysis. Surg Laparosc Endosc Percutan Tech. 2012;22(2):95–101.
27. Papadia F. Effect of standard versus extended Roux limb length on weight loss outcomes after laparoscopic Roux-en-Y gastric bypass. Surg Endosc. 2004;18(11):1683.
28. Brolin RE, Kenler HA, Gorman JH, Cody RP. Long-limb gastric bypass in the superobese. A prospective randomized study. Ann Surg. 1992;215(4):387–95.
29. Choban PS, Flancbaum L. The effect of Roux limb lengths on outcome after Roux-en-Y gastric bypass: a prospective. Randomized clinical trial. Obes Surg. 2002;12(4):540–5.
30. Inabnet WB, Quinn T, Gagner M, Urban M, Pomp A. Laparoscopic Roux-en-Y gastric bypass in patients with BMI <50: a prospective randomized trial comparing short and long limb lengths. Obes Surg. 2005;15(1):51–7.
31. Christou NV, Look D, Maclean LD. Weight gain after short- and long-limb gastric bypass in patients followed for longer than 10 years. Ann Surg. 2006;244(5):734–40.

32. Savassi-Rocha AL, Diniz MTC, Savassi-Rocha PR, Ferreira JT, Rodrigues de Almeida Sanches S, Diniz Mde FHS, et al. Influence of jejunoileal and common limb length on weight loss following Roux-en-Y gastric bypass. Obes Surg. 2008;18(11):1364–8.
33. Nelson WK, Fatima J, Houghton SG, Thompson GB, Kendrick ML, Mai JL, et al. The malabsorptive very, very long limb Roux-en-Y gastric bypass for super obesity: results in 257 patients. Surgery. 2006;140(4):517–22; discussion 522–3.
34. Brolin RE, Cody RP. Adding malabsorption for weight loss failure after gastric bypass. Surg Endosc. 2007;21(11):1924–6.
35. Garza E, Kuhn J, Arnold D, Nicholson W, Reddy S, McCarty T. Internal hernias after laparoscopic Roux-en-Y gastric bypass. Am J Surg. 2004;188(6):796–800.
36. Higa K, Boone K, Arteaga González I, López-Tomassetti Fernández E. Mesenteric closure in laparoscopic gastric bypass: surgical technique and literature review. Cir Esp. 2007;82(2):77–88.
37. Iannelli A, Facchiano E, Gugenheim J. Internal hernia after laparoscopic Roux-en-Y gastric bypass for morbid obesity. Obes Surg. 2006;16(10):1265–71.
38. Comeau E, Gagner M, Inabnet WB, Herron DM, Quinn TM, Pomp A. Symptomatic internal hernias after laparoscopic bariatric surgery. Surg Endosc. 2005;19(1):34–9.
39. Champion JK, Williams M. Small bowel obstruction and internal hernias after laparoscopic Roux-en-Y gastric bypass. Obes Surg. 2003;13(4):596–600.
40. Higa KD, Ho T, Boone KB. Internal hernias after laparoscopic Roux-en-Y gastric bypass: incidence, treatment and prevention. Obes Surg. 2003;13(3):350–4.
41. Miyashiro LA, Fuller WD, Ali MR. Favorable internal hernia rate achieved using retrocolic, retrogastric alimentary limb in laparoscopic Roux-en-Y gastric bypass. Surg Obes Relat Dis. 2010;6(2):158–62.
42. Carmody B, DeMaria EJ, Jamal M, Johnson J, Carbonell A, Kellum J, et al. Internal hernia after laparoscopic Roux-en-Y gastric bypass. Surg Obes Relat Dis. 2005;1(6):543–8.
43. Cho M, Carrodeguas L, Pinto D, Lascano C, Soto F, Whipple O, et al. Diagnosis and management of partial small bowel obstruction after laparoscopic antecolic antegastric Roux-en-Y gastric bypass for morbid obesity. J Am Coll Surg. 2006;202(2):262–8.
44. Linner JH. Gastric operations. In: Linner JH, editor. Surgery for morbid obesity. New York: Springer; 1984. p. 65–107.
45. Fobi MAL, Lee H, Flemming AW. The surgical techniqueof the banded gastric bypass. J Obes Weight Regulation. 1989;8:99–102.
46. Bessler M, Daud A, Kim T, DiGiorgi M. Prospective randomized trial of banded versus nonbanded gastric bypass for the super obese: early results. Surg Obes Relat Dis. 2007;3(4):480–4; discussion 484–5.
47. Fobi M, 2004 ABS Consensus Conference. Banded gastric bypass: combining two principles. Surg Obes Relat Dis. 2005;1(3):304–9.
48. Heneghan HM, Annaberdyev S, Eldar S, Rogula T, Brethauer S, Schauer P. Banded Roux-en-Y gastric bypass for the treatment of morbid obesity. Surg Obes Relat Dis. 2014;10(2):210–6.
49. Awad W, Garay A, Martínez C. Ten years experience of banded gastric bypass: does it make a difference? Obes Surg. 2012;22(2):271–8.
50. Al-Mansour MR, Mundy R, Canoy JM, Dulaimy K, Kuhn JN, Romanelli J. Internal hernia after laparoscopic antecolic Roux-en-Y gastric bypass. Obes Surg. 2015;25(11):2106–11.
51. Quartararo G, Facchiano E, Scaringi S, Liscia G, Lucchese M. Upper gastrointestinal series after Roux-en-Y gastric bypass for morbid obesity: effectiveness in leakage detection. a systematic review of the literature. Obes Surg. 2014;24(7):1096–101.

Technical Considerations of Duodenal Switch and Its Variants

11

Kazunori Kasama and Praveen Raj Palanivelu

11.1 Introduction

Most modern bariatric operations are now based upon the performance of a gastric restriction procedure, responsible for the short-term weight loss, and a gastrointestinal bypass, which should warrant the maintenance of weight loss over time. But due to concerns of nutritional deficiencies, the more malabsorptive operations have declined in numbers with the restrictive varieties becoming more popular [1]. But there still remains a definite role for more malabsorption even as we try to become more conservative in the choice of procedure. This is applicable, more so in super obese patients and in patients with a severe metabolic syndrome [2].

Nicola Scopinaro is credited with describing the original bilio-pancreatic diversion (BPD) [3]. His procedure was a modification of the jejuno-ileal bypass (JIB) (anastomoses of the proximal jejunum to the distal ileum without any excision resulting in a long blind loop). He performed a distal gastrectomy anastomosing to a 250 cm roux limb and a short common channel of 50 cm (distal gastrectomy with exclusion of the first half of the small bowel with a gastro-ileostomy with reconnection of the bypassed bowel). This procedure thus abandoned the long blind loop of a JIB but maintained the malabsorption. However this was associated with a relatively high rate of dumping and marginal ulcers.

The stand-alone duodenal switch procedure (without bypass) was described by DeMeester in the 1980s to treat bile-reflux gastritis as a roux-en-Y duodenojejunostomy [4]. The modified duodenal switch (DS) was later introduced as a modification

K. Kasama, MD, FACS
Weight Loss and Metabolic Surgery Center, Yotsuya Medical Cube, Tokyo, Japan
e-mail: kazukasama@gmail.com

P.R. Palanivelu, MS, DNB, DNB(SGE), FALS, FMAS (✉)
Bariatric Division, Upper Gastrointestinal Surgery and Minimal Access Surgery Unit, GEM Hospital and Research Centre, Coimbatore, India
e-mail: drraj@geminstitute.in

P.R. Palanivelu et al. (eds.), *Bariatric Surgical Practice Guide*,
DOI 10.1007/978-981-10-2705-5_11

of Scopinaros BPD, first described by Marceau in 1993 which combined the Scopinaro procedure and the DeMeester's DS (vertical gastrectomy with exclusion of the first half of the small bowel with a duodeno-ileostomy with reconnection of the bypassed bowel) [5]. A vertical gastrectomy was performed rather than a distal gastrectomy anastomosing the roux limb to the stapled proximal duodenum thus reducing the parietal cell mass, eliminating the distensible fundus, preserving the pylorus valve and the duodenum. In 1998, Hess and Hess further modified this with the diversion of the duodenum, leading to the modern day biliopancreatic diversion with duodenal switch (BPD/DS) [6]. Gagner et al. described the first laparoscopic BPD/DS, which represents the current standard technique widely followed [7].

Laparoscopic BPD/DS is the most commonly performed malabsorptive operation worldwide [1]. But different modifications have been made to this to make it more technically simpler and also to reduce the extent of malabsorption. This includes the Sleeve gastrectomy with duodenal jejunal bypass (Sleeve DJB) or Sleeve gastrectomy with loop DJB and Single anastomosis duodeno-ileal bypass (SADI-S), the latter two with advantage of a single anastomosis [8–10]. Although they have been described as separate procedures in literature, for better understanding we refer to this as variants of the more standardized BPD/DS.

In this chapter we aim to describe the standard steps in the technical creation of BPD/DS with necessary variations of the variant techniques. The different variants are named according to the length of limb and/or method of reconstruction (roux-en-Y or loop anastomosis). BPD/DS and SADI-S have a short common limb, Sleeve DJB and Sleeve with loop DJB have a long common limb for avoiding malnutrition. BPD/DS and Sleeve DJB are provided with roux-en-Y reconstruction, SADI-S and loop DJB are with loop (Billroth-II) reconstruction to avoid technical difficulty of a roux-en-Y reconstruction. The procedures are routinely done laparoscopically, but in difficult situations, hand assisted techniques have also been described [11].

11.2 Technical Considerations of Duodenal Switch and Its Variants

11.2.1 Standardized Biliopancreatic Diversion with Duodenal Switch (BPD/DS)

The major steps of BPD/DS consist of a vertical gastrectomy or the sleeve gastrectomy, duodenoileostomy and enteroenterostomy and a concomitant cholecystectomy. The sleeve is usually created over a 60F bougie. The common channel varies between 50 and 100 cm, the alimentary limb length is around 250 cm [7]. The long biliopancreatic limb is not measured and is the longest. Hess and Hess had used alimentary limb lengths of 250 cm, 275 cm or 300 cm with occasional 225 cm or 325 cm in patients with an unusually short or long small bowel respectively [6]. They also recommended that the total length of the alimentary limb (from the cecum to the stomach) to be approximately 40 % of the total small bowel length and that the common channel (the distal portion of the alimentary limb just beyond the anastomosis of the biliary limb) to be around 10 % of the total small bowel length [6]. Similar lengths were used by Gagner et al. where the sleeve was created over a 60F bougie which is now considered to be the standard [4, 7].

11.2.2 Single Anastomosis Duodeno-Ileal Bypass with Sleeve Gastrectomy" (SADI-S)

Trying to simplify this Torres et al. developed a new technique based on the duodenal switch (DS), in which only one anastomosis is performed, and named it the 'Single anastomosis duodeno-ileal bypass with sleeve gastrectomy' or SADI-S reducing the number of anastomosis to one. This consists of a sleeve gastrectomy over a 60F bougie with the duodeno-ileal anastomosis performed at 200 cm proximal to the IC junction [9]. The procedure has shown promising outcomes in terms of weight loss outcomes and resolution of co-morbidities [12].

11.2.3 Sleeve Gastrectomy with Duodeno-Jejunal Bypass (Sleeve DJB)

In an attempt to find an alternative to the more popular RYGB in carcinoma stomach in endemic regions and also to reduce the chances of malabsorption, Kasama et al. proposed the sleeve gastrectomy with duodeno-jejunal bypass (Sleeve DJB) constructed in a roux-en-Y fashion, which is similar to the duodenal switch but with significantly longer common channel [8]. Unlike the DS, the common channel length is variable with the BP limb of 50–100 cm and alimentary limb of 150–200 cm. This is similar to the conventional LRYGB but with an intact pylorus and avoiding a gastric remnant [8, 13]. Praveen Raj et al. have compared this with the LRYGB in a randomised controlled trial and have demonstrated similar results in terms of weight loss and resolution of comorbidities among both the procedures [14].

11.2.4 Sleeve Gastrectomy with Loop Duodeno-Jejunal Bypass (Sleeve with Loop DJB)

This is similar to the Sleeve-DJB, but a loop duodeno-jejunostomy instead of the roux-en-Y configuration is performed. This works similar to SADI-S (a variant of DS) with a single anastomosis but with the measurements based on the DJ flexure. WJ Lee et al. used 150 cm of biliopancreatic limb in patients with <35 BMI and 200 cm for patients with >35 BMI [10]. When compared with the conventional LRYGB, the outcomes were comparable. CK Huang et al. had reported 2 cases of revision of RYGB to loop-DJB for intractable marginal ulcer [15].

11.3 Key Operative Steps of Duodenal Switch and Its Variants

The patient position could be supine or split leg. The trocars can be positioned based on surgeon preferences. The position of trocars is usually the same as when performing a LSG as this is the initial step and then additional trocars are placed as needed. The major steps of duodenal switch and its variants include

(1) Sleeve gastrectomy with dissection and division of the duodenum
(2) the entero-enterostomy and
(3) the duodeno-enterostomy.

11.3.1 Sleeve Gastrectomy with Dissection and Division of the Duodenum

For LSG, devascularization of the right gastroepiploic artery is usually started from 4 to 5 cm proximal of the pyloric ring. Here dissection needs to be continued distally to approximately 1.5 cm beyond the pylorus. The retro-duodenal and supraduodenal tissues are dissected free in order to facilitate transection of the duodenum at this point with a linear stapler with a blue or purple cartridge. The right gastric artery should be preserved to maintain the blood supply to the anastomosis. Extra care must be taken during this step because an injury to the pancreas posterior to this point is a possible complication. The wall of the duodenum is thinner than that of the stomach, so the surgeon must avoid a cavitation injury when using the laparoscopic coagulating shears (LCS).

11.3.2 Entero-Enterostomy

This step will not be required in SADI-S and Sleeve with Loop DJB. The limbs should be appropriately measured and the anastomosis can be created using stapled, handsewn anastomosis or a combination of both. The mesenteric defects should be closed with a continuous, non-absorbable suture to limit the possibility of internal hernia.

11.3.3 Duodenojejunostomy/Duodenoileostomy

In BPD/DS and SADI-S, this anastomosis would be a duodenoileostomy, and in Sleeve DJB and Sleeve with loop DJB, this will be a duodenojejunostomy. The duodenojejunostomy and duodenoileostomy is commonly performed using the antecolic method. The omentum can be bisected if needed to avoid the tension to the anastomosis. Duodenojejunostomy is the most important part of this surgery. This anastomosis can be fashioned in several ways similar to the gastrojejunostomy in LRYGB, such as using a circular stapler, linear stapler, and hand suturing.

The authors prefer to perform the hand suturing method with double layer anastomosis. A hand sewn anastomosis can be performed with a smaller length of duodenum from the pylorus in comparison with other stapler using methods.

Conclusion

Biliopancreatic diversion with duodenal switch is the most effective surgical procedure, both in terms of weight loss and resolution of comorbidities. However, the popularity has been on the decline considering the increased technical complexity and perceived risk of long term nutritional complications. Thus the variants of this procedure have been increasingly becoming popular and in selected situations with adequate experience, appropriate patient selection this can be safely offered to patients, making knowledge of the principles and technique important.

Recommendations

- Laparoscopic BPD/DS can be modified to make it more technically simpler and to reduce the malabsorption and associated nutritional complications.
- These procedures have the advantage of preserving the pylorus
- The modifications include a SADI-S (a short common limb), Sleeve DJB and Sleeve with loop DJB (long common limb). BPD/DS and Sleeve DJB are provided with roux-en-Y reconstruction and SADI-S and loop DJB are with loop reconstruction.

References

1. Buchwald H, Oien DM. Metabolic/bariatric surgery worldwide 2011. Obes Surg. 2013;23(4):427–36.
2. Silecchia G, Rizzello M, Casella G, et al. Two-stage laparoscopic biliopancreatic diversion with duodenal switch as treatment of high-risk super-obese patients: analysis of complications. Surg Endosc. 2009;23:1032–7.
3. Scopinaro N, Gianetta E, Pandolfo N, et al. Bilio-pancreatic bypass. Proposal and preliminary experimental study of a new type of operation for the functional surgical treatment of obesity. Minerva Chir. 1976;31(10):560–6 [Article in Italian].
4. DeMeester TR, Fuchs KH, Ball CS, Albertucci M, Smyrk TC, Marcus JN. Experimental and clinical results with proximal end-to-end duodenojejunostomy for pathologic duodenogastric reflux. Ann Surg. 1987;206(4):414–26.
5. Marceau P, Hould FS, Simard S, et al. Biliopancreatic diversion with duodenal switch. World J Surg. 1998;22(9):947–54.
6. Hess DS, Hess DW. Biliopancreatic diversion with a duodenal switch. Obes Surg. 1998;8(3):267–82.
7. Ren CJ, Patterson E, Gagner M. Early results of laparoscopic biliopancreatic diversion with duodenal switch: a case series of 40 consecutive patients. Obes Surg. 2000;10(6):514–23.
8. Kasama K, Tagaya N, Kanehira E, et al. Laparoscopic sleeve gastrectomy with duodenojejunal bypass: technique and preliminary results. Obes Surg. 2009;19(10):1341–5.

9. Sánchez-Pernaute A, Rubio Herrera MA, Pérez-Aguirre E, et al. Proximal duodenal-ileal end-to-side bypass with sleeve gastrecto- my: proposed technique. Obes Surg. 2007;17:1614–8.
10. Lee WJ, Lee KT, Kasama K, et al. Laparoscopic single-anastomosis duodenal-jejunal bypass with sleeve gastrectomy (SADJB-SG): short-term result and comparison with gastric bypass. Obes Surg. 2014;24(1):109–13.
11. Rabkin RA, Rabkin JM, Metcalf B, et al. Laparoscopic technique for performing duodenal switch with gastric reduction. Obes Surg. 2003;13(2):263–8.
12. Sánchez-Pernaute A, Herrera MA, Pérez-Aguirre ME, et al. Single anastomosis duodeno-ileal bypass with sleeve gastrectomy (SADI-S). One to three-year follow-up. Obes Surg. 2010;20(12):1720–6.
13. Raj PP, Kumaravel R, Chandramaliteeswaran C, et al. Laparoscopic duodenojejunal bypass with sleeve gastrectomy: preliminary results of a prospective series from India. Surg Endosc. 2012;26(3):688–92.
14. Praveen Raj P, Kumaravel R, Chandramaliteeswaran C, et al. Is laparoscopic duodenojejunal bypass with sleeve an effective alternative to Roux en Y gastric bypass in morbidly obese patients: preliminary results of a randomized trial. Obes Surg. 2012;22(3):422–6.
15. Huang CK, Wang MY, Das SS, et al. Laparoscopic conversion to loop duodenojejunal bypass with sleeve gastrectomy for intractable dumping syndrome after Roux-en-Y gastric bypass – two case reports. Obes Surg. 2015;25(5):947.

Part IV

Specific Situations in Bariatric Surgery

Gastroesophageal Reflux and Bariatric Surgery

12

Satish Pattanchetti and Sivalingam Perumal

12.1 Introduction

Gastroesophageal Reflux Disease (GERD) is a disorder of the upper gastrointestinal tract that is characterized by heartburn and acid regurgitation. According to the evidence-based consensus GERD is defined as 'a disease that is associated with troublesome symptoms and/or complications on account of reflux of stomach contents into the esophagus'. GERD is a disorder of the upper gastrointestinal tract that is defined by heartburn and acid regurgitation [1, 2].

There are many factors responsible for occurrence of GERD. These include transient lower esophageal sphincter (LES) relaxations, hypotensive LES and/or anatomic disruption of the esophageal hiatus or the phreno-esophageal membrane at the gastroesophageal junction (GEJ) like a hiatus hernia (HH).

The most common symptoms associated with GERD include heartburn, regurgitation, laryngitis, chronic cough, water brash, aspiration, wheezing, night time awakening with choking, belching or burping more than normal, and difficulty in swallowing.

S. Pattanchetti, MS, FMAS, FBMS (Taiwan) (✉)
Bariatric Surgery, Ruby Hall Clinic, Pune, India
e-mail: drsatishpattan@gmail.com

S. Perumal, MS, FMAS
Department of Upper GI Surgery and Minimal Access Surgery, GEM Hospital and Research Centre, Coimbatore, India
e-mail: dr.avps@gmail.com

P.R. Palanivelu et al. (eds.), *Bariatric Surgical Practice Guide*,
DOI 10.1007/978-981-10-2705-5_12

12.2 GERD and Obesity

The prevalence of GERD is estimated to be between 10 and 20% in the Western world, with a lower frequency in Asia [3]. Obesity is a very important risk factor for development of GERD which has been increasing in prevalence and is strongly associated with adverse metabolic, cardiovascular, chronic inflammatory and malignant health outcomes [4]. It has been shown that increasing weight leads to both increased esophageal reflux of acid and mechanical dysfunction of LES [5]. The other factors that influence the raised gastroesophageal gradient seen in obesity include raised intra-abdominal pressure (IAP), raised intra gastric pressure (IGP), raised negative inspiratory intra-thoracic pressure, oesophageal motor and sensory abnormalities, increase in prevalence of HH, increase in serum female hormonal levels, increase in comorbidities and a mechanical separation between the LES and the extrinsic compression provide by the diaphragmatic crura [6, 7]. Obese patients have also been reported to have higher rates of esophageal motility disorders and bolus transit impairments compared to normal BMI patients with GERD [8, 9].

It has also been shown that people who are obese are six times more likely to develop GERD than normal BMI people, being more common among pre-menopausal women and women on hormone therapy (including birth control pills), suggesting the possibility of estrogen to be a factor in GERD pathogenesis. Morbidly obese men (BMI >35 kg/m^2) are 3.3 times more likely to have reflux symptoms than men of normal weight with morbidly obese women being 6.3 times more likely to have these same symptoms compared to normal weighted women. It is being speculated that estrogen stimulates the production of nitrous oxide which relaxes smooth muscle fibers such as in the LES [10]. Brian et al. had observed a relationship between increasing BMI and the frequency of reflux symptoms and noted that for those who had a reduction in BMI of 3.5 or more there was nearly a 40% reduction in heartburn and other GERD symptoms than for women who did not lose weight [11].

It is also important to understand that the long-term effectiveness of fundoplication in the treatment of GERD in obese individuals (BMI >30) been questioned due to higher failure rates compared to normal weight counterparts [12, 13]. Although there is only limited evidence suggesting that obesity diminishes the efficacy of Nissen fundoplication, several other factors may impede the outcome of the procedure. Firstly, obesity can create several technical difficulties precipitating higher rates of surgical failures. For instance, an enlarged left lobe of the liver can interfere with visualization of the hiatus. Fatty deposition at the esophagogastric junction can impede proper suture placement. Lastly, a thick abdominal wall may hinder manipulation of laparoscopic instruments [4].

12.3 GERD and Laparoscopic Sleeve Gastrectomy (LSG)

Laparoscopic Sleeve Gastrectomy (LSG) has emerged as a popular bariatric procedure worldwide due to its relative operative simplicity, lack of anastomoses, retention of normal gastrointestinal continuity and absence of a malabsorptive component

[14–16]. But, it is generally believed that LSG increases the incidence/severity of GERD and is considered a contraindication in patients with pre-existing GERD.

The increasing incidence of de-novo GERD could be related to lack of gastric compliance, increased intraluminal pressure, removal of the gastric fundus, alteration in the angle of His, lower LES pressure, hiatal herniation, narrowing at the junction of the vertical and horizontal parts of the sleeve (incisura), twisting of the sleeve, dilation of the remnant fundus etc [17–20].

Arias et al. in his retrospective review of 130 patients who had undergone LSG noted an 2.1 % incidence of de novo GERD [21]. Carter et al. had reported the results of 176 patients who had undergone LSG with 34.6 % having preoperative GERD. Postoperatively, 49 % complained of immediate (within 30 days) GERD symptoms, 47.2 % had persistent GERD symptoms that lasted >1 month, and 33.8 % of patients were taking medications specifically for GERD. The most common symptoms were heartburn (46 %), followed by heartburn with regurgitation (29.2 %) [22].

Himpens et al. in 2006 did the only prospective study comparing LSG with gastric band and concluded that at the end of 1 year 21.8 % of patients developed de-novo GERD which decreased to 3.1 % at end of 3 years possibly due to restoration of Angle of His [19]. DuPree et al. in 2014 in their retrospective review of the Bariatric Outcomes Longitudinal Database (BOLD), a total of 4832 patients underwent LSG and 33,867 underwent laparoscopic roux-en-Y gastric bypass (LRYGB), with preexisting GERD present in 44.5 % of the LSG cohort and 50.4 % of the LRYGB cohort. Most LSG patients (84.1 %) continued to have GERD symptoms postoperatively, with only 15.9 % demonstrating GERD resolution. Of LSG patients who did not demonstrate preoperative GERD, 8.6 % developed GERD postoperatively [23].

It has also been reported by a few authors that LSG leads to improvement in GERD. The possible explanation could be reduced intra-abdominal pressure after weight reduction, reduced acid production, accelerated gastric emptying and reduced gastric volume [17]. It has been noted that during LSG if the anatomy of the esophago-gastric junction (EGJ) flap valve is maintained without axial separation of the crura and LES, an elevation of IGP would be transmitted to the intra-abdominal LES thus closing the EGJ. However, if the EGJ flap valve is obliterated, elevations in IGP may increase the volume of refluxate once the EGJ is forced open. Daes et al., in their prospective evaluation of 382 patients, showed a 94 % resolution of symptoms and emphasized the need for careful attention to surgical technique, such as avoiding relative narrowing at the level of incisura, and the importance of placing the anterior stomach wall and posterior stomach wall in an equal and flat position when firing the stapler, in order to prevent the sleeve from rotating [24]. A prospective database from Pallati et al., which included 585 patients, showed a 41 % improvement in GERD symptoms, thus indicating that LSG may be performed in obese patients suffering from GERD [25]. Chiu et al. in a systematic review on GERD and its effects following LSG showed that four studies demonstrated an increase in prevalence with seven studies showing a reduced prevalence of GERD following LSG [26].

Interestingly, there are some studies demonstrating positive outcomes after concomitant LSG and hiatal hernia (HH) repair. Soricelli et al. reported significant improvement of GERD symptoms after a LSG with concomitant HH repair [27]. They described repair of a posterior crural defect with two interrupted non-absorbable sutures, approximating the right and left diaphragmatic pillars. HH repair was shown to be feasible and safe with no postoperative complications related to this procedure. The exposure of the hiatal area in the presence of a HH implies complete freeing of the posterior stomach wall and facilitates complete resection of the gastric fundus. This in turn is of great importance for the success of a LSG in terms of weight loss but also avoids de novo GERD caused by acid secretion and regurgitation of the persistent gastric fundus content into the esophagus. In addition, the postoperative development of de novo reflux symptoms was significantly greater in patients who underwent a LSG without an HH repair compared to those with an HH repair. Similar results have also been shown by Daes et al. and Soliman et al. who had favorable outcomes in the improvements of GERD by combining LSG with HH repair [24, 28]. Gibson et al. had also shown favorable outcomes even with an anterior crural closure [29].

Cheung et al. reported the results from revisional surgery after a LSG (Re-LSG and LRYGB) and found that both procedures were effective in achieving weight loss following a failed LSG. As weight loss may influence GERD symptoms, a Re-SG may also work as an effective tool to reduce GERD [30].

Silecchia et al. reported on the safety and efficacy of Re-LSG (also referred to as laparoscopic fundectomy) in cases where a residual fundus or neofundus is responsible for GERD symptoms. A Re-LSG was done in 19 patients when a residual fundus or neofundus was found in patients with severe GERD symptoms. Of note is that cruroplasty was concomitantly done when a HH was found in this series. All patients had improved GERD symptoms and discontinued proton pump inhibitors (PPIs) [31]. HH is not only responsible for GERD but contributes to the incomplete removal of the gastric fundus, which is often missed at the time of a LSG. The latter is responsible for acid secretion, which is then regurgitated back into the esophagus, especially if there are other factors such as a HH or an impaired LES, and if increased transient relaxation is present. Thus, Re-LSG may be an option for patients with a persistent gastric fundus and or a HH responsible for GERD that is non-responsive to PPIs. However, this procedure should remain limited to patients in whom a relationship between GERD and a persistent gastric fundus is clear, and should be conducted by a specialized bariatric surgeon. If a HH is present, it should be fixed during the same procedure [17].

12.4 GERD and LRYGB

The LRYGB is considered to be the most effective treatment option for GERD in the morbidly obese patient, since it treats GERD effectively and provides the additional benefit of weight loss and improvement in comorbidities [32]. Its efficacy in treating GERD is possibly related to the relatively low acid production of the small-volume (15–30 mL) gastric pouch, reduction of esophageal biliopancreatic refluxate by use of a roux limb measuring at least 100 cm in length and weight loss. The physiological effects of the anatomic configuration of LRYGB, and specifically, the configuration of the gastric pouch, might in fact be a more important contributor to reflux improvement than reducing alkaline bile reflux or weight loss. The cardia region of the stomach, where the pouch is created, has also been shown to relatively lack parietal cells [33].

Frezza et al. conducted a study on a total of 152 patients with pre-existing GERD, on changes in GERD symptoms, quality of life, and patient satisfaction after LRYGB. There was a significant decrease in GERD-related symptoms, including heartburn (from 87 to 22 %), water brash (from 18 to 7 %), wheezing (from 40 to 5 %), laryngitis (from 17 to 7 %) and aspiration (from 14 to 2 %) following LRYGB and the overall patient satisfaction was 97 % [33].

A prospective study based on the Montreal Consensus by Madalasso et al. on the impact of gastric bypass on gastroesophageal reflux disease in patients with morbid obesity showed that the prevalence of GERD reduced from 64 % before LRYGB to 33 % after LRYGB. GERD-related well-being and use of PPIs were both improved after LRYGB. Typical reflux syndrome (TRS) was present in 47 patients (55 %) preoperatively and disappeared in 39 of them (79 %) post-LRYGB. Extraesophageal symptoms in 16 patients resolved in all [34].

Perry and colleagues assessed 57 patients who underwent a LRYGB for patients with gastroesophageal reflux disease pre- and postoperatively. Hiatal hernias or esophagitis were present in 48 patients and Barretts esophagus was present in 2 patients preoperatively. Patients were followed up at a mean of 18 months, and they attained a mean weight loss of 40 kg. In follow-up all patients reported improvement or no symptoms of GERD [35].

Raftoupoulous and colleagues assessed seven morbidly patients with previous Nissen fundoplications with recurrent/persistent GERD who underwent revision LRYGB. Assessment with the Gastroesophageal Reflux Disease–Health Related Quality of Life (GERD-HRQL) scale preoperatively and postoperatively showed a significant reduction in GERD scores [20].

Most patients with hiatal hernias do not undergo hernia repair during their LRYGB, as most surgeons consider the procedure unnecessary owing to the alleviation of GERD symptoms after significant weight loss but some suggest repair to fully alleviate GERD following LRYGB. A recent retrospective analysis by Kothari and colleagues compared the results of LRYGB and LRYGB combined with laparoscopic hiatal hernia repair (LHHR). Their study involved three groups of patients: the first group (n = 33 717) did not have hiatal hernias and underwent LRYGB alone, the second group (n = 644) had hiatal hernias and underwent both LRYGB and LHHR, and the final group (n = 1589) had hiatal hernias but did not undergo LHHR. On comparison of patients with HH who underwent LRYGB and simultaneous LHHR with those who had LRYGB without LHHR, no significant difference with regards to all the outcome measures was noted [36].

A recent variation on the RYGB is the omega-loop gastric bypass, also known as the mini-gastric bypass or one-anastomosis gastric bypass. There have been concerns about the effects of biliary reflux into the gastric tube in this procedure unlike LRYGB. In a small study of 15 patients receiving omega- loop gastric bypass were compared with a control group of LSG. High-resolution impedance manometry and 24-h pH-impedance monitoring, both before and 1 year after the procedures were performed. At 1 year after surgery, none of the patients reported de novo heartburn or regurgitation. Dramatic decrease in episodes of reflux was reported. On endoscopy esophagitis was absent in all patients and no biliary gastritis or presence of bile was recorded. Manometric features and patterns did not vary significantly after surgery. In contrast, LSG resulted in increased reflux epiosodes, significant elevation in intragastric pressures (IGP) and gastroesophageal pressure gradient (GEPG) However, long- term data on the risk of GERD developing after this particular procedure is required [37].

Conclusion

With regards to bariatric surgery and its effect on GERD, studies have shown inconsistencies with different types of bariatric surgery. LRYGB has been consistently shown to provide good improvement in GERD in morbidly obese patients. Hence it is considered the gold standard for the treatment of GERD in morbidly obese patients. LSG has had inconsistent results with regards to GERD improvement. Although, the improvement of symptoms have been clearly documented, the long term effects of non-acid reflux and associated long term complications has not been clearly studied. Hence, although LSG cannot be considered as an absolute contraindication, caution has to be exerted while choosing the procedure with more closer follow-up.

As bariatric surgeries affect anatomy and physiology of the gastrointestinal tract in different ways, it is important to assess patient's comorbidities when considering the different types of bariatric surgeries. A careful assessment and discussion with the patient along with a very close follow up for the long term is mandatory.

Recommendation

- Laparoscopic Roux-en-Y gastric bypass is considered to be the gold standard treatment option for GERD in morbidly obese patients
- Laparoscopic Roux-en-Y gastric bypass is preferable to fundoplication in morbidly obese patients with GERD.
- Laparoscopic sleeve gastrectomy is a relative contraindication in the presence of clinical GERD.
- Laparoscopic sleeve gastrectomy can be combined with cruroplasty in the presence of hiatus hernia without GERD.
- Refractory GERD following laparoscopic sleeve gastrectomy would benefit from a revision to roux-en-Y gastric bypass

References

1. Vakil N, van Zanten SV, Kahrilas P, Dent J, Jones R, Consensus Group Global. The Montreal definition and classification of gastroesophageal reflux disease: a global evidence-based consensus. Am J Gastroenterol. 2006;101(8):1900–20; quiz 1943.
2. Vakil N, van Zanten SV, Kahrilas P, Dent J, Jones R, Globale Konsensusgruppe. The Montreal definition and classification of gastroesophageal reflux disease: a global, evidence-based consensus paper. Am J Gastroenterol. 2007;45(11):1125–40.
3. Katz PO, Gerson LB, Vela MF. Guidelines for the diagnosis and management of gastroesophageal reflux disease. Am J Gastroenterol. 2013;108(3):308–28; quiz 329.
4. Khan A, Kim A, Sanossian C, Francois F. Impact of obesity treatment on gastroesophageal reflux disease. World J Gastroenterol. 2016;22(4):1627–38.
5. Ayazi S, Hagen JA, Chan LS, DeMeester SR, Lin MW, Ayazi A, et al. Obesity and gastroesophageal reflux: quantifying the association between body mass index, esophageal acid exposure, and lower esophageal sphincter status in a large series of patients with reflux symptoms. J Gastrointest Surg. 2009;13(8):1440–7.
6. Pandolfino JE, El-Serag HB, Zhang Q, Shah N, Ghosh SK, Kahrilas PJ. Obesity: a challenge to esophagogastric junction integrity. Gastroenterology. 2006;130(3):639–49.
7. De Vries DR, van Herwaarden MA, Smout AJPM, Samsom M. Gastroesophageal pressure gradients in gastroesophageal reflux disease: relations with hiatal hernia, body mass index, and esophageal acid exposure. Am J Gastroenterol. 2008;103(6):1349–54.
8. Roman S, Pandolfino JE. Environmental – lifestyle related factors. Best Pract Res Clin Gastroenterol. 2010;24(6):847–59.
9. Wu JC-Y, Mui L-M, Cheung CM-Y, Chan Y, Sung JJ-Y. Obesity is associated with increased transient lower esophageal sphincter relaxation. Gastroenterology. 2007;132(3):883–9.
10. Close H, Mason JM, Wilson D, Hungin APS. Hormone replacement therapy is associated with gastro-oesophageal reflux disease: a retrospective cohort study. BMC Gastroenterol. 2012;12:56.
11. Jacobson BC, Somers SC, Fuchs CS, Kelly CP, Camargo CA. Body-mass index and symptoms of gastroesophageal reflux in women. N Engl J Med. 2006;354(22):2340–8.
12. Morgenthal CB, Lin E, Shane MD, Hunter JG, Smith CD. Who will fail laparoscopic Nissen fundoplication? Preoperative prediction of long-term outcomes. Surg Endosc. 2007;21(11):1978–84.
13. Perez AR, Moncure AC, Rattner DW. Obesity adversely affects the outcome of antireflux operations. Surg Endosc. 2001;15(9):986–9.
14. Eid GM, Brethauer S, Mattar SG, Titchner RL, Gourash W, Schauer PR. Laparoscopic sleeve gastrectomy for super obese patients: forty-eight percent excess weight loss after 6 to 8 years with 93 % follow-up. Ann Surg. 2012;256(2):262–5.
15. Sánchez-Santos R, Masdevall C, Baltasar A, Martínez-Blázquez C, García Ruiz de Gordejuela A, Ponsi E, et al. Short- and mid-term outcomes of sleeve gastrectomy for morbid obesity: the experience of the Spanish National Registry. Obes Surg. 2009;19(9):1203–10.
16. Baltasar A, Serra C, Pérez N, Bou R, Bengochea M, Ferri L. Laparoscopic sleeve gastrectomy: a multi-purpose bariatric operation. Obes Surg. 2005;15(8):1124–8.
17. Stenard F, Iannelli A. Laparoscopic sleeve gastrectomy and gastroesophageal reflux. World J Gastroenterol. 2015;21(36):10348–57.
18. Burgerhart JS, Schotborgh CAI, Schoon EJ, Smulders JF, van de Meeberg PC, Siersema PD, et al. Effect of sleeve gastrectomy on gastroesophageal reflux. Obes Surg. 2014;24(9):1436–41.
19. Himpens J, Dapri G, Cadière GB. A prospective randomized study between laparoscopic gastric banding and laparoscopic isolated sleeve gastrectomy: results after 1 and 3 years. Obes Surg. 2006;16(11):1450–6.

20. Braghetto I, Lanzarini E, Korn O, Valladares H, Molina JC, Henriquez A. Manometric changes of the lower esophageal sphincter after sleeve gastrectomy in obese patients. Obes Surg. 2010;20(3):357–62.
21. Arias E, Martínez PR, Ka Ming Li V, Szomstein S, Rosenthal RJ. Mid-term follow-up after sleeve gastrectomy as a final approach for morbid obesity. Obes Surg. 2009;19(5):544–8.
22. Carter PR, LeBlanc KA, Hausmann MG, Kleinpeter KP, deBarros SN, Jones SM. Association between gastroesophageal reflux disease and laparoscopic sleeve gastrectomy. Surg Obes Relat Dis. 2011;7(5):569–72.
23. DuPree CE, Blair K, Steele SR, Martin MJ. Laparoscopic sleeve gastrectomy in patients with preexisting gastroesophageal reflux disease : a national analysis. JAMA Surg. 2014;149(4):328–34.
24. Daes J, Jimenez ME, Said N, Daza JC, Dennis R. Laparoscopic sleeve gastrectomy: symptoms of gastroesophageal reflux can be reduced by changes in surgical technique. Obes Surg. 2012;22(12):1874–9.
25. Pallati PK, Shaligram A, Shostrom VK, Oleynikov D, McBride CL, Goede MR. Improvement in gastroesophageal reflux disease symptoms after various bariatric procedures: review of the Bariatric Outcomes Longitudinal Database. Surg Obes Relat Dis. 2014;10(3):502–7.
26. Chiu S, Birch DW, Shi X, Sharma AM, Karmali S. Effect of sleeve gastrectomy on gastroesophageal reflux disease: a systematic review. Surg Obes Relat Dis. 2011;7(4):510–5.
27. Soricelli E, Iossa A, Casella G, Abbatini F, Calì B, Basso N. Sleeve gastrectomy and crural repair in obese patients with gastroesophageal reflux disease and/or hiatal hernia. Surg Obes Relat Dis. 2013;9(3):356–61.
28. Soliman A, Maged H, Awad A, El-Shiekh O. Laparoscopic crural repair with simultaneous sleeve gastrectomy: a way in gastroesophageal reflux disease treatment associated with morbid obesity. J Minim Invasive Surg Sci. 2012;1(2):67–73.
29. Gibson SC, Le Page PA, Taylor CJ. Laparoscopic sleeve gastrectomy: review of 500 cases in single surgeon Australian practice. ANZ J Surg. 2015;85(9):673–7.
30. Cheung D, Switzer NJ, Gill RS, Shi X, Karmali S. Revisional bariatric surgery following failed primary laparoscopic sleeve gastrectomy: a systematic review. Obes Surg. 2014;24(10):1757–63.
31. Silecchia G, De Angelis F, Rizzello M, Albanese A, Longo F, Foletto M. Residual fundus or neofundus after laparoscopic sleeve gastrectomy: is fundectomy safe and effective as revision surgery? Surg Endosc. 2015;29(10):2899–903.
32. Patterson EJ, Davis DG, Khajanchee Y, Swanström LL. Comparison of objective outcomes following laparoscopic Nissen fundoplication versus laparoscopic gastric bypass in the morbidly obese with heartburn. Surg Endosc. 2003;17(10):1561–5.
33. Frezza EE, Ikramuddin S, Gourash W, Rakitt T, Kingston A, Luketich J, et al. Symptomatic improvement in gastroesophageal reflux disease (GERD) following laparoscopic Roux-en-Y gastric bypass. Surg Endosc. 2002;16(7):1027–31.
34. Madalosso CAS, Gurski RR, Callegari-Jacques SM, Navarini D, Thiesen V, Fornari F. The impact of gastric bypass on gastroesophageal reflux disease in patients with morbid obesity: a prospective study based on the Montreal Consensus. Ann Surg. 2010;251(2):244–8.
35. Perry Y, Courcoulas AP, Fernando HC, Buenaventura PO, McCaughan JS, Luketich JD. Laparoscopic Roux-en-Y gastric bypass for recalcitrant gastroesophageal reflux disease in morbidly obese patients. JSLS. 2004;8(1):19–23.
36. Kothari V, Shaligram A, Reynoso J, Schmidt E, McBride CL, Oleynikov D. Impact on perioperative outcomes of concomitant hiatal hernia repair with laparoscopic gastric bypass. Obes Surg. 2012;22(10):1607–10.
37. Tolone S, Cristiano S, Savarino E, Lucido FS, Fico DI, Docimo L. Effects of omega-loop bypass on esophagogastric junction function. Surg Obes Relat Dis. 2016;12(1):62–9.

Ventral Hernia Repair in the Morbidly Obese

13

Rachel Maria Gomes and Praveen Raj Palanivelu

13.1 Introduction

Ventral hernias either spontaneous or incisional and both primary and recurrent are more prevalent in the morbidly obese population. Patients coming for bariatric consultations hence often have hernias or history of hernia repairs being performed. Datta et al. reported that 8 % of patients who presented for a gastric bypass procedure had a ventral hernia [1].

Morbid obesity with its associated comorbidities has been shown to be a significant factor predisposing to the occurrence of ventral hernias. Sugerman et al. reported in their series that incisional hernias occurred in 20 % of the open gastric bypass patients, with an even greater rate in those with previous incisional hernias [2]. Several factors have been implicated for this increased incidence. Morbid obesity is associated with chronically elevated intra-abdominal pressures [3, 4]. Excess fat deposition leads to defects in fascial structure [5, 6]. In those undergoing surgeries thick subcutaneous layers lead to suboptimal fascial approximation. Healing is reduced secondary to fat deposition as well as presence of comorbidities. There is an increased rate of postoperative wound infections [7].

A ventral hernia in a bariatric surgery candidate is an important influencing factor for the operative approach. The aim of this chapter was to review the pros and cons of the various possible operative approaches in a patient with ventral hernia needing bariatric surgery.

R.M. Gomes, MS, FMAS (✉) • P.R. Palanivelu, MS, DNB, DNB (SGE), FALS, FMAS
Bariatric Division, Upper Gastrointestinal Surgery and Minimal Access Surgery Unit, GEM Hospital and Research Centre, Coimbatore, India
e-mail: dr.gomes@rediffmail.com; drraj@geminstitute.in

P.R. Palanivelu et al. (eds.), *Bariatric Surgical Practice Guide*,
DOI 10.1007/978-981-10-2705-5_13

The options for management of the bariatric patient with a ventral hernia include

- (i) Two stage procedures
  - (a) First perform the bariatric surgery and postpone the ventral hernia repair until weight loss
  - (b) First perform the ventral hernia repair and postpone the bariatric surgery until recovery
- (ii) Concomitant bariatric surgery with ventral hernia repair
  - (a) Primary sutured repair
  - (b) Mesh repair
    - (a) Biological meshes
    - (b) Permanent meshes

13.2 Two Stage Procedures

13.2.1 First Perform the Bariatric Surgery and Postpone the Ventral Hernia Repair Until Weight Loss

In a preoperatively detected ventral hernia, the patient can undergo repair of the hernia after bariatric surgery. Two main advantages of this approach exist. Firstly, a lengthy and difficult primary combined procedure is avoided. Secondly, at the time of subsequent surgery patient will be optimized by weight loss and resolution of co-morbid conditions decreasing both operative risk and possibly risk of recurrence.

Though some suggest that subsequent hernia repair may be easier, studies have shown that patients who were once morbidly obese then become a unique challenge to hernia repair, because of larger fascial defects and extreme amounts of abdominal wall laxity [8]. Post-bariatric surgery ventral hernia repair can be done during abdominoplasty as an open procedure or can also be done laparoscopically when body contouring procedures have not been planned. The superiority of laparoscopic ventral hernias is already known from existing literature. Abdominoplasty can be also be safely combined with ventral hernia repairs. Downey et al. reported a series of 50 patients who had undergone fascial plication and midline mesh placement. They found only minor wound problems and no recurrence [8]. Borud et al. reported a series of 50 patients with ventral hernias after bariatric surgery. Twelve had large hernias and underwent a component separation technique with abdominal wall plication and onlay mesh placement. Borud et al. reported a high rate of major and minor wound complications but only one recurrence [9]. Saxe et al. reported 71 patients who underwent concomitant ventral hernia repair with abdominoplasty, 40 with prosthetic mesh. Wound complications were increased but no patient sustained a wound complication that required mesh removal [10].

This approach conforms to the basic teaching of 'treating the precipitating factor before a hernia is repaired to avoid recurrence'. Though this principle may hold good for precipitating factors like chronic bronchitis, benign prostatic hypertrophy

(BPH), or chronic constipation, as these are correctable in a few days to few weeks it may not be scientifically right to postpone the hernia repair for months until the obesity factor is addressed by surgical means. Also the risk of leaving a hernia unrepaired is the development of small bowel obstruction. Reducing the hernia without repair resulted in 33 % of the patients developing obstruction in the series by Eid et al. [6]. In cases where laparoscopic roux-en-Y gastric bypass (LRYGB)/anastomotic techniques are performed the risk of delayed diagnosis exists if the biliopancreatic limb is obstructed [11]. Thus when no repair has been done, the patient should be closely followed up to detect obstructive symptoms. Another possible option will be to leave the hernia unrepaired with incarcerated omentum plugged in at the time of bariatric surgery and plan for a mesh repair at a later date. In the series by Datta et al., incarcerated asymptomatic hernias confirmed to contain only omentum and outside the operating field were left untouched. This was shown to have no complications after an average follow-up of 14 months. But, this may not always be possible as it will be required to reduce the contents of the hernial sac to facilitate the bariatric procedure especially where a LRYGB is undertaken and for upper abdominal hernias. Another option as was suggested by Datta et al. for hernia contents blocking the operative field, was to maintain the plug of omentum but transect the omentum using ultrasonic shears starting at the mid-transverse colon and lift the free "leaf" of the omentum over the transverse colon to access the bowel. Newcomb et al. preferred to leave large hernias untouched, without reducing even the small bowel because they believed that the risk of bowel obstruction was reduced if the bowel did not need to reorganize during the period of rapid weight loss [12].

In a recent study Eid et al. attempted to recommend an approach based on patient and hernia characteristics. Hernias were classified based on anatomy into favourable anatomy (BMI <50 kg/m^2, gynecoid body habitus, reducible hernias found in a central location, abdominal wall thickness less than 4 cm, and the defect <8 cm). and unfavourable anatomy (BMI >50 kg/m^2, android body habitus, irreducible hernias, hernias in a lateral location, abdominal wall thickness more than 4 cm, and the defects >8 cm) and based on symptoms into symptomatic and asymptomatic. Unfavourable anatomy were those who were more likely to need an open approach to repair of hernia. They recommended that patients who were asymptomatic with unfavourable anatomy were the patients who were likely to benefit from bariatric surgery followed by ventral hernia repair. All symptomatic hernias should have their hernias addressed first [13].

13.2.2 First Perform the Ventral Hernia Repair and Postpone the Bariatric Surgery Until Recovery

Conventional open ventral hernia repairs (OVHRs) in the obese population has traditionally been marked by high failure rates exclusive of other factors [14]. Studies have reported improved results with laparoscopic ventral hernia repairs (LVHRs) perhaps because of tension free repairs with intra-peritoneal prosthetic meshes with a low rate of wound complications [15]. A study by Ching et al. showed that the morbidly obese did not have a significant difference in the complication rate, including recurrence after laparoscopic ventral hernia repair, compared with the non-morbidly obese. The median follow-up period was 19 months (range 6–62) [16]. A study by Birginsson et al. showed that though the operative times were longer in morbidly obese patients, surgery can be performed with minimal morbidity and had no recurrences at a follow-up period ranging from 1 to 35 months comparable to non-obese patients [17]. A study by Novitsky et al. showed that the operative time, hospital stay, and incidence of complications were not influenced by the BMI when the patients undergoing ventral hernia repair were stratified according to the BMI [18].

However a study by Heniford et al. showed that morbidly obese patients had higher recurrence rates and higher incidence of complications [19]. Raftopolous et al. reported hernia repairs have higher recurrence rates in morbidly obese patients [20]. A study by Tsereteli et al. reported that the complication rates were not greater although the rate of recurrence was significantly greater in the morbidly obese [21]. Therefore there is no consensus found in the literature as to the long-term effectiveness and durability of laparoscopic ventral hernia repair (LVHR) in morbidly obese patients. Additional randomized controlled studies are needed to prove the safety and efficacy of ventral hernia repair in the morbidly obese before weight loss.

Eid et al. attempted to recommend approach based on patient and hernia characteristics by classifying hernias based on anatomy into favourable and unfavourable as described before. They recommended that all symptomatic hernias should have their ventral hernias repaired first followed by bariatric surgery. In those with unfavourable anatomy who were more likely to need complex repair of hernias this should be preceded by medically supervised low calorie diet and preoperative weight loss to optimize the patients [13].

This approach has the advantage that a lengthy and difficult primary combined procedure is avoided. A possible disadvantage is that subsequent surgery may be posed a difficulty by occurrence of adhesions. However Eid et al. reported that the level of adhesion formation encountered during the subsequent bariatric procedure is very manageable and does not increase the risk of converting to an open approach [13] Though studies showed improved results with laparoscopic ventral hernia repairs (LVHRs) in obese patients more data is needed to confidently conclude that safety and efficacy of ventral hernia repair in the morbidly obese is equal to non-obese patients. Till then if this approach is used in morbidly obese patients it should be followed by bariatric surgery as early as possible after recovery to avoid recurrence.

13.3 Concomitant Bariatric Surgery with Ventral Hernia Repair

Two types of strategies can be used for concomitant bariatric surgery with ventral hernia repair

(a) Primary repair
(b) Mesh repair

13.3.1 Primary Repair

For intra-operatively detected ventral hernias in the morbidly obese bariatric patient, it would be best to repair the hernia if the hernia contents have been reduced. Reducing the hernia without repair resulted in 33 % of the patients developing obstruction in the series shown by Eid et al. [11]. Primary repair seems to be the preferred approach for many bariatric surgeons today because of the fear of mesh infection. Although this temporarily protects against obstruction or incarceration, the rate of recurrence has been high. The recurrence rate has been reported to be 22 % by Eid et al. [11]. Newcomb et al. repaired small defects in his series. All these small defects recurred and were repaired electively [12].

In a recent series by Eid et al. they suggested that a fairly large number of bariatric patients present with asymptomatic small hernias with greatest diameter of less than 2 cm which are often incidental findings during laparoscopic bariatric surgery. This subset is perhaps the group that can undergo repair primarily with the use of permanent sutures [13].

13.3.2 Concomitant Mesh Repair

Although it has been shown that clean procedures like gastric banding can be combined with mesh repairs, the controversy is in combining gastric bypass and sleeve gastrectomy for the fear of infection of the mesh. Roux en Y gastric bypass involves voluntary creation of enterotomies and in case of sleeve gastrectomy there is presence of exposed gastric mucosa. Because enterotomies are not created in a gastric banding procedure, it is possible to use synthetic mesh for the primary, or staged, repair of hernias, such as was shown by Bonnati et al. [22]. No recurrence or infection had developed after a median follow-up of 34 months.

The placement of absorbable meshes may be opted in the setting of sleeve gastrectomy/roux-en-Y or other anastomotic techniques. Eid et al. initially reported that the use of Surgisis (Cook, Bloomington, IN) mesh resulted in no hernia recurrence in patients undergoing LRYGB with a secondary diagnosis of ventral hernia [11]. Wound infection occurred in 25 % and seroma in 33 % of patients who had undergone mesh repair. However they later reported that with longer-term follow-up rates (mean of 30 months and 50 % follow-up) that all patients presented back with hernia recurrences [13]. In the series by Newcomb et al., also all defects recurred when repaired with a biologic mesh [12]. Thus though it may be considered as a temporary fix to avoid bowel strangulation albeit an expensive choice, it cannot be considered as permanent option.

We now have enough evidence to show that placement of prosthetic mesh in contaminated cases does not increase the risk of wound infections or other mesh-related complications [23–29]. Enough data has been published over time proving the safety of concomitant bariatric surgery and LVHRs. Datta et al. compared primary ventral hernia repair with sutures against primary ventral hernia repair with a prosthetic mesh with concomitant gastric bypass (ten patients) and showed usage of a mesh reduced the recurrence rates drastically without any incidence of mesh infection. Schuster and colleagues reported concomitant LRYGB and ventral hernia repair in 12 patients using polyester/collagen or polypropylene/cellulose with no mesh infections and two recurrences [30]. Chan et al. reported their series of 45 patients undergoing synchronous bariatric surgery and ventral hernia repair, (36 gastric bypass or sleeve gastrectomy and 9 gastric banding). Two patients developed infected seromas that responded to simple drainage (mesh infection 4.44 %) with no recurrences at a median follow-up of 13 months [31]. Raziel et al. reported 54 patients with synchronous bariatric surgery and ventral hernia repair (48 LSG 4 LRYGB and 2 LAGB) and reported no mesh infections with recurrence in 1 patient [32]. Praveenraj et al. reported 36 patients (11 LRYGB, 25 LSG) with synchronous bariatric surgery and ventral hernia repair without mesh infection or recurrence. In the largest study to date Spaniolas et al. identified 503 patients (433 LRYGB and 70 LSG) with synchronous bariatric surgery and ventral hernia repair by querying the American College of Surgeons National Surgical Quality Improvement Program (ACS-NSQIP) database and reported an increase in surgical site infection (SSI) but not overall morbidity and no significant difference in the SSI rate between LRYGB and LSG.

Hence a mesh repair is a feasible option however it needs utmost care to prevent any undue gross contamination in the operating field and skill in managing these procedures concomitantly. A low threshold for deferral of mesh repair has to be followed in case of any concerns. Cozacov et al. prospectively assessed with intraoperative peritoneal aspirates, patients undergoing LRYGB and LSG and found bacterial growth in 15 % of the LRYGB aspirates and none in the LSG samples, suggesting that the use of synthetic mesh may be safer in patients undergoing LSG. Though data has not demonstrated an effect of type of procedure on mesh infection a LSG may be a preferred option when feasible.

Recommendations

- Weight loss is an important consideration for successful treatment of ventral hernias in obese patients
- Primary bariatric surgery followed by ventral hernia repair after adequate weight loss is a treatment option, but hernia related complications in the interval period have to be closely monitored.
- Primary hernia repair followed by bariatric surgery is another option especially in symptomatic hernias.
- In experienced centers composite mesh hernia repair can be concomitantly performed with bariatric surgery

References

1. Datta T, Eid G, Nahmias N, Dallal RM. Management of ventral hernias during laparoscopic gastric bypass. Surg Obes Relat Dis Off J Am Soc Bariatr Surg. 2008;4(6):754–7.

2. Sugerman HJ, Kellum JM, Reines HD, DeMaria EJ, Newsome HH, Lowry JW. Greater risk of incisional hernia with morbidly obese than steroid-dependent patients and low recurrence with prefascial polypropylene mesh. Am J Surg. 1996;171(1):80–4.
3. Varela JE, Hinojosa M, Nguyen N. Correlations between intra-abdominal pressure and obesity-related co-morbidities. Surg Obes Relat Dis. 2009;5(5):524–8.
4. Sugerman HJ. Effects of increased intra-abdominal pressure in severe obesity. Surg Clin North Am. 2001;81(5):1063–75, vi.
5. Szczesny W, Bodnar M, Dabrowiecki S, Szmytkowski J, Marszałek A. Histologic and immunohistochemical studies of rectus sheath in obese patients. J Surg Res. 2013;180(2):260–5.
6. Klinge U, Si ZY, Zheng H, Schumpelick V, Bhardwaj RS, Klosterhalfen B. Collagen I/III and matrix metalloproteinases (MMP) 1 and 13 in the fascia of patients with incisional hernias. J Investig Surg Off J Acad Surg Res. 2001;14(1):47–54.
7. Veljkovic R, Protic M, Gluhovic A, Potic Z, Milosevic Z, Stojadinovic A. Prospective clinical trial of factors predicting the early development of incisional hernia after midline laparotomy. J Am Coll Surg. 2010;210(2):210–9.
8. Downey SE, Morales C, Kelso RL, Anthone G. Review of technique for combined closed incisional hernia repair and panniculectomy status post-open bariatric surgery. Surg Obes Relat Dis Off J Am Soc Bariatr Surg. 2005;1(5):458–61.
9. Borud LJ, Grunwaldt L, Janz B, Mun E, Slavin SA. Components separation combined with abdominal wall plication for repair of large abdominal wall hernias following bariatric surgery. Plast Reconstr Surg. 2007;119(6):1792–8.
10. Saxe A, Schwartz S, Gallardo L, Yassa E, Alghanem A. Simultaneous panniculectomy and ventral hernia repair following weight reduction after gastric bypass surgery: is it safe? Obes Surg. 2008;18(2):192–5; discussion 196.
11. Eid GM, Prince JM, Mattar SG, Hamad G, Ikrammudin S, Schauer PR. Medium-term follow-up confirms the safety and durability of laparoscopic ventral hernia repair with PTFE. Surgery. 2003;134(4):599–603; discussion 603–4.
12. Eid GM, Wikiel KJ, Entabi F, Saleem M. Ventral hernias in morbidly obese patients: a suggested algorithm for operative repair. Obes Surg. 2013;23(5):703–9.
13. Manninen MJ, Lavonius M, Perhoniemi VJ. Results of incisional hernia repair. A retrospective study of 172 unselected hernioplasties. Eur J Surg Acta Chir. 1991;157(1):29–31.
14. Heniford BT, Ramshaw BJ. Laparoscopic ventral hernia repair: a report of 100 consecutive cases. Surg Endosc. 2000;14(5):419–23.
15. Ching SS, Sarela AI, Dexter SPL, Hayden JD, McMahon MJ. Comparison of early outcomes for laparoscopic ventral hernia repair between nonobese and morbidly obese patient populations. Surg Endosc. 2008;22(10):2244–50.
16. Birgisson G, Park AE, Mastrangelo MJ, Witzke DB, Chu UB. Obesity and laparoscopic repair of ventral hernias. Surg Endosc. 2001;15(12):1419–22.
17. Novitsky YW, Cobb WS, Kercher KW, Matthews BD, Sing RF, Heniford BT. Laparoscopic ventral hernia repair in obese patients: a new standard of care. Arch Surg. 2006;141(1):57–61.
18. Heniford BT, Park A, Ramshaw BJ, Voeller G. Laparoscopic repair of ventral hernias. Ann Surg. 2003;238(3):391–400.
19. Raftopoulos I, Vanuno D, Khorsand J, Ninos J, Kouraklis G, Lasky P. Outcome of laparoscopic ventral hernia repair in correlation with obesity, type of hernia, and hernia size. J Laparoendosc Adv Surg Tech A. 2002;12(6):425–9.
20. Tsereteli Z, Pryor BA, Heniford BT, Park A, Voeller G, Ramshaw BJ. Laparoscopic ventral hernia repair (LVHR) in morbidly obese patients. Hernia J Hernias Abdom Wall Surg. 2008;12(3):233–8.
21. Newcomb WL, Polhill JL, Chen AY, Kuwada TS, Gersin KS, Getz SB, et al. Staged hernia repair preceded by gastric bypass for the treatment of morbidly obese patients with complex ventral hernias. Hernia J Hernias Abdom Wall Surg. 2008;12(5):465–9.
22. Bonatti H, Hoeller E, Kirchmayr W, Muhlmann G, Zitt M, Aigner F, et al. Ventral hernia repair in bariatric surgery. Obes Surg. 2004;14(5):655–8.

23. Palanivelu C, Rangarajan M, Parthasarathi R, Madankumar MV, Senthilkumar K. Laparoscopic repair of suprapubic incisional hernias: suturing and intraperitoneal composite mesh onlay. A retrospective study. Hernia J Hernias Abdom Wall Surg. 2008;12(3):251–6.
24. Palanivelu C, Rangarajan M, Jategaonkar PA, Amar V, Gokul KS, Srikanth B. Laparoscopic repair of diastasis recti using the "Venetian blinds" technique of plication with prosthetic reinforcement: a retrospective study. Hernia J Hernias Abdom Wall Surg. 2009;13(3):287–92.
25. Geisler DJ, Reilly JC, Vaughan SG, Glennon EJ, Kondylis PD. Safety and outcome of use of nonabsorbable mesh for repair of fascial defects in the presence of open bowel. Dis Colon Rectum. 2003;46(8):1118–23.
26. Birolini C, Utiyama EM, Rodrigues AJ, Birolini D. Elective colonic operation and prosthetic repair of incisional hernia: does contamination contraindicate abdominal wall prosthesis use? J Am Coll Surg. 2000;191(4):366–72.
27. Simon E, Kelemen O, Knausz J, Bodnár S, Bátorfi J. Synchronically performed laparoscopic cholecystectomy and hernioplasty. Acta Chir Hung. 1999;38(2):205–7.
28. Stringer RA, Salameh JR. Mesh herniorrhaphy during elective colorectal surgery. Hernia J Hernias Abdom Wall Surg. 2005;9(1):26–8.
29. De Biasi A, Lumpkins K, Turner PL. Laparoscopic ventral hernia repair with acute perforated cholecystitis and no short- or long-term evidence of prosthesis infection. Am Surg. 2011;77(4):510–1.
30. Schuster R, Curet MJ, Alami RS, Morton JM, Wren SM, Safadi BY. Concurrent gastric bypass and repair of anterior abdominal wall hernias. Obes Surg. 2006;16(9):1205–8.
31. Chan DL, Talbot ML, Chen Z, Kwon SCM. Simultaneous ventral hernia repair in bariatric surgery. ANZ J Surg. 2014;84(7–8):581–3.
32. Raziel A, Sakran N, Szold A, Goitein D. Concomitant bariatric and ventral/incisional hernia surgery in morbidly obese patients. Surg Endosc. 2014;28(4):1209–12.

Gallstone Disease Before and After Bariatric Surgery

14

Saravana Kumar

14.1 Introduction

Prevalence of gall stones in the general population is 5–10 % and among them 30 % need surgery subsequently for symptomatic disease. Obese patients are at increased risk for biliary disease [1]. The prevalence of gallstones in the obese is 13.6–47.9 % [1, 2]. Ultrasonogram (USG) is the most sensitive investigation for diagnosis of GSD but its use in obese individuals is limited due to increased adipose tissue mass. In obese individuals USG may miss 8–12 % gall stones [2]. There is an increased incidence of gall stone disease after bariatric surgery associated with the rapid weight loss period [3].

14.2 Cholelithiasis in Obesity

Bile secretion results from the active transport of solutes into the canaliculus followed by passive flow of water. The major organic solutes are bilirubin, bile salts, phospholipids and cholesterol. Water constitutes approximately 85 % of the volume of bile.

Bilirubin is conjugated with glucuronic acid by glucuronyl transferase and is excreted actively into the adjacent canaliculus. Bile salts are steroid molecules synthesized by the hepatocyte. The primary bile salts, cholic and chenodeoxycholic acid, account for more than 80 % of those produced. They are then conjugated with either taurine or glycine, can undergo bacterial alteration in the intestine to form the secondary bile salts, deoxycholate and lithocholate. The purpose of bile salts is to

S. Kumar, MS, FMAS, DNB (Gen. Surgery)
Bariatric Division, Upper Gastrointestinal Surgery and Minimal Access Surgery Unit, GEM Hospital and Research Centre, Coimbatore, India
e-mail: drsakubariatric@gmail.com

P.R. Palanivelu et al. (eds.), *Bariatric Surgical Practice Guide*,
DOI 10.1007/978-981-10-2705-5_14

solubilize lipids and facilitate their absorption. Phospholipids and cholesterol are synthesized in liver. The normal volume of bile secreted daily by the liver is 750–1000 ml.

Cholesterol is highly non polar and insoluble in bile. Key to maintaining cholesterol in solution is the formation of micelles, a bile salt-phospholipid-cholesterol complex. Cholesterol solubility depends on the relative concentration of cholesterol, bile salts and phospholipids. When cholesterol saturation index (lithogenic index) is greater than 1.0, cholesterol is supersturated and crystallization occurs. Gall stones are common in obesity because of elevated biliary cholesterol secretion, incremented nucleation factors, and impaired gallbladder contractility [4] In obese patients, cholesterol secretion is greatly increased without any absolute reduction in bile salt or phospholipid secretion unlike non-obese individuals who have decreased bile salt and phospholipid secretion [4].

14.3 Cholelithiasis After Bariatric Surgery

Incidence of gall stones increases after bariatric surgery. Probable causes for increased incidence are rapid weight loss, increased bile cholesterol saturation, increased gallbladder secretion of mucin and reduced gallbladder motility due to injury of the vagal nerve [3, 4]. Patients are transiently at risk for gall stone formation during active weight reduction phase, usually during the first 6–12 months and the risk is very less after 2 years [3, 4]. Gustafsson et al. found that crystallization promoting compounds like mucin are of great importance in the development of cholesterol crystals and gallstones in obese subjects during weight reduction, probably because of defective gallbladder emptying [5].

Incidence differs among various types of bariatric surgeries. Incidence of gallstones is reported to be 26.5 % in gastric banding patients though only 6.8 % of patients become symptomatic postoperatively [6]. Asymptomatic gallstones ranged from 30 to 52.8 % after 6 to 12 months postoperatively whilst symptomatic gallstones occurred in 7–16 % of roux-en-Y gastric bypass (RYGB) patients [7–11]. Coupaye et al. found out that the incidence of cholelithiasis after sleeve gastrectomy (SG) and RYGB were similar (28 % Vs 34 %) with most cases occurring in first year and 12 % and 13 % of patient who underwent SG & RYGB, respectively, became symptomatic [12].

Coupaye et al. identified weight loss of >30 kg at 6 months as a risk factor for post-operative cholelithiasis [12]. Melmer et al. followed up 190 patients over 10 years after bariatric surgery and identified female sex and rapid weight loss as major risk factors for post-operative cholelithiasis [7]. Frequency was highest in the first 6 months but declined over time to <1 % per year after 3 years. An excess weight loss of >25 % within the first 3 months was the strongest predictor [8]. Similar results were shown by Li et al. who concluded that a weight loss of more than 25 % of original weight was the only factor that help selecting patients for post-operative USG surveillance and subsequent cholecystectomy once gallstones were identified [13].

14.4 Cholecystectomy in Obese Patients

Cholecystectomy in patients undergoing bariatric surgery is a controversial area with lots of ongoing debate. There is no uniform consensus among surgeons regarding the optimal management strategies. Traditionally cholecystectomy was indicated only in the presence of both gallstones and symptoms, but some surgeons have advocated cholecystectomy even in the absence of symptoms and sometimes even in the absence of gallstones [14].

Cholecystectomy in patients undergoing bariatric surgery is technically demanding due to suboptimal port placement and difficult body habitus [3]. It is also less popular with some surgeons due to increased operative time (adds ~18 min to laparoscopic roux-en-Y gastric bypass (LRYGB)), morbidity, prolonged hospitalization and surgeons concern of removing a normal organ if preoperative investigation shows no cholelithiasis [3, 4]. Serious complications can occur in 2–3 % of patients [3].

The various strategies for management include a prophylactic approach, an elective/selective approach and a conventional approach which is discussed below.

14.4.1 Prophylactic Approach

This approach refers to performing laparoscopic cholecystectomy in all patients at the time of initial surgery, regardless of the presence or absence of gallstones [3]. The rationale behind this approach is based on the increased incidence of gallstones after bariatric surgery compared to the normal population and the low sensitivity and specificity of USG in morbid obesity [14]. The main concern is that the diagnosis of microlithiasis is difficult and incidence might be higher than expected [4].

This is supported by the findings of Fobi et al. who found abnormal findings in gall bladder specimens including gall stones, cholesterolosis and cholecystitis in 75 % of surgical specimens despite negative pre-operative USG. He reported additional time of 15 min with no specific morbidity [2]. Similarly Nougou et al. found some pathology in almost 82 % of specimens with additional 19 min for lap cholecystectomy and no specific morbidity related to it [15]. Liem et al. found gallbladder pathology in 80 % specimens [16]. Guadalajara et al. found gallstones in 24 % of the specimens while pre-operative USG was positive for stones in only 16 % [17]. Obeid et al. did a study to assess the safety of laparoscopic adjustable gastric banding with concurrent cholecystectomy for symptomatic cholelithiasis and found that it is as safe as laparoscopic adjustable gastric banding (LAGB) alone [8].

14.4.2 Elective/Selective Approach

This approach involves performing simultaneous laparoscopic cholecystectomy only in patients with gallstones diagnosed pre/intra-operatively, even if asymptomatic [3, 14]. The rationale behind this is an assumed higher incidence of symptomatic disease as compared to patients without gallstones.

Hamad et al. performed simultaneous cholecystectomy in 16.9 % patients during RYGB and compared outcomes in those who did not have concomitant surgery. These had significantly longer operative time, longer hospital stay and higher major morbidity. There was however no specific morbidity directly related to cholecystectomy [18]. In the series of open gastric bypass of Caruana et al., cholecystectomy was performed after the diagnosis of gallstones by intraoperative palpation of the gallbladder with no significant increase in morbidity but with longer operative time [19]. Ahmed et al. in his series of 400 patients found significant increase in operative time of 29 min with no additional morbidity [20].

Villegas et al. performed simultaneous cholecystectomy on 14 % of patients after intraoperative diagnosis of gallstones or sludge with the aid of laparoscopic ultrasound and patients were adviced prophylactic ursodeoxycholic acid at discharge. On follow up there was a low incidence of symptomatic gallstones requiring cholecystectomy after LRYGB and they concluded that selective cholecystectomy with close patient follow-up is a rational approach [21]. Nagem et al. prospectively followed LRYGB patients and found that 28.9 % patients developed gallstones and 15.8 % patients developed symptoms (biliary pain, acute biliary pancreatitis) [4]. They concluded that it is reasonable to perform cholecystectomy during RYGB in the presence of cholelithiasis or if gallstones develop after the procedure. Thus this approach reduces the potential for future gallbladder-related morbidity and the need for further surgery. Hence this can be a preferred option for patients with simultaneous gallstone disease whether symptomatic or asymptomatic.

14.4.3 Conventional Approach

This involves expectant management with or without prophylactic administration of ursodeoxycholic acid (UDCA) until symptoms develop. Thus cholecystectomy is performed only when symptoms arise [3, 14]. The advantage of this approach is that the surgery is performed after a significant weight loss is achieved, i.e., on leaner and healthier patient which may be relatively simpler.

Swartz et al. found an incidence of subsequent cholecystectomy of 14.7 %, with a significant lower incidence for patients completing prophylactic ursodeoxycholic acid treatment [23]. Fuller and co-workers noted the need for subsequent cholecystectomy in patients completing prophylactic ursodeoxycholic acid treatment was only 7.69 % [22]. Similarly, Papasavas et al. in a restrospective study has shown that the need for a subsequent cholecystectomy in patients with gallstones present at the time of gastric bypass was 8.3 %, which is similar to the incidence observed for patients without gallstones (6.9 %).

Ellner et al. did not administer prophylactic ursodeoxycholic acid treatment and found an incidence of subsequent cholecystectomy of 9 % [23]. In the series by Bernabe et al., 9.84 % patients after RYGB without prophylactic UDCA required subsequent cholecystectomy and they concluded that natural history of patients with asymptomatic gallstones undergoing gastric bypass is very much like the natural history of asymptomatic gallstones in the general population [14]. This approach can be reserved for patients who develop symptomatic gallstone disease after bariatric surgery irrespective of whether they had it during the primary surgery.

14.5 UDCA After Bariatric Surgery

While reserving cholecystectomy for symptomatic disease is a safe approach, management of asymptomatic gallstones/gall stone prophylaxis is still not clear. The natural history of asymptomatic gallstones suggests that many affected individuals will remain asymptomatic [3].

Gallstones rapidly develop in first few months after surgery during the period of rapid weight loss. During this time cholesterol saturation of bile increases due to decreased output of bile acids, phospholipids and mobilization of cholesterol from adipose tissue. This led to the concept of using UDCA, which is a bile acid, during the first 6 months after bariatric surgery. This reduces stone formation by decreasing the supersaturation of bile with cholesterol (acts on cholesterol and mucin levels in bile), improving gallbladder emptying and reduces the incidence of gallstones from 32 to 2 % [4].

A RCT by Sugerman et al. showed that UDCA is significantly better than placebo in preventing gallstone formation. A daily dose of 600 mg was associated with the lowest rate of gallstone formation and the lowest incidence of adverse events. Also patients who developed gallstones showed a lower complication rate [24]. In a meta-analysis by Uy et al., five RCTs including 521 patients were assessed and it was found that 8.8 % of those taking UDCA developed gallstones compared to 27.7 % for placebo [25]. Hence it's a reasonable approach to prescribe patients with UDCA during the initial months of rapid weight loss in all patients with/without gallstones reserving cholecystecomy for patients with symptomatic disease.

14.6 Management of Choledocholithiasis After RYGB

After LRYGB, the new gastrointestinal configuration does not permit easy endoscopic access to the biliary system in standard fashion [26]. Management of choledocholithiasis is a challenge for both the surgeon and endoscopist. Management options include percutaneous transhepatic instrumentation of the common bile duct (CBD), percutaneous or laparoscopic assisted transgastric endoscopic retrograde changiopancreaticography (ERCP), transenteric ERCP using specialized endoscopes and laparoscopic or open CBD exploration/choledochoduodenostomy [26].

(A) **Laparoscopic Choledochoduodenostomy** – DuCoin et al. in their study, performed laparoscopic choledochodudenostomy in 11 patients and concluded that this is a viable option for management of choledocholithiasis after RYGB with less morbidity in experienced hands [27].

(B) **Laparoscopic assisted ERCP** – Schreiner et al. in their retrospective study compared balloon endoscopic assisted ERCP (BEA-ERCP) with laparoscopic assisted ERCP (LA-ERCP) and showed that LA-ERCP was superior in papilla identification, cannulation rate and therapeutic success (100% vs 59%) with no difference in hospital stay and complication rate. They also stated that if alimentary limb length is <150 cm patients can be offered BEA-ERCP first due to high success rate and if length is more than 150 cm, LA-ERCP can be the preferred approach because of the lack of need for a second procedure [28]. Lopes et al. in his study performed LA-ERCP in ten patients, and endoscopic access was obtained to the gastric remnant or biliopancreatic limb. Biliary cannulation was successfully achieved in nine patients, mean duration was 89 min, mean hospital stay was 2 days and concluded that LA-ERCP is a safe option [29].

(C) **Percutaneous transhepatic instrumentation of CBD:** Ahmed et al. described percutaneous transhepatic access to the CBD for management of choledocholithiasis where in percutaneous choledochoscopy was used for endoluminal visualization of CBD [26].

Recommendations

- Prophylactic cholecystectomy in patients undergoing bariatric surgery is not recommended, but may be considered in severe malabsorptive procedures like duodenal switch.
- Elective approach may be employed in patients undergoing RYGB/anastomotic techniques wherein altered anatomy may render management of subsequent choledocholithiasis difficult.
- Conventional approach of management may be employed in patients undergoing SG/other restrictive procedures. Such patients may be advised UDCA 600 mg for 6 months and should be followed up regularly during the period of active weight loss. Laparoscopic cholecystectomy should be offered if the patient develops symptomatic cholelithiasis.

References

1. Dittrick GW, Thompson JS, Campos D, Bremers D, Sudan D. Gallbladder pathology in morbid obesity. Obes Surg. 2005;15(2):238–42.
2. Fobi M, Lee H, Igwe D, Felahy B, James E, Stanczyk M, et al. Prophylactic cholecystectomy with gastric bypass operation: incidence of gallbladder disease. Obes Surg. 2002; 12(3):350–3.
3. Sioka E, Zacharoulis D, Zachari E, Papamargaritis D, Pinaka O, Katsogridaki G, et al. Complicated gallstones after laparoscopic sleeve gastrectomy. J Obes. 2014;2014:468203.
4. Nagem RG, Lázaro-da-Silva A, de Oliveira RM, Morato VG. Gallstone-related complications after Roux-en-Y gastric bypass: a prospective study. Hepatobiliary Pancreat Dis Int. 2012;11(6):630–5.
5. Gustafsson U, Benthin L, Granström L, Groen AK, Sahlin S, Einarsson C. Changes in gallbladder bile composition and crystal detection time in morbidly obese subjects after bariatric surgery. Hepatology. 2005;41(6):1322–8.

6. Kiewiet RM, Durian MF, van Leersum M, Hesp FLEM, van Vliet ACM. Gallstone formation after weight loss following gastric banding in morbidly obese Dutch patients. Obes Surg. 2006;16(5):592–6.
7. Melmer A, Sturm W, Kuhnert B, Engl-Prosch J, Ress C, Tschoner A, et al. Incidence of gallstone formation and cholecystectomy 10 years after bariatric surgery. Obes Surg. 2015;25(7):1171–6.
8. Obeid NR, Kurian MS, Ren-Fielding CJ, Fielding GA, Schwack BF. Safety of laparoscopic adjustable gastric banding with concurrent cholecystectomy for symptomatic cholelithiasis. Surg Endosc. 2015;29(5):1192–7.
9. Tsirline VB, Keilani ZM, El Djouzi S, Phillips RC, Kuwada TS, Gersin K, et al. How frequently and when do patients undergo cholecystectomy after bariatric surgery? Surg Obes Relat Dis Off J Am Soc Bariatr Surg. 2014;10(2):313–21.
10. Stokes CS, Gluud LL, Casper M, Lammert F. Ursodeoxycholic acid and diets higher in fat prevent gallbladder stones during weight loss: a meta-analysis of randomized controlled trials. Clin Gastroenterol Hepatol Off Clin Pract J Am Gastroenterol Assoc. 2014;12(7):1090–100. e2; quiz e61.
11. Moon RC, Teixeira AF, DuCoin C, Varnadore S, Jawad MA. Comparison of cholecystectomy cases after Roux-en-Y gastric bypass, sleeve gastrectomy, and gastric banding. Surg Obes Relat Dis Off J Am Soc Bariatr Surg. 2014;10(1):64–8.
12. Coupaye M, Castel B, Sami O, Tuyeras G, Msika S, Ledoux S. Comparison of the incidence of cholelithiasis after sleeve gastrectomy and Roux-en-Y gastric bypass in obese patients: a prospective study. Surg Obes Relat Dis Off J Am Soc Bariatr Surg. 2015;11(4):779–84.
13. Li VKM, Pulido N, Fajnwaks P, Szomstein S, Rosenthal R, Martinez-Duartez P. Predictors of gallstone formation after bariatric surgery: a multivariate analysis of risk factors comparing gastric bypass, gastric banding, and sleeve gastrectomy. Surg Endosc. 2009;23(7):1640–4.
14. Quesada BM, Kohan G, Roff HE, Canullán CM, Porras LTC. Management of gallstones and gallbladder disease in patients undergoing gastric bypass. World J Gastroenterol. 2010;16(17):2075–9.
15. Nougou A, Suter M. Almost routine prophylactic cholecystectomy during laparoscopic gastric bypass is safe. Obes Surg. 2008;18(5):535–9.
16. Liem RK, Niloff PH. Prophylactic cholecystectomy with open gastric bypass operation. Obes Surg. 2004;14(6):763–5.
17. Guadalajara H, Sanz Baro R, Pascual I, Blesa I, Rotundo GS, López JMG, et al. Is prophylactic cholecystectomy useful in obese patients undergoing gastric bypass? Obes Surg. 2006; 16(7):883–5.
18. Hamad GG, Ikramuddin S, Gourash WF, Schauer PR. Elective cholecystectomy during laparoscopic Roux-en-Y gastric bypass: is it worth the wait? Obes Surg. 2003;13(1):76–81.
19. Caruana JA, McCabe MN, Smith AD, Camara DS, Mercer MA, Gillespie JA. Incidence of symptomatic gallstones after gastric bypass: is prophylactic treatment really necessary? Surg Obes Relat Dis Off J Am Soc Bariatr Surg. 2005;1(6):564–7; discussion 567–8.
20. Ahmed AR, O'Malley W, Johnson J, Boss T. Cholecystectomy during laparoscopic gastric bypass has no effect on duration of hospital stay. Obes Surg. 2007;17(8):1075–9.
21. Villegas L, Schneider B, Provost D, Chang C, Scott D, Sims T, et al. Is routine cholecystectomy required during laparoscopic gastric bypass? Obes Surg. 2004;14(2):206–11.
22. Fuller W, Rasmussen JJ, Ghosh J, Ali MR. Is routine cholecystectomy indicated for asymptomatic cholelithiasis in patients undergoing gastric bypass? Obes Surg. 2007;17(6):747–51.
23. Ellner SJ, Myers TT, Piorkowski JR, Mavanur AA, Barba CA. Routine cholecystectomy is not mandatory during morbid obesity surgery. Surg Obes Relat Dis Off J Am Soc Bariatr Surg. 2007;3(4):456–60.
24. Sugerman HJ, Brewer WH, Shiffman ML, Brolin RE, Fobi MA, Linner JH, et al. A multicenter, placebo-controlled, randomized, double-blind, prospective trial of prophylactic ursodiol for the prevention of gallstone formation following gastric-bypass-induced rapid weight loss. Am J Surg. 1995;169(1):91–6; discussion 96–7.

25. Uy MC, Talingdan-Te MC, Espinosa WZ, Daez MLO, Ong JP. Ursodeoxycholic acid in the prevention of gallstone formation after bariatric surgery: a meta-analysis. Obes Surg. 2008;18(12):1532–8.
26. Ahmed AR, Husain S, Saad N, Patel NC, Waldman DL, O'Malley W. Accessing the common bile duct after Roux-en-Y gastric bypass. Surg Obes Relat Dis Off J Am Soc Bariatr Surg. 2007;3(6):640–3.
27. DuCoin C, Moon RC, Teixeira AF, Jawad MA. Laparoscopic choledochoduodenostomy as an alternate treatment for common bile duct stones after Roux-en-Y gastric bypass. Surg Obes Relat Dis Off J Am Soc Bariatr Surg. 2014;10(4):647–52.
28. Schreiner MA, Chang L, Gluck M, Irani S, Gan SI, Brandabur JJ, et al. Laparoscopy-assisted versus balloon enteroscopy-assisted ERCP in bariatric post-Roux-en-Y gastric bypass patients. Gastrointest Endosc. 2012;75(4):748–56.
29. Lopes TL, Clements RH, Wilcox CM. Laparoscopy-assisted ERCP: experience of a high-volume bariatric surgery center (with video). Gastrointest Endosc. 2009;70(6):1254–9.

Polycystic Ovarian Syndrome, Pregnancy and Bariatric Surgery

15

Praveen Raj Palanivelu

15.1 Introduction

Polycystic ovarian syndrome (PCOS) is a common endocrine disorder with a prevalence of about 6–10% in women of reproductive age [1]. Since PCOS is commonly associated with obesity, this chapter aims to understand the role of bariatric surgery in patients with PCOS and also the precautions that needs to be taken in patients with subsequent pregnancy after bariatric surgery.

15.2 Definition of PCOS

According to the American Society for Reproductive Medicine Criteria, presence of any two of the following refers to PCOS and not just visualization of polycysts on imaging [2].

1. oligomenorrhea and/or anovulation
2. clinical and/or biochemical signs of hyperandrogenism
3. polycystic ovaries in imaging

The currently accepted definition of a polycystic ovary is the presence of ≥12 follicles in each ovary, measuring 2–9 mm in diameter and/or increased ovarian volume (>10 mL) [2]. It is also important that the other etiologies (congenital adrenal hyperplasia, androgen-secreting tumors, or Cushing syndrome), potentially resulting in a hyper-androgenic state are excluded [2].

P.R. Palanivelu, MS, DNB, DNB (SGE), FALS, FMAS
Bariatric Division, Upper Gastrointestinal Surgery and Minimal Access Surgery Unit, GEM Hospital and Research Centre, Coimbatore, India
e-mail: drraj@geminstitute.in

P.R. Palanivelu et al. (eds.), *Bariatric Surgical Practice Guide*,
DOI 10.1007/978-981-10-2705-5_15

15.3 Pathophysiology

The pathophysiology is complex, multifactorial and incompletely understood. Chronic elevated levels of luteinizing hormone (LH) and insulin resistance are the hallmarks of PCOS [3, 4]. Insulin resistance with type 2 diabetes mellitus (T2DM) and compensatory hyperinsulinemia have been consistently documented in obese women with PCOS [5]. Insulin resistance is related to the chronic visceral fat inflammation seen in patients with metabolic syndrome [6, 7]. Insulin resistance leads to increased production of insulin levels, hence the hyperinsulinemia [8]. It is also interesting to note that the severity of insulin resistance correlates with the severity of the clinical and metabolic phenotype of PCOS [9].

The reason behind elevated levels of LH is not clear. This could probably be the result of relatively high and unchanging concentrations of estrogens that might alter the control of this hormone by the hypothalamic- pituitary axis [10]. This high LH levels along with hyperinsulinemia work synergistically causing ovarian growth, androgen production and cysts formation in the ovaries. High insulin levels also cause decrease of sex hormone binding globulin (SHBG). SHBG binds to sex steroids, especially androgens which then contribute to hyperandrogenism which further inhibits normal follicular maturation. Also, only 50–65 % of PCOS patients are obese. The non-obese groups of patients with PCOS also have been shown to have insulin resistance but the levels of insulin have been lower compared to their obese counterparts. Still they will have evidence of hyperandrogenism and oligo-ovulation/anovulation similar to their obese counterparts [3]. Only a few patients classically present with the triad of hyperandrogenism, insulin resistance and acanthosis nigiricans [11].

15.4 Evaluation

The evaluation in obese patients with PCOS referred for bariatric consultation should include an endocrinologist evaluation to rule out pituitary or thyroid disease as the cause of anovulation and premature ovarian failure which is characterized by high FSH levels.

As mentioned previously the other causes of hyperandrogenic state like androgen producing neoplasms, congenital adrenal hyperplasia (high 17-OH progesterone) and Cushings syndrome should be excluded by appropriate evaluation [2].

Diabetic evaluation is important as it is noted that 35–45 % of patients with PCOS will have impaired glucose tolerance and 7–10 % will actually be diabetic. Hence a complete T2DM profile has to be done which includes GTT, HbA1C and HOMA-IR [12, 13]. It is also noted that patients with PCOS have higher chances of developing cardiovascular events. Hence a cardiac evaluation is also important [14].

Endometrial aspiration can be considered in patients above 35 years to rule out endometrial carcinoma. Imaging in the form of ultrasonogram needs to be done to assess the ovaries for polycysts. But it needs to be understood that many PCOS patients may not have cysts and cysts may also be seen in 25 % of healthy women [15].

15.5 Bariatric Surgery and PCOS

Sustained weight loss is the only currently available definitive intervention expected to have a lifelong effect on reducing the long-term complications of PCOS. Eventually, any intervention directed at reducing obesity will not only improve the quality of life, but also correct the hyperinsulinism and improve fertility and the lipid and androgen profiles [16]. It has been shown that a modest 5–10 % weight loss can lead to the resumption of ovulation within weeks and improving many features of PCOS [17].

Bariatric surgery is the most effective approach for sustained weight loss in the morbidly obese with effectiveness confirmed in large prospective trials with substantial weight loss and improvements in metabolic effects [18, 19]. Bariatric surgery resulted in improved fertility especially in patients with PCOS where biochemical studies showed normalization of hormones after surgery [20]. In the study by Jaamal M et al., it was shown that weight loss after roux-en-Y bypass (RYGB) had a dramatic effect on several manifestations of PCOS, with a 100 % successful conception rate, even without hormonal therapy. Regulation of the menstrual cycle and remission of T2DM occurred immediately, and improvement in hirsutism occurred relatively slowly. In fact >40 % improvement in the menstrual cycle and T2DM was noted within the first month with an approximate 25 % excess weight loss [10].

15.6 Bariatric Surgery and Artificial Reproductive Techniques (ART)

It is quite clear that weight loss by both non-surgical means and bariatric surgery has shown better outcomes for successful artificial reproduction technique in obese patients. This has been by improved pregnancy rates and live birth. It has also been shown that following bariatric surgery there is better regularization of menstrual pattern, a decrease in cancellation rates, increase in the number of embryos available for transfer, reduced numbers of ART cycles and decreased miscarriage rates. There was an increased number of natural conceptions noted [21]. Following RYGB, significant improvements were seen in testosterone, fasting glucose, insulin, cholesterol, and triglyceride at 12 months. The improvements in biomarkers, menstrual cycles and hirsutism did not correlate with degree of weight change [22].

15.7 Timing of Pregnancy After Bariatric Surgery

No guidelines or consensus exist with the exact timing of pregnancy after a bariatric procedure. Most surgeons generally prefer a minimum of 12 months before pregnancy, as rapid weight loss (relative starvation phase) may be unhealthy for the mother and a baby [23]. Hence it is advisable to delay pregnancy for 12–18 months following the bariatric procedure to avoid nutritional deficiencies [24].

15.8 Obesity and Pregnancy

Obesity increases the risk of both maternal and infant morbidity. Obese women who become pregnant face higher risk of developing gestational diabetes (GDM), pregnancy-induced hypertension, and pre-eclampsia [30]. In obese women complicated by GDM, the pregnancy outcome is definitely compromised regardless of the severity of obesity or the treatment modality [25]. They also have a greater incidence of having preterm labor, higher rates of cesarean sections and perioperative morbidity. Infants born to obese women are also expected to have increased rates of macrosomia and congenital anomalies, as well as life-long complications of obesity associated co-morbidities like T2DM, hypertension etc. [26].

15.9 Bariatric Surgery and Pregnancy

Bariatric surgery reduces the above mentioned risks both to the mother and the infant [26–30, 32–34]. In fact the rates of caesarean section were lower after bariatric surgery [28, 29]. The same was stressed by Willis K et al., who emphasized that pregnancy after bariatric surgery appears to be safe and is effective in reducing complications such as GDM, gestational hypertensive disorders and fetal macrosomia, but with the possibility of having neonates born small-for-gestational-age [30].

A recent review of literature by Kajer et al. on pregnancy after bariatric surgery and its associated risks and benefits, has suggested that there is a possible risk of lower birth weight, although the data has been conflicting [31].

15.10 Nutrition in Post Bariatric Patients with Pregnancy

Although pregnancy after bariatric surgery appears to be safe, health care providers should take extra care to properly monitor their post-operative pregnant patients for appropriate weight gain and nourishment [32]. Women with pregnancy after bariatric surgery were diagnosed with micronutrient deficiencies more frequently than those with pregnancy before surgery. Hence increased testing may help identify nutrient deficiencies and prevent consequences for maternal and child health [33, 34]. Deficiencies in iron, vitamin A, vitamin B12, vitamin K, folate and calcium can result in both maternal complications, such as severe anaemia, and fetal complications, such as congenital abnormalities, IUGR and failure to thrive [35].

Hence postoperative nutrient supplementation and close supervision before, during, and after pregnancy adjusted as per individual requirements of a woman will help preventing nutrition-related complications such as deficiencies in iron, vitamin A, vitamin B12, vitamin K, folate and calcium, and improving maternal and fetal health [23].

Recommendations

- Weight loss is the key to improvement of PCOS.
- In those with PCOS and infertility artificial reproductive techniques have been more successful after weight loss.
- Bariatric surgery significantly improves all features of PCOS.
- Pregnancy has to be delayed at least from 12 to 18 months after the bariatric surgery
- All the health consequences associated with obesity in pregnancy is diminishes after bariatric surgery however the chance of IUGR has been higher in pregnancies after bariatric surgery necessitating close supervision.
- Regular followup and adequate nutrient supplementation before, during and after pregnancy is important to prevent nutrition related complications

References

1. Hart R, Hickey M, Franks S. Definitions, prevalence and symptoms of polycystic ovaries and polycystic ovary syndrome. Best Pract Res Clin Obstet Gynaecol. 2004;18(5):671–83.
2. Stankiewicz M, Norman R. Diagnosis and management of polycystic ovary syndrome: a practical guide. Drugs. 2006;66(7):903–12.
3. Poretsky L, Piper B. Insulin resistance, hypersecretion of LH, and a dual-defect hypothesis for the pathogenesis of polycystic ovary syndrome. Obstet Gynecol. 1994;84(4):613–21.
4. Barbieri RL. Induction of ovulation in infertile women with hyperandrogenism and insulin resistance. Am J Obstet Gynecol. 2000;183(6):1412–8.
5. Dunaif A. Insulin resistance and the polycystic ovary syndrome: mechanism and implications for pathogenesis. Endocr Rev. 1997;18(6):774–800.
6. Hotamisligil GS. Inflammation and metabolic disorders. Nature. 2006;444(7121):860–7.
7. Kahn SE, Hull RL, Utzschneider KM. Mechanisms linking obesity to insulin resistance and type 2 diabetes. Nature. 2006;444(7121):840–6.
8. Shanik MH, Xu Y, Skrha J, Dankner R, Zick Y, Roth J. Insulin resistance and hyperinsulinemia: is hyperinsulinemia the cart or the horse? Diabetes Care. 2008;31 Suppl 2:S262–8.
9. Robinson S, Kiddy D, Gelding SV, Willis D, Niththyananthan R, Bush A, et al. The relationship of insulin insensitivity to menstrual pattern in women with hyperandrogenism and polycystic ovaries. Clin Endocrinol (Oxf). 1993;39(3):351–5.
10. Jamal M, Gunay Y, Capper A, Eid A, Heitshusen D, Samuel I. Roux-en-Y gastric bypass ameliorates polycystic ovary syndrome and dramatically improves conception rates: a 9-year analysis. Surg Obes Relat Dis Off J Am Soc Bariatr Surg. 2012;8(4):440–4.
11. Barbieri RL, Ryan KJ. Hyperandrogenism, insulin resistance, and acanthosis nigricans syndrome: a common endocrinopathy with distinct pathophysiologic features. Am J Obstet Gynecol. 1983;147(1):90–101.
12. Dahlgren E, Janson PO, Johansson S, Lapidus L, Odén A. Polycystic ovary syndrome and risk for myocardial infarction. Evaluated from a risk factor model based on a prospective population study of women. Acta Obstet Gynecol Scand. 1992;71(8):599–604.
13. Ehrmann DA, Barnes RB, Rosenfield RL, Cavaghan MK, Imperial J. Prevalence of impaired glucose tolerance and diabetes in women with polycystic ovary syndrome. Diabetes Care. 1999;22(1):141–6.
14. Okoroh EM, Boulet SL, George MG, Craig Hooper W. Assessing the intersection of cardiovascular disease, venous thromboembolism, and polycystic ovary syndrome. Thromb Res. 2015;136(6):1165–8.

15. Lobo RA, Carmina E. The importance of diagnosing the polycystic ovary syndrome. Ann Intern Med. 2000;132(12):989–93.
16. Trent M, Austin SB, Rich M, Gordon CM. Overweight status of adolescent girls with polycystic ovary syndrome: body mass index as mediator of quality of life. Ambul Pediatr Off J Ambul Pediatr Assoc. 2005;5(2):107–11.
17. Teede H, Deeks A, Moran L. Polycystic ovary syndrome: a complex condition with psychological, reproductive and metabolic manifestations that impacts on health across the lifespan. BMC Med. 2010;8:41.
18. Buchwald H, Avidor Y, Braunwald E, Jensen MD, Pories W, Fahrbach K, et al. Bariatric surgery: a systematic review and meta-analysis. JAMA. 2004;292(14):1724–37.
19. Eid GM, Cottam DR, Velcu LM, Mattar SG, Korytkowski MT, Gosman G, et al. Effective treatment of polycystic ovarian syndrome with Roux-en-Y gastric bypass. Surg Obes Relat Dis Off J Am Soc Bariatr Surg. 2005;1(2):77–80.
20. Maggard M, Li Z, Yermilov I, Maglione M, Suttorp M, Carter J, et al. Bariatric surgery in women of reproductive age. Rockville: Agency for Healthcare Research and Quality; 2008.
21. Sim KA, Partridge SR, Sainsbury A. Does weight loss in overweight or obese women improve fertility treatment outcomes? A systematic review. Obes Rev Off J Int Assoc Study Obes. 2014;15(10):839–50.
22. Eid GM, McCloskey C, Titchner R, Korytkowski M, Gross D, Grabowski C, et al. Changes in hormones and biomarkers in polycystic ovarian syndrome treated with gastric bypass. Surg Obes Relat Dis Off J Am Soc Bariatr Surg. 2014;10(5):787–91.
23. Kanadys WM, Leszczyńska-Gorzelak B, Oleszczuk J. Obesity among women. Pregnancy after bariatric surgery: a qualitative review. Ginekol Pol. 2010;81(3):215–23.
24. Tan O, Carr BR. The impact of bariatric surgery on obesity-related infertility and in vitro fertilization outcomes. Semin Reprod Med. 2012;30(6):517–28.
25. Yogev Y, Langer O. Pregnancy outcome in obese and morbidly obese gestational diabetic women. Eur J Obstet Gynecol Reprod Biol. 2008;137(1):21–6.
26. Abodeely A, Roye GD, Harrington DT, Cioffi WG. Pregnancy outcomes after bariatric surgery: maternal, fetal, and infant implications. Surg Obes Relat Dis Off J Am Soc Bariatr Surg. 2008;4(3):464–71.
27. Weintraub AY, Levy A, Levi I, Mazor M, Wiznitzer A, Sheiner E. Effect of bariatric surgery on pregnancy outcome. Int J Gynaecol Obstet Off Organ Int Fed Gynaecol Obstet. 2008;103(3):246–51.
28. Aricha-Tamir B, Weintraub AY, Levi I, Sheiner E. Downsizing pregnancy complications: a study of paired pregnancy outcomes before and after bariatric surgery. Surg Obes Relat Dis Off J Am Soc Bariatr Surg. 2012;8(4):434–9.
29. Burke AE, Bennett WL, Jamshidi RM, Gilson MM, Clark JM, Segal JB, et al. Reduced incidence of gestational diabetes with bariatric surgery. J Am Coll Surg. 2010;211(2):169–75.
30. Willis K, Sheiner E. Bariatric surgery and pregnancy: the magical solution? J Perinat Med. 2013;41(2):133–40.
31. Kjaer MM, Nilas L. Pregnancy after bariatric surgery – a review of benefits and risks. Acta Obstet Gynecol Scand. 2013;92(3):264–71.
32. Karmon A, Sheiner E. Pregnancy after bariatric surgery: a comprehensive review. Arch Gynecol Obstet. 2008;277(5):381–8.
33. Devlieger R, Guelinckx I, Jans G, Voets W, Vanholsbeke C, Vansant G. Micronutrient levels and supplement intake in pregnancy after bariatric surgery: a prospective cohort study. PLoS One. 2014;9(12):e114192.
34. Gadgil MD, Chang H-Y, Richards TM, Gudzune KA, Huizinga MM, Clark JM, et al. Laboratory testing for and diagnosis of nutritional deficiencies in pregnancy before and after bariatric surgery. J Womens Health. 2014;23(2):129–37.
35. Guelinckx I, Devlieger R, Vansant G. Reproductive outcome after bariatric surgery: a critical review. Hum Reprod Update. 2009;15(2):189–201.

Non-alcoholic Fatty Liver Disease and the Effects of Bariatric Surgery

16

Rachel Maria Gomes and Praveen Raj Palanivelu

16.1 Introduction

Non-alcoholic fatty liver disease (NAFLD) is one of the most common causes of chronic liver disease in India and worldwide and is strongly linked to obesity and the metabolic syndrome. NAFLD is now recognized as the most common cause of cryptogenic cirrhosis [1]. The reported prevalence of NAFLD and Non-alcoholic steatohepatitis (NASH) is 10–30 % and 3–5 % respectively [2–6]. However in morbidly obese patients from bariatric surgery series the incidence of NAFLD is as high as 65–95 % and that of NASH is around 30–40 % [7–12].

NAFLD can be classified as primary NAFLD and secondary NAFLD. If it occurs in the absence of secondary causes it is called primary NAFLD. Classically primary NAFLD is associated with one or more features of metabolic syndrome which includes obesity, diabetes mellitus, raised TGs and low HDL. The clinical course of most patients with NAFLD is benign but patients who develop fibrosis have a high incidence of progression to cirrhosis.

Nonalcoholic fatty liver disease (NAFLD) is a pathologically defined entity comprising of a spectrum of lesions ranging from simple steatosis to steatohepatitis to fibrosis and cirrhosis. The key histological features in the diagnosis of NAFLD are steatosis, ballooning, lobular inflammation and peri-sinusoidal fibrosis with zone 3 predominance. Patients with NAFLD are largely asymptomatic and liver enzymes are normal in 80 % of patients with NAFLD at any given time [13]. Steatosis can be

R.M Gomes, MS, FMAS (✉) • P.R. Palanivelu, MS, DNB, DNB (SGE), FALS, FMAS
Bariatric Division, Upper Gastrointestinal Surgery and Minimal Access Surgery Unit, GEM Hospital and Research Centre, Coimbatore, India
e-mail: dr.gomes@rediffmail.com; drraj@geminstitute.in

P.R. Palanivelu et al. (eds.), *Bariatric Surgical Practice Guide*,
DOI 10.1007/978-981-10-2705-5_16

detected in the liver by radiological methods, only when more than one-third of the liver is involved. Hence there is a poor correlation between NAFLD and clinical, biochemical and radiological findings. Even if detected, staging is not reliably possible. Liver biopsy is thus the gold standard for diagnosing and staging NAFLD which is most commonly procured by an imaging guided percutaneous method in the general population [14]. However the cost and possible risks of an imaging guided percutaneous liver biopsy makes this impractical for use [14]. But unlike people from the general population, the liver can be visualized in patients undergoing bariatric surgery and can be easily subjected to a laparoscopic guided percutaneous biopsy under vision with confirmation of hemostasis without any additional cost [11].

16.2 Pathogenesis

The increased adipose tissue associated with obesity has been recognized to secrete numerous substances that induce insulin resistance. Distribution of adipose tissue is more important than total adipose mass. Many investigators have suggested that visceral adipose tissue is a major contributor to insulin resistance [15, 16]. It is now realized that NAFLD is a consequence of insulin resistance [17]. The exact pathogenesis of NAFLD is not fully understood, however it is hypothesized that the starting point is hepatic steatosis and further progression occurs by the multiple hit hypothesis. Different pathogenic factors lead firstly to hepatic steatosis, "the first hit" and secondly to hepatic damage, "the second hit" [18] (Fig. 16.1).

Insulin resistance increases lipolysis of peripheral adipose tissue. Insulin resistance also leads to increased fatty acid influx, de novo triglyceride synthesis and decreased fatty acid oxidation within the liver thereby promoting triglyceride accumulation in the hepatocytes. It is unknown what "second hit" leads to the development of liver damage and fibrogenesis, although several factors have been implicated including oxidative stress, mitochondrial abnormalities, tumour necrosis factor and hormones leptin and adiponectin [17].

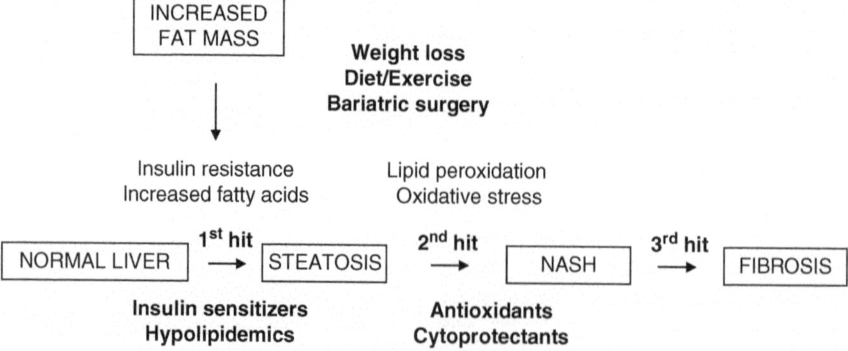

Fig. 16.1 Pathogenesis of NAFLD and possible treatment strategies directed at the different steps of pathogenesis

Simple steatosis is comparatively benign with a 0–4 % risk of developing cirrhosis over a one to two decade period. In contrast, 5–8 % of patients with NASH may develop cirrhosis over approximately 5 years. Assessment of fibrosis stage is also valuable in prognosticating risk of developing liver related morbidity, with patients with advanced fibrosis (bridging fibrosis and cirrhosis) at most risk [19].

16.3 Treatment of NAFLD

Several strategies directed at the different steps of pathogenesis can be used for the treatment of NAFLD. Key drugs used are insulin sensitizers, hypolipidemics, antioxidants and cytoprotectants. Weight loss is the only measure that acts at the source of the pathogenesis and can offer complete cure versus drugs. This can be achieved by diet, exercise and bariatric surgery. NAFLD per se is not an indication for bariatric surgery. Bariatric surgery is the best alternative option for weight reduction if diet/exercise fails [20].

16.4 Effects of Bariatric Surgery on NAFLD

Numerous studies have reported significant histological improvement after roux-en Y gastric bypass (RYGB) [21–33]. Few studies have reported improvement after vertical banded gastroplasty (VBG) and adjustable gastric banding (AGB) [34–40]. Keshshian et al. and Kral et al. reported improvement after duodenal switch (DS) and bilio-pancreatic diversion (BPD) respectively [41, 42]. The authors have reported improvement after sleeve gastrectomy (SG) [12]. Though majority of studies report a consistent beneficial effect on liver histology, some studies have reported a few cases of worsening or new onset steatosis, inflammation or fibrosis. Silverman et al., Mattar et al., Mottin et al., Csendes et al. and Furuya et al. reported a few cases of worsening or new fibrosis after RYGB [21, 23, 25, 28, 29]. Luyckx et al. found significant regression of hepatic steatosis but an increase in the incidence of hepatocellular inflammation after gastroplasty [38]. Stratopoulos et al. found significant improvement in steatosis and steatohepatitis with an overall decrease in fibrosis but 11.7 % had increased fibrosis after gastroplasty [34]. AGB was one of three interventions used by Mathurin et al., the other two being RYGB and biliointestinal bypass [36]. Percentage of steatosis fell but inflammation remained unchanged and a significant increase in fibrosis was seen in 20 % of patients. Kral et al. after biliopancreatic diversion showed decreased steatosis but postoperative increase in fibrosis in 40 % [42]. Some showed decreasing mild inflammation, whereas some developed new onset mild inflammation. Keshishian et al. after duodenal switch (DS) operation showed improved steatosis and inflammation but liver function tests/inflammation had slightly worsened by the 6-month period, but then normalized by 12 months [41]. Fibrosis was not examined in this study. Most data on effects of bariatric surgery on NAFLD is from western literature. Two histological studies from Asia exist. In 2008 Huang et al. in 21 RYGB patients and in 2015

Praveenraj et al. in 20 SG and 10 RYGB patients demonstrated dramatic histological improvement in steatosis, steatohepatitis and fibrosis.

Histologic studies comparing the effects of the various bariatric interventions are lacking in literature. Caiazzo et al. recently reported superior NAFLD improvement after RYGB versus AGB. This favorable liver outcome occurred earlier and was more profound after RYGB which was suggested to be related to better weight loss outcomes after RYGB. Other potential influencing factors suggested were greater improvement in insulin sensitivity and other hormonal changes as AGB is an exclusively restrictive operation [43]. The authors reported better NAFLD improvement after sleeve gastrectomy versus a RYGB though comparison did not reveal statistically significant difference [11]. Further studies are needed to confirm superiority of the various bariatric procedures. While most studies demonstrated improvement by repeating liver biopsy at 1–2 years after surgery we demonstrated improvement as early as 6 months after surgery [11].

16.5 Mechanism of Bariatric Surgery Causing Improvement or Worsening

The mechanism of how bariatric surgery plays a role as potential treatment of NAFLD is complex and not fully understood. Bariatric surgery is associated with sustained and significant weight loss. It leads to improvement of insulin sensitivity. It leads to improvement/resolution of hyperglycemia, dyslipidemia and hypertension. It reduces obesity-related low-grade chronic inflammation resulting from excess production tumor necrosis factor-α, interleukin-1, interleukin-8, interleukin-18, monocyte chemoattractant protein-1, C-reactive protein etc. Last, it acts by producing complex hormonal changes in ghrelin, glucagon-likepeptide-1, peptide YY, oxyntomodulin, adiponectin, etc. [44].

Though a majority of studies report a consistently beneficial effect on liver histologic examination, the exact mechanism of worsening reported in some series is unclear. This could probably be related to the rapid weight loss resulting in increased free fatty acid levels derived from extensive fat mobilization causing liver injury. Exposure to toxins from bacterial overgrowth from intestinal diversion, nutritional deficiencies, and protein malnutrition from malabsorption probably could act as a "second hit". Another possibility that has been suggested is a 'misdiagnosis' of worsening in many reported cases that may occur as steatosis is a prominent feature in specimens obtained before weight loss and careful assessment and reporting of necro-inflammatory and portal tract changes may often not be done by the pathologist if the latter is minimal [35]. A dramatic reduction in steatosis post-surgery may enhance or unmask the view of these inflammatory cells which would then be reported [35].

16.6 Bariatric Surgery in Established Cirrhosis

There is exists few series in literature that suggests that bariatric surgery can be performed safely in selected patients with Childs A cirrhosis. They can be safely subjected to a sleeve gastrectomy or a RYGB. These patients may have a greater incidence of transient renal dysfunction (acute tubular necrosis) and an increased potential for blood loss. Patients achieved excellent weight loss and improvement in obesity-related co-morbidities [45–47]. Several issues however need to be taken into consideration in day to day practice. RYGB is the most widely accepted bariatric procedure with good effect on metabolic syndrome and minimal degree of malabsorption. Although we have ourselves reported that it can be safely done even in cirrhotics, one of the main concerns of its use in patients with cirrhosis is that the bypassed stomach will be inaccessible should variceal bleeding develop [12]. Biliopancreatic diversion/duodenal switch (BPD/DS) is a less commonly used bariatric procedure which has a high risk of complications by induced malabsorption and there are a few reports about hepatic dysfunction. Restrictive operations – LAGB and SG are quick procedures and less invasive than a RYGB or BPD/DS which makes these more practical options.

There may be two scenarios in which such a choice needs to be made –unexpected cirrhosis at bariatric surgery and patients with known cirrhosis and medically complicated obesity. The intraoperative decision making for unexpected cirrhosis (found in 1–2 % cases) may involve changing the planned procedure to a different one e.g. a RYGB or BPD/DS to a SG if cirrhosis was suspected preoperatively and this was discussed with the patient. If extent of cirrhosis or portal hypertension is not known or if the patient had not consented to have an alternative procedure, it would be right to perform only a liver biopsy and defer the operation until full workup.

In referred patients with known cirrhosis and medically complicated obesity the cause of cirrhosis should be elucidated (i.e. NASH, hepatitis, alpha 1-antitrypsin deficiency). Childs A cirrhosis with normal synthetic function can be safely subjected to a sleeve gastrectomy or a RYGB. The recommendation would be preferably a restrictive procedure, such as SG. However if liver disease is secondary to steatohepatitis, and there is no portal hypertension, a RYGB should be considered because of the added benefits to the metabolic syndrome. Patients who have decompensated liver function or severe portal HT should be managed in partnership with the liver transplant service. In severe portal hypertension. with an otherwise preserved liver function, some consideration can be given to placement of transjugular intrahepatic posrtosystemic shunts (TIPSS) to decrease the portal pressure and then proceed to a safer, technically possible surgical procedure possibly as a bridge to liver transplantation. Most surgeons would not consider a RYGB in these circumstances because of the possibility of variceal bleeding.

Recommendations

- Surgically induced weight loss improves nonalcoholic fatty liver disease (NAFLD) in morbidly obese patients
- Restrictive procedures and lesser malabsorptive procedures like roux en Y bypass are safe procedures with excellent outcomes in all stages of NAFLD
- Malabsorptive procedures can likely precipitate liver failure.
- Bariatric surgery can be safely performed even in patients with Child A cirrhosis without portal hypertension.

References

1. Maheshwari A, Thuluvath PJ. Cryptogenic cirrhosis and NAFLD: are they related? Am J Gastroenterol. 2006;101(3):664–8.
2. Siraj P, Kohli N, Srivastava VK, Singh SK, Natu SM, Mehrotra R. Relationship of nonalcoholic fatty liver disease with anthropometric measurement among patients attending a tertiary care hospital of Northern India. Indian J Community Health. 2013;25(3):208–12.
3. Singh SP, Nayak S, Swain M, Rout N, Mallik RN, Agrawal O, et al. Prevalence of nonalcoholic fatty liver disease in coastal eastern India: a preliminary ultrasonographic survey. Trop Gastroenterol Off J Dig Dis Found. 2004;25(2):76–9.
4. Singh SP, Kar SK, Panigrahi MK, Misra B, Pattnaik K, Bhuyan P, et al. Profile of patients with incidentally detected nonalcoholic fatty liver disease (IDNAFLD) in coastal eastern India. Trop Gastroenterol Off J Dig Dis Found. 2013;34(3):144–52.
5. Mohan V, Farooq S, Deepa M, Ravikumar R, Pitchumoni CS. Prevalence of non-alcoholic fatty liver disease in urban south Indians in relation to different grades of glucose intolerance and metabolic syndrome. Diabetes Res Clin Pract. 2009;84(1):84–91.
6. Amarapurkar D, Kamani P, Patel N, Gupte P, Kumar P, Agal S, et al. Prevalence of non-alcoholic fatty liver disease: population based study. Ann Hepatol. 2007;6(3):161–3.
7. Dixon JB, Bhathal PS, O'Brien PE. Nonalcoholic fatty liver disease: predictors of nonalcoholic steatohepatitis and liver fibrosis in the severely obese. Gastroenterology. 2001;121(1):91–100.
8. Beymer C, Kowdley KV, Larson A, Edmonson P, Dellinger EP, Flum DR. Prevalence and predictors of asymptomatic liver disease in patients undergoing gastric bypass surgery. Arch Surg. 2003;138(11):1240–4.
9. Gholam PM, Kotler DP, Flancbaum LJ. Liver pathology in morbidly obese patients undergoing Roux-en-Y gastric bypass surgery. Obes Surg. 2002;12(1):49–51.
10. Ong JP, Elariny H, Collantes R, Younoszai A, Chandhoke V, Reines HD, et al. Predictors of nonalcoholic steatohepatitis and advanced fibrosis in morbidly obese patients. Obes Surg. 2005;15(3):310–5.
11. Praveenraj P, Gomes RM, Kumar S, Karthikeyan P, Shankar A, Parthasarathi R, et al. Prevalence and predictors of non-alcoholic fatty liver disease in morbidly obese south Indian patients undergoing bariatric surgery. Obes Surg. 2015;25(11):2078–87.
12. Praveen Raj P, Gomes RM, Kumar S, Senthilnathan P, Karthikeyan P, Shankar A, et al. The effect of surgically induced weight loss on nonalcoholic fatty liver disease in morbidly obese Indians: "NASHOST" prospective observational trial. Surg Obes Relat Dis Off J Am Soc Bariatr Surg. 2015;11(6):1315–22.
13. Chang Y, Ryu S, Sung E, Jang Y. Higher concentrations of alanine aminotransferase within the reference interval predict nonalcoholic fatty liver disease. Clin Chem. 2007;53(4):686–92.

14. Sumida Y, Nakajima A, Itoh Y. Limitations of liver biopsy and non-invasive diagnostic tests for the diagnosis of nonalcoholic fatty liver disease/nonalcoholic steatohepatitis. World J Gastroenterol. 2014;20(2):475–85.
15. Matsuzawa Y, Shimomura I, Nakamura T, Keno Y, Kotani K, Tokunaga K. Pathophysiology and pathogenesis of visceral fat obesity. Obes Res. 1995;3 Suppl 2:187S–94.
16. Yamashita S, Nakamura T, Shimomura I, Nishida M, Yoshida S, Kotani K, et al. Insulin resistance and body fat distribution. Diabetes Care. 1996;19(3):287–91.
17. Polyzos SA, Kountouras J, Zavos C. Nonalcoholic fatty liver disease: the pathogenetic roles of insulin resistance and adipocytokines. Curr Mol Med. 2009;9(3):299–314.
18. Day CP, James OF. Steatohepatitis: a tale of two "hits"? Gastroenterology. 1998;114(4):842–5.
19. Teli MR, James OF, Burt AD, Bennett MK, Day CP. The natural history of nonalcoholic fatty liver: a follow-up study. Hepatology. 1995;22(6):1714–9.
20. Sjöström L, Lindroos A-K, Peltonen M, Torgerson J, Bouchard C, Carlsson B, et al. Lifestyle, diabetes, and cardiovascular risk factors 10 years after bariatric surgery. N Engl J Med. 2004;351(26):2683–93.
21. Mottin CC, Moretto M, Padoin AV, Kupski C, Swarowsky AM, Glock L, et al. Histological behavior of hepatic steatosis in morbidly obese patients after weight loss induced by bariatric surgery. Obes Surg. 2005;15(6):788–93.
22. Clark JM, Alkhuraishi ARA, Solga SF, Alli P, Diehl AM, Magnuson TH. Roux-en-Y gastric bypass improves liver histology in patients with non-alcoholic fatty liver disease. Obes Res. 2005;13(7):1180–6.
23. Mattar SG, Velcu LM, Rabinovitz M, Demetris AJ, Krasinskas AM, Barinas-Mitchell E, et al. Surgically-induced weight loss significantly improves nonalcoholic fatty liver disease and the metabolic syndrome. Ann Surg. 2005;242(4):610–7; discussion 618–20.
24. De Almeida SR, Rocha PRS, Sanches MD, Leite VHR, da Silva RAP, Diniz MTC, et al. Roux-en-Y gastric bypass improves the nonalcoholic steatohepatitis (NASH) of morbid obesity. Obes Surg. 2006;16(3):270–8.
25. Furuya CK, de Oliveira CPMS, de Mello ES, Faintuch J, Raskovski A, Matsuda M, et al. Effects of bariatric surgery on nonalcoholic fatty liver disease: preliminary findings after 2 years. J Gastroenterol Hepatol. 2007;22(4):510–4.
26. Weiner RA. Surgical treatment of non-alcoholic steatohepatitis and non-alcoholic fatty liver disease. Dig Dis Basel Switz. 2010;28(1):274–9.
27. Barker KB, Palekar NA, Bowers SP, Goldberg JE, Pulcini JP, Harrison SA. Non-alcoholic steatohepatitis: effect of Roux-en-Y gastric bypass surgery. Am J Gastroenterol. 2006;101(2):368–73.
28. Silverman EM, Sapala JA, Appelman HD. Regression of hepatic steatosis in morbidly obese persons after gastric bypass. Am J Clin Pathol. 1995;104(1):23–31.
29. Csendes A, Smok G, Burgos AM. Histological findings in the liver before and after gastric bypass. Obes Surg. 2006;16(5):607–11.
30. Liu X, Lazenby AJ, Clements RH, Jhala N, Abrams GA. Resolution of nonalcoholic steatohepatits after gastric bypass surgery. Obes Surg. 2007;17(4):486–92.
31. Moretto M, Kupski C, da Silva VD, Padoin AV, Mottin CC. Effect of bariatric surgery on liver fibrosis. Obes Surg. 2012;22(7):1044–9.
32. Klein S, Mittendorfer B, Eagon JC, Patterson B, Grant L, Feirt N, et al. Gastric bypass surgery improves metabolic and hepatic abnormalities associated with nonalcoholic fatty liver disease. Gastroenterology. 2006;130(6):1564–72.
33. Tai C-M, Huang C-K, Hwang J-C, Chiang H, Chang C-Y, Lee C-T, et al. Improvement of nonalcoholic fatty liver disease after bariatric surgery in morbidly obese Chinese patients. Obes Surg. 2012;22(7):1016–21.
34. Stratopoulos C, Papakonstantinou A, Terzis I, Spiliadi C, Dimitriades G, Komesidou V, et al. Changes in liver histology accompanying massive weight loss after gastroplasty for morbid obesity. Obes Surg. 2005;15(8):1154–60.

35. Dixon JB, Bhathal PS, Hughes NR, O'Brien PE. Nonalcoholic fatty liver disease: improvement in liver histological analysis with weight loss. Hepatology. 2004;39(6):1647–54.
36. Mathurin P, Hollebecque A, Arnalsteen L, Buob D, Leteurtre E, Caiazzo R, et al. Prospective study of the long-term effects of bariatric surgery on liver injury in patients without advanced disease. Gastroenterology. 2009;137(2):532–40.
37. Ranløv I, Hardt F. Regression of liver steatosis following gastroplasty or gastric bypass for morbid obesity. Digestion. 1990;47(4):208–14.
38. Luyckx FH, Desaive C, Thiry A, Dewé W, Scheen AJ, Gielen JE, et al. Liver abnormalities in severely obese subjects: effect of drastic weight loss after gastroplasty. Int J Obes Relat Metab Disord J Int Assoc Study Obes. 1998;22(3):222–6.
39. Dixon JB, Bhathal PS, O'Brien PE. Weight loss and non-alcoholic fatty liver disease: falls in gamma-glutamyl transferase concentrations are associated with histologic improvement. Obes Surg. 2006;16(10):1278–86.
40. Jaskiewicz K, Raczynska S, Rzepko R, Sledziński Z. Nonalcoholic fatty liver disease treated by gastroplasty. Dig Dis Sci. 2006;51(1):21–6.
41. Keshishian A, Zahriya K, Willes EB. Duodenal switch has no detrimental effects on hepatic function and improves hepatic steatohepatitis after 6 months. Obes Surg. 2005;15(10):1418–23.
42. Kral JG, Thung SN, Biron S, Hould F-S, Lebel S, Marceau S, et al. Effects of surgical treatment of the metabolic syndrome on liver fibrosis and cirrhosis. Surgery. 2004;135(1):48–58.
43. Caiazzo R, Lassailly G, Leteurtre E, Baud G, Verkindt H, Raverdy V, et al. Roux-en-Y gastric bypass versus adjustable gastric banding to reduce nonalcoholic fatty liver disease: a 5-year controlled longitudinal study. Ann Surg. 2014;260(5):893–8; discussion 898–9.
44. Hafeez S, Ahmed MH. Bariatric surgery as potential treatment for nonalcoholic fatty liver disease: a future treatment by choice or by chance? J Obes. 2013;2013:839275.
45. Takata MC, Campos GM, Ciovica R, Rabl C, Rogers SJ, Cello JP, et al. Laparoscopic bariatric surgery improves candidacy in morbidly obese patients awaiting transplantation. Surg Obes Relat Dis Off J Am Soc Bariatr Surg. 2008;4(2):159–64; discussion 164–5.
46. Shimizu H, Phuong V, Maia M, Kroh M, Chand B, Schauer PR, et al. Bariatric surgery in patients with liver cirrhosis. Surg Obes Relat Dis Off J Am Soc Bariatr Surg. 2013;9(1):1–6.
47. Dallal RM, Mattar SG, Lord JL, Watson AR, Cottam DR, Eid GM, et al. Results of laparoscopic gastric bypass in patients with cirrhosis. Obes Surg. 2004;14(1):47–53.

Outcomes of Diabetic Microvascular Complications After Bariatric Surgery

17

Helen M. Heneghan and Carel W. le Roux

17.1 Introduction

The recent obesity pandemic has been paralleled by an equally dramatic rise in the prevalence of type 2 diabetes mellitus (T2DM), which is of major concern to healthcare providers globally. The metabolic dysregulation characteristic of T2DM gives rise to a host of macrovascular and microvascular complications, specifically cardiovascular, cerebrovascular and peripheral vascular diseases, as well as retinopathy, nephropathy and neuropathy. The mechanisms underlying development of these complications are multifactorial, and incompletely understood. In addition to the direct injurious effect of hyperglycemia, other purported factors include hypertension, the endocrine activity of adipose tissue, the pro-inflammatory state induced by obesity, and the increased intra-abdominal pressure imposed by central adiposity.

The cost of treating these complications, to patients and society, is exorbitant. The American Diabetes Association's most recent estimate of the annual economic cost of diabetes was $245 billion (2012 data), a 41 % increase from their previous estimate of $174 billion in 2007 [1]. Much of this (72 %) is accounted for by healthcare costs, the remainder by loss of productivity. With regard to healthcare costs, almost half of this is spent treating microvascular disease complications, particularly diabetic kidney disease(DKD) which accounts for 44 % of cases of renal failure in the US and is the leading indication for renal replacement therapy at present.

H.M. Heneghan, MD, PhD, FRCSI
C.W. le Roux, MBChB, MSc, FRCP, FRCPath, PhD (✉)
Diabetes Complications Research Centre, Conway Institute,
University College Dublin, Belfield, Ireland
e-mail: helenheneghan@hotmail.com; carel.leroux@ucd.ie

P.R. Palanivelu et al. (eds.), *Bariatric Surgical Practice Guide*,
DOI 10.1007/978-981-10-2705-5_17

Furthermore, data from the Third National Health and Nutrition Examination Survey (NHANES III) in the US highlights the mortality risk associated with diabetic kidney disease (DKD) by demonstrating that there is a 400 % increase in 10-year all-cause mortality for patients with DKD relative to the non-diabetic populations, largely attributable to death from associated cardiovascular disease [2].

Hitherto, clinicians have focused on attaining tight glycemic control through pharmacological interventions to prevent and/or arrest the macrovascular and microvascular complications of T2DM. While this is certainly effective, as evidenced by the intensive treatment arms of the first United Kingdom prospective diabetes study (UKPDS) glycemic control study, the Action in Diabetes and Vascular Disease Preterax and Diamicron Modified Release Controlled Evaluation (ADVANCE) randomized controlled trial and the Action to Control Cardiovascular Risk in Diabetes (ACCORD) trial, the benefits are marginal [3–5]. At most, a 33 % reduction in the progression of diabetic retinopathy was observed in the ACCORD trial, and although minor reductions in the incidence and progression of albuminuria were noted in this study, they were counter-intuitively coincident with a higher rate of doubling of serum creatinine in the intensified treatment group. The ADVANCE study reported a 10 % decrease in a composite end-point of macrovascular and microvascular disease that was not significant after adjusting for a 21 % decrease in new or worsening nephropathy, and no significant difference in retinopathy was observed following treatment intensification. Synthesis of data from these and similar studies indicates that a multimodal approach targeting both blood pressure and glycemic control is optimal in relation to providing for an effective reduction in microvascular complications in combination with reductions in all-cause mortality and cardiovascular events, neither of which are well met by individual treatment intensification strategies.

Metabolic (bariatric) surgery has revolutionized the management of severe obesity and obesity-related comorbidities in recent years. In addition to substantial weight loss, it leads to dramatic improvements in glycemic control, insulin sensitivity, and cardiovascular disease risk. To date, 11 randomized controlled trials have directly compared medical versus surgical treatment for T2DM [6]. The first of these, by Dixon et al. compared the two year outcomes of conventional medical treatment with gastric banding for the management of T2DM, in 60 obese patients [7]. More recently, Schauer et al. and Mingrone et al. evaluated the 12, 24 and 36 month effects of bariatric surgery (gastric bypass, sleeve gastrectomy, or biliopancreatic diversion) compared to intensive medical therapy on diabetes management [8–10]. All 3 groups demonstrated that weight loss surgery was far more effective than medical therapy at inducing remission or improvement of diabetes. Meta-analysis of the data from the 11 RCTs comparing multimodal medical therapy with bariatric surgery for management of T2DM indicates that weight loss was significantly greater in the surgical groups and bariatric surgery patients had a higher remission rate of T2DM (relative risk 22.1 (3.2–154.3)) and metabolic syndrome (relative risk 2.4 (1.6–3.6)), greater improvements in quality of life and reductions in medicine use. Other notable benefits in the surgical arms of these trials included significant decrease in plasma triglyceride concentrations, and increase in high density lipoprotein cholesterol concentrations [6]. Although not included in this meta-analysis because it was not a randomized trial, the noteworthy Swedish Obese Subjects (SOS) case-control study demonstrated a hazard ratio of 0.17 for diabetes incidence following assorted bariatric surgical interventions illustrating how effectively bariatric surgery reduces progression from the pre-diabetic state [11]. The SOS studies have also shown that bariatric surgery is associated with a decreased incidence of diabetic microvascular complications (HR 0.44; 95 % CI, 0.34–0.56; $p<0.001$) and macrovascular complications (HR 0.68; 95 % CI, 0.54–0.85; $p<.001$) [12]. These benefits are obviously not without risk. Whilst there were no deaths reported after bariatric surgery in any of the RCTs included in this meta-analysis, common adverse events after bariatric surgery were iron deficiency anemia (15 % of individuals undergoing malabsorptive bariatric surgery) and reoperations (8 %).

17.1.1 Improvement in Diabetic Kidney Disease (DKD) After Bariatric Surgery

The pathophysiology of diabetic and obesity-related kidney disease, although complex and multifactorial, is important to understand in order to elucidate how surgically-induced weight loss and glycaemic changes affect nephropathy. Hyperglycemia initiates a cascade of events which are injurious to the kidney, including the production of vasodilatory prostaglandins, inflammatory cytokines, advanced glycosylation products and reactive oxygen species. In obesity-related kidney disease, the increase in intra-abdominal pressure causes an increase in renal venous pressure, systemic blood pressure, and vascular resistance, all of which impairs renal perfusion, activates the juxtaglomerular apparatus (JGA) and the renin-angiotensin-aldosterone system (RAAS), causing increased release of renin, angiotensin and aldosterone. This in turn causes hypertension, glomerulopathy and proteinuria [13, 14]. Whilst surgically-induced weight loss correlates well with a decrease in intra-abdominal pressure, improved glycemic control and the improved metabolic milieu after bariatric surgical procedures is believed in part to be a consequence of weight-independent optimization of insulin secretion and hepatic insulin sensitivity [15, 16].

To date, 3 prospective studies and 7 retrospective studies have evaluated the effects of bariatric surgery on diabetic kidney disease. The most compelling evidence regarding the effect of bariatric surgery versus conventional medical therapy on microvascular outcomes is an unblinded, case-controlled prospective study by Iaconelli et al. examining the effects of biliopancreatic diversion (BPD) on urinary albumin excretion and glomerular filtration rate (GFR) in 50 patients with obesity and newly diagnosed T2DM. BPD patients were followed for 10 years, and compared to a 'control' group who received conventional medical treatment for T2DM and obesity [17]. The 10-year prevalence of hypercreatininemia was 39.3 % in conventionally managed subjects versus 9 % in BPD subjects and the 10-year variation in GFR was −45.7 ± 18.8 % in the conventionally managed group versus +13.6 ± 24.5 %, reflecting preservation of GFR in the surgical group. While 14.3 % of the control patients versus 31.8 % of the BPD patients had microalbuminuria at baseline, at 2-year follow-up, the situation was reversed with the control group percentage increased to 28.6 % and the BPD group percentage decreased to 9.1 %. After 10-years, all subjects in the BPD group recovered from microalbuminuria, whereas in the control group, albuminuria was uniformly worsened.

Several retrospective studies also support these findings; the largest by Johnson et al. who conducted a population-based survey of patients with obesity and T2DM, between 1996 and 2009, and compared microvascular outcomes in 2,580 patients who underwent bariatric surgery with 13,371 non-operated obese diabetic controls meeting the same inclusion criteria [18]. Microvascular outcomes were a composite measure of nephropathy, retinopathy, neuropathy and peripheral vascular disease (defined as a new diagnosis of blindness in at least one eye, laser eye or retinal surgery, non-traumatic amputation or creation of permanent arteriovenous access for dialysis). Bariatric surgery was associated with a significant reduction in microvascular events (adjusted HR of 0.22, 95 % CI 0.09–0.49). Navaneethan et al. have shown that urinary albumin excretion decreases in obese diabetics after roux-en-Y gastric bypass (RYGB) [19]. This reduction in albuminuria correlated with an improvement in insulin sensitivity and was related to a significant improvement in the anti-inflammatory adipokine, adiponectin. Interestingly, these effects were independent of the degree of weight loss. A retrospective review conducted by Brethauer et al. detailing results of a 5-year follow-up in a series of patients with T2DM undergoing bariatric surgery (RYGB n = 162, LAGB n = 32 and VSG n = 23) between 2004 and 2007, showed that diabetic kidney disease regressed in 53 % of patients and stabilized in the remaining 47 % [20]. Miras et al. compared 70 patients after RYGB with best medical care received by another 25 patients in a case-control study and showed that urinary albumin-creatinine ratio (ACR) decreased significantly in the surgical group but increased in the medical group [21].

Thus bariatric surgery consistently helps improve early changes of diabetic kidney disease and also helps in preventing further progression. The role of bariatric surgery now becomes even more important with these changes setting in.

17.1.2 Improvement in Diabetic Retinopathy After Bariatric Surgery

Retinopathy occurs in almost 35 % of patients with T2DM and its development correlates with the duration of diabetes, HbA1C level and blood pressure control [22]. Concerns have previously been raised that very rapid tightening of blood glucose control, achieved with medications, could paradoxically cause an acute deterioration in diabetic retinopathy [23]. However, available data suggests that bariatric surgery is safe in this regard for the majority of T2DM patients. Miras et al. demonstrated that mean retinal grading scores of 67 patients with T2DM were stable 12 months after surgery, but improved significantly in the sub-group of patients with pre-operative retinopathy [24]. Similar results were obtained by Varadhan et al. in a smaller retrospective study evaluating the effects of bariatric surgery on diabetic retinopathy [25]. Of 23 patients who had undergone RYGB or laparoscopic sleeve gastrectomy (LSG) and were followed for 3-years postoperatively, retinopathy regressed in two patients (9 %), developed in two patients (9 %), while a further two patients (9 %) had progression of pre-existing retinopathy. Thirteen patients (59 %) did not have retinopathy before or after surgery, and in three patients (14 %), retinopathy remained stable. In the aforementioned retrospective population-based study by Johnson et al. which reported on macrovascular and microvascular outcomes in 2,580 obese diabetic patients who underwent bariatric surgery (compared to a large number of non-operated obese diabetic controls) the proportion of patients who developed a new diagnosis of blindness, or needed laser-eye or retinal surgery, was lower after bariatric surgery than in the control group [18]. Lammert et al. also investigated the effect of bariatric surgery on endothelial dysfunction in retinal vessels as a marker of metabolic and cardiovascular risk in severely obese patients [26]. They found that the retinal arteriole-to-venule ratio, a surrogate marker of retinal inflammation and endothelial dysfunction, significantly improved 9 months after bariatric surgery. Schauer et al. randomized controlled STAMPEDE (Surgical Treatment and Medications Potentially Eradicate Diabetes Efficiently) trial included ophthalmic outcomes as one of its secondary endpoints. At 24 months, despite the dramatic improvements in glycemic control in the surgical arms of this trial, bariatric surgery did not appear to accelerate or improve retinopathy outcomes when compared to intensive medical treatment [27].

Thus, although bariatric surgery has shown to have good outcomes on the changes of retinopathy, due to the variability in findings cannot be considered as a treatment modality for this complication.

17.1.3 Improvement in Diabetic Peripheral Neuropathy After Bariatric Surgery

There is currently a paucity of data with regard to the effect of bariatric surgery on peripheral neuropathy in patients with T2DM. Most studies have focused on reporting the development of new symptoms or signs of peripheral neuropathy as a result of micronutrient deficiencies consequent to malabsorptive procedures, rather than that due to pre-existing peripheral neuropathy or progression of microvascular disease. The most common forms are sensory neuropathies, mononeuropathies, and radiculopathies that develop because of deficiencies in vitamin B1, B6, B12, E, or copper [28]. However, these complications are largely preventable or treatable when diagnosed. In terms of diabetes-related peripheral neuropathy, Miras et al. reported in their prospective case–control study of 70 obese diabetic surgical patients and 25 carefully matched medical patients, on peripheral neuropathy outcomes along with other microvascular complications of T2DM 12 months after intervention [21]. Peripheral nerve conduction studies were utilized to assess for the presence and severity of neuropathy. There were no clinically significant changes in any of the nerve conduction variables at 1-year, which is reassuring considering the progressive nature of this microvascular complication. Schauer et al. also reported that most patients noticed a subjective improvement or stability of their neuropathy symptoms after RYGB surgery, although this was per a self-reported questionnaire completed by patients themselves [29].

Conclusion

Bariatric surgery appears to be able to address microvascular complications of diabetes. Diabetic kidney disease is the most sensitive of these complications and shows improvements in urinary albumin creatinine ratios early, while changes in retinopathy and neuropathy do not appear to worsen, but equally do not improve as quickly as diabetic kidney disease. Bariatric surgery can thus be considered for the treatment of the diabetic kidney complications of diabetes, but more work is needed to determine which patients may benefit most.

Recommendations

- Bariatric surgery shows improvements in microalbuminuria and creatinine and can thus be considered for the treatment of the early diabetic kidney disease
- Bariatric surgery shows variable outcomes in diabetic retinopathy and neuropathy and cannot be recommended as a treatment modality.

References

1. American Diabetes Association. Economic costs of diabetes in the U.S. in 2012. Diabetes Care. 2013;36(4):1033–46.
2. Afkarian M, Sachs MC, Kestenbaum B, Hirsch IB, Tuttle KR, Himmelfarb J, et al. Kidney disease and increased mortality risk in type 2 diabetes. J Am Soc Nephrol. 2013;24(2): 302–8.
3. Intensive blood-glucose control with sulphonylureas or insulin compared with conventional treatment and risk of complications in patients with type 2 diabetes (UKPDS 33). UK Prospective Diabetes Study (UKPDS) Group. Lancet. 1998;352(9131):837–53.
4. ADVANCE Collaborative Group; Patel A, MacMahon S, Chalmers J, Neal B, Billot L, et al. Intensive blood glucose control and vascular outcomes in patients with type 2 diabetes. N Engl J Med. 2008;358(24):2560–72.
5. Action to Control Cardiovascular Risk in Diabetes Study Group, Gerstein HC, Miller ME, Byington RP, Goff DC, Bigger JT, et al. Effects of intensive glucose lowering in type 2 diabetes. N Engl J Med. 2008;358(24):2545–59.
6. Gloy VL, Briel M, Bhatt DL, Kashyap SR, Schauer PR, Mingrone G, et al. Bariatric surgery versus non-surgical treatment for obesity: a systematic review and meta-analysis of randomised controlled trials. BMJ. 2013;347:f5934.
7. Dixon JB, O'Brien PE, Playfair J, Chapman L, Schachter LM, Skinner S, et al. Adjustable gastric banding and conventional therapy for type 2 diabetes: a randomized controlled trial. JAMA. 2008;299(3):316–23.

8. Schauer PR, Kashyap SR, Wolski K, Brethauer SA, Kirwan JP, Pothier CE, et al. Bariatric surgery versus intensive medical therapy in obese patients with diabetes. N Engl J Med. 2012;366(17):1567–76.
9. Schauer PR, Bhatt DL, Kirwan JP, Wolski K, Brethauer SA, Navaneethan SD, et al. Bariatric surgery versus intensive medical therapy for diabetes – 3-year outcomes. N Engl J Med. 2014;370(21):2002–13.
10. Mingrone G, Panunzi S, De Gaetano A, Guidone C, Iaconelli A, Leccesi L, et al. Bariatric surgery versus conventional medical therapy for type 2 diabetes. N Engl J Med. 2012;366(17):1577–85.
11. Carlsson LMS, Peltonen M, Ahlin S, Anveden Å, Bouchard C, Carlsson B, et al. Bariatric surgery and prevention of type 2 diabetes in Swedish obese subjects. N Engl J Med. 2012;367(8):695–704.
12. Sjöström L, Peltonen M, Jacobson P, Ahlin S, Andersson-Assarsson J, Anveden Å, et al. Association of bariatric surgery with long-term remission of type 2 diabetes and with microvascular and macrovascular complications. JAMA. 2014;311(22):2297–304.
13. Sugerman HJ. Increased intra-abdominal pressure in obesity. Int J Obes Relat Metab Disord J Int Assoc Study Obes. 1998;22(11):1138.
14. Bloomfield GL, Blocher CR, Fakhry IF, Sica DA, Sugerman HJ. Elevated intra-abdominal pressure increases plasma renin activity and aldosterone levels. J Trauma. 1997;42(6):997–1004; discussion 1004–5.
15. Sugerman H, Windsor A, Bessos M, Kellum J, Reines H, DeMaria E. Effects of surgically induced weight loss on urinary bladder pressure, sagittal abdominal diameter and obesity comorbidity. Int J Obes Relat Metab Disord J Int Assoc Study Obes. 1998;22(3):230–5.
16. Laferrère B. Diabetes remission after bariatric surgery: is it just the incretins? Int J Obes (Lond). 2011;35 Suppl 3:S22–5.
17. Iaconelli A, Panunzi S, De Gaetano A, Manco M, Guidone C, Leccesi L, et al. Effects of biliopancreatic diversion on diabetic complications: a 10-year follow-up. Diabetes Care. 2011;34(3):561–7.
18. Johnson BL, Blackhurst DW, Latham BB, Cull DL, Bour ES, Oliver TL, et al. Bariatric surgery is associated with a reduction in major macrovascular and microvascular complications in moderately to severely obese patients with type 2 diabetes mellitus. J Am Coll Surg. 2013;216(4):545–56; discussion 556–8.
19. Navaneethan SD, Kelly KR, Sabbagh F, Schauer PR, Kirwan JP, Kashyap SR. Urinary albumin excretion, HMW adiponectin, and insulin sensitivity in type 2 diabetic patients undergoing bariatric surgery. Obes Surg. 2010;20(3):308–15.
20. Brethauer SA, Harris JL, Kroh M, Schauer PR. Laparoscopic gastric plication for treatment of severe obesity. Surg Obes Relat Dis Off J Am Soc Bariatr Surg. 2011;7(1):15–22.
21. Miras AD, Chuah LL, Khalil N, Nicotra A, Vusirikala A, Baqai N, et al. Type 2 diabetes mellitus and microvascular complications 1 year after Roux-en-Y gastric bypass: a case-control study. Diabetologia. 2015;58(7):1443–7.
22. Yau JWY, Rogers SL, Kawasaki R, Lamoureux EL, Kowalski JW, Bek T, et al. Global prevalence and major risk factors of diabetic retinopathy. Diabetes Care. 2012;35(3):556–64.
23. Dahl-Jørgensen K, Brinchmann-Hansen O, Hanssen KF, Sandvik L, Aagenaes O. Rapid tightening of blood glucose control leads to transient deterioration of retinopathy in insulin dependent diabetes mellitus: the Oslo study. Br Med J (Clin Res Ed). 1985;290(6471):811–5.
24. Miras AD, Chuah LL, Lascaratos G, Faruq S, Mohite AA, Shah PR, et al. Bariatric surgery does not exacerbate and may be beneficial for the microvascular complications of type 2 diabetes. Diabetes Care. 2012;35(12):e81.
25. Varadhan L, Humphreys T, Walker AB, Cheruvu CVN, Varughese GI. Bariatric surgery and diabetic retinopathy: a pilot analysis. Obes Surg. 2012;22(3):515–6.
26. Lammert A, Hasenberg T, Kräupner C, Schnülle P, Hammes H-P. Improved arteriole-to-venule ratio of retinal vessels resulting from bariatric surgery. Obesity (Silver Spring). 2012;20(11):2262–7.

27. Singh RP, Gans R, Kashyap SR, Bedi R, Wolski K, Brethauer SA, et al. Effect of bariatric surgery versus intensive medical management on diabetic ophthalmic outcomes. Diabetes Care. 2015;38(3):e32–3.
28. Becker DA, Balcer LJ, Galetta SL. The neurological complications of nutritional deficiency following bariatric surgery. J Obes. 2012;2012:608534.
29. Schauer PR, Burguera B, Ikramuddin S, Cottam D, Gourash W, Hamad G, et al. Effect of laparoscopic Roux-en Y gastric bypass on type 2 diabetes mellitus. Ann Surg. 2003;238(4):467–84; discussion 84–5.

Role of Bariatric Surgery in End-Stage Organ Failure

18

Rachel Maria Gomes

18.1 Introduction

As the prevalence of obesity is increasing with time, the presentation of morbid obesity with end-stage organ dysfunction is also increasing. Obesity related co-morbidities of hypertension and diabetes are inter-linked to chronic renal disease and cardiovascular disease, and the obesity related co-morbidity of non-alcoholic steatoheaptitis (NASH) is interlinked to cirrhosis. Morbid obesity presents a high risk to transplantation, as these patients have been found to have increased risk of complications and allograft loss [1–5]. In addition morbid obesity increases the technical complexity of surgery. Weight loss is necessary to improve outcomes, help improve or resolve obesity-related comorbidities and make patients become eligible for transplantation based on strict body mass index (BMI) criteria existent in many centers [1–5]. Management of morbid obesity is important even in the post-transplant setting. However reduction of weight when contemplated in these high risk patients before transplantation is limited by time with lifestyle measures and increased risk of morbidity/mortality related to bariatric surgery. The aim of this chapter is to review the current literature on the role of surgically induced weight loss in patients with end stage organ dysfunction in a peri-transplant setting.

R.M. Gomes, MS, FMAS
Bariatric Division, Upper Gastrointestinal Surgery and Minimal Access Surgery Unit, GEM Hospital and Research Centre, Coimbatore, India
e-mail: dr.gomes@rediffmail.com

P.R. Palanivelu et al. (eds.), *Bariatric Surgical Practice Guide*,
DOI 10.1007/978-981-10-2705-5_18

18.2 Bariatric Surgery for Morbid Obesity in End-Stage Renal Disease

The effective and long-term sustained outcomes of bariatric surgery in the general population have led many to consider bariatric surgery in morbidly obese patients with chronic kidney disease (CKD). As most transplant centers have strict criteria for listing patients based on BMI, patients with BMI>35 become ineligible for transplant. Hence, most series on CKD includes these patients who were subjected to bariatric surgery. Bariatric surgery with its effect on weight reduction and reduction of comorbidities could help these patients become eligible and also improve associated comorbidities. In a small series by Koshy et al. three patients with end-stage renal disease (ESRD) underwent adjustable gastric banding (AGB) to qualify for renal transplantation. All underwent uncomplicated kidney transplantations. There was no change in post-operative renal function. All 3 had an excess weight loss ranging from 35 to 41 %, at 12 and 15 months with resolution of co-morbidities later meeting the BMI criterion for transplantation allowing for renal transplantation. Long –term success was however not assessed [6]. In another series by Newcomb et al. three patients with end stage renal disease (ESRD) underwent AGB to qualify for renal transplantation. All underwent uncomplicated kidney transplantations. All lost weight at follow-up, meeting the BMI criterion for transplantation allowing for renal transplantation to proceed and in addition had resolution/improvement of obesity related co-morbidities with stable renal function. Again this series did not report long –term success [7]. In a series by Alexander et al. 30 morbidly obese patients with chronic renal failure/post-transplantation underwent gastric bypass. 19 patients had CRF at the time of Roux en Y gastric bypass (RYGB), eight had transplantation followed by RYGB, and three had RYGB and then transplantation. The reduction in excess BMI and resolution of co-morbid conditions was similar to patients without transplantation or chronic renal failure. The only perioperative complication among the group was a wound separation. No patients required blood transfusions in the perioperative period. One patient died 7.9 years after a RYGB and 6.1 years after transplantation from cardiovascular disease related to longstanding diabetes [8]. Takata et al. reported 7 morbidly obese patients with ESRD needing transplantation who underwent RYGB without morbidity and mortality with a mean percentage of excess weight loss at ≥9 months of 61 % with improvement or resolution obesity-associated co-morbidities in all patients. All eventually qualified for renal transplantation [9]. In a recent series by Lin et al. six pre-transplant patients with end-stage renal disease underwent sleeve gastrectomy (SG). All patients met the institution's BMI cutoffs for transplantation by 12 months after the procedure. There were no deaths, and there was 1 temporary renal insufficiency. The mean percentage of excess weight loss was 50 % at 1 year. One patient's renal function stabilized, and he was taken off the transplant list. One patient received a combined liver and kidney transplant and 1 received a kidney transplant [10].

Thus a SG or a RYGB can be performed safely in patients with CKD/ESRD. Also the risk of worsening renal function in the post-operative period is low with low morbidity. They achieve excellent weight loss and improvement in obesity-related co-morbidities with improved candidacy for renal transplantation.

18.3 Bariatric Surgery for Morbid Obesity in Post-transplant End-Stage Renal Disease

Kidney transplant recipients are at increased risk for developing or worsening obesity after transplantation [11]. Postoperative weight gain following organ transplantation may in part be explained by a direct corticosteroid effect, reduction of leptin synthesis/release and significantly elevated neuropeptide levels as well as lifestyle changes related to psychosocial factors [11]. There may be a need for surgical intervention in post-renal transplant weight gain with new onset or worsening of obesity and obesity-related comorbidities such as diabetes and hypertension.

In the series by Alexander et al. eight had transplantation followed by RYGB. The reduction in excess BMI and resolution of co-morbid conditions was similar to patients without transplantation or chronic renal failure with no major peri-operative morbidity. There was no death in the group who had RYGB after renal transplantation [8]. A small pharmacokinetic study showed that mycophenolic acid, tacrolimus, and sirolimus after gastric bypass would need higher dosing levels to account for the differences in pharmacokinetics, than in the non-bypass population [12]. However in a series by Szomstein et al. five renal transplant patients underwent bariatric surgery. Four patients had RYGB and one had SG. Percent of excess weight loss (%EWL) at 2 years was over 50 % for all patients with resolution or improvement of co-morbidities. There were no postoperative complications in any patients, and no alteration to the dosages of the immunosuppressant drugs after bariatric surgery [13]. In another series by Arias et al. five had transplantation followed by RYGB. One had an anastomotic leak at the gastrojejunal anastomosis that healed with conservative treatment. The remaining four patients did not have any postoperative complications. Three of the patients had diabetes and achieved good control after the surgery. The absorption of immune suppressors was not altered; and some of the patients were even able to reduce their doses.

Hence bariatric surgery can be considered as a treatment option in kidney transplant recipients with weight gain with new onset or worsening of obesity and related comorbidities such as diabetes and hypertension. There is no requirement for alteration in the dosages of the immunosuppressant drugs after bariatric surgery.

18.4 Bariatric Surgery in Cirrhotic or Pre-transplant Patients

Considering the excellent outcomes of bariatric surgery in the general population and CKD patients in a pre-transplant setting have led many to further consider bariatric surgery in morbidly obese patients with cirrhosis. Obese liver transplant candidates showed higher wound infection rates, had increased intraoperative blood transfusion, longer operating times, reduced early graft survival and increased early deaths from multi-organ failure in comparison to non-obese candidates [2, 4, 14]. Thus most transplant centers based on established criteria prevent patients with morbid obesity to be listed for transplantation. Thus the definitive treatment of obesity will be of great benefit to transplant recipients. However the perioperative risk for cirrhotic patients with decompensated liver disease and significant portal hypertension for any surgical intervention is very high. Most series of bariatric surgery in cirrhotics in pre-transplant setting are therefore restricted to bariatric surgery performed in Childs A and selected Childs B cirrhosis without portal hypertension or after transjugular intrahepatic intrabdominal shunt (TIPS).

In a series by Takata et al. six morbidly obese patients with cirrhosis (4 Child A and 2 Child B) underwent SG. There was no mortality. Two developed complications, 1 postoperative bleeding and the other encephalopathy which recovered. There was no liver decompensation. At a mean follow-up of 12.4 months, the mean percentage of excess weight loss at >9 months was 33 % Five of the 6 patients subsequently became candidates for liver transplantation [9]. In another series by Shimizu et al. colleagues 23 patients (22 with Child-Pugh class A and 1 with Child-Pugh class B) underwent bariatric surgery [15]. Fourteen patients underwent a RYGB, eight patients an SG, and one patient an AGB. Two patients had a SG after TIPS. There was no perioperative mortality. There was 1 leak each in the RYGB and SG groups. There was no liver decompensation. Mean excess weight loss was 67 % at 12 months' follow up [16]. In a series by Dallal and colleagues, 30 patients, 90 % of whom were diagnosed intraoperatively with cirrhosis underwent bariatric surgery. All were Child's A without obvious portal hypertension [17]. Twenty-seven patients underwent a RYGB and three patients underwent an SG. There were no perioperative deaths. There was no liver decompensation. Early complications occurred in nine patients and included 1 anastomotic leak, 4 acute tubular necrosis, 2 prolonged intubation, 1 ileus, and 2 needing blood transfusion. There was one late unrelated death and one patient with prolonged nausea and protein malnutrition at an average follow-up time of 16 months. The average percent excess weight loss was $63 \pm 15\,\%$ at >12 months.

Thus there exists a few series in literature that suggests that a SG or a RYGB can be performed safely in Childs A and selected patients with Childs B cirrhosis without portal HT or after TIPS. These patients may have an increased incidence of complications without much fear of liver decompensation and mortality. Patients achieved excellent weight loss and improvement in obesity-related co-morbidities with improved candidacy for liver transplantation. However because of small series and limited follow-up it is not entirely clear which surgical modality is safest in cirrhotics. SG is a less-invasive approach but may pose a significant bleeding risk and RYGB may make the fundus inaccessible if further varices should develop. RYGB may benefit some patients with metabolic syndrome better than a SG but it remains unknown whether it may complicate a future liver transplant because of lack of endoscopic access to biliary tree and malabsorption.

18.5 Bariatric Surgery During Liver Transplant in Cirrhotic Patients

Definitive treatment of obesity should be of benefit to obese liver transplant recipients. In cirrhotic patients with decompensated liver disease and significant portal hypertension who cannot be subjected to bariatric surgery because of prohibitive risk and who fail a preoperative medical weight loss program, may be subjected to bariatric procedures at the time of the liver transplant. Advantages are that as the patient is already subjected to surgery, the additional procedure can be done in the same sitting and the added time to complete the bariatric procedure would be minimal. Also after the liver transplant the portal system would be decompressed. Campsen and colleagues reported a case of placement of an adjustable gastric band performed at the time of liver transplantation in a morbidly obese patient with hypertension, diabetes, sleep apnea, and venous stasis who did well postoperatively and lost approximately 45 % of excess weight by 6 months [18]. In a recent series from the Mayo Clinic, a total of 7 patients underwent a liver transplant combined with sleeve gastrectomy. (RYGB was avoided to prevent malabsorption and to maintain endoscopic access to the biliary tree). There were no mortalities in this series, and no graft losses. Two developed complications. One patient developed a severe early graft dysfunction followed by leak from the gastric staple line with multiple re-operations and prolonged hospital stay and one had excess weight loss to a BMI of 20 with late hepatic artery thrombosis and multiple hepatic abscesses. Both patients recovered from complications and were doing well at follow up. All had substantial weight loss with mean BMI 29 at follow-up. None of the patients had steatosis on follow-up. All patients received standard post-transplant immunosuppression and experienced no difficulty with tacrolimus dosing [19].

Though data is limited it can be concluded that it is feasible to combine liver transplant with a restrictive bariatric procedure. It may be considered in cirrhotic patients with decompensated liver disease and significant portal hypertension who cannot be subjected to bariatric surgery because of prohibitive risk and who fail a preoperative medical weight loss program. At present feasibility of a RYGB is not known and is perhaps better avoided to maintain easy endoscopic access to the biliary tree post liver transplant.

18.6 Bariatric Surgery After Liver Transplant in Cirrhotic Patients

Liver transplant recipients are at increased risk of developing or worsening obesity after transplantation [20, 21]. Of concern in an obese patient is the prevention of non-alcoholic steatohepatitis (NASH) and the treatment of recurrent NASH which has the associated risk of development of fibrosis [22]. The feasibility of bariatric surgery in a post-liver transplant setting has been reported in several small series. Duchini and Brunson reported two patients undergoing an open RYGB for recurrent steatohepatitis after liver transplant without complications with good weight loss and eventual resolution of steatohepatitis. Both did not require changes in tacrolimus or immunosuppression dosing [23]. Tichansky and Madan reported one patient with RYGB in a post–liver transplant patient whose BMI was 54 without complications with good weight loss [24]. Butte et al. reported a patient who was diagnosed intraoperatively at the time of bariatric surgery with cirrhosis with mild portal hypertension and a planned RYGB was deferred [25]. After few months he developed variceal bleeding and decompensated liver cirrhosis. He was listed and placed on intragastric balloon to qualify for transplantation with a loss of 18 kgs. He then underwent liver transplantation. He subsequently developed a biliary stricture that required a revision to a Roux-en-Y biliary bypass. He had by this time regained weight with a BMI of 37.9. He then underwent a simultaneous open biliary bypass and a sleeve gastrectomy uneventfully. Postoperatively, his BMI decreased to 29.8 at 6 months' follow-up and no changes in post-operative cyclosporine levels were seen. A larger recent series by Lin and colleagues described SGs in 9 patients with prior liver transplantation [26]. There were three complications in three patients. One patient developed a bile leak from the liver surface, which subsequently resolved with drainage and argon-beam coagulation. Another patient had a simultaneous repair of a large incisional hernia and experienced a dehiscence on postoperative day two. The third patient had persistent dysphagia. Manometry was performed, which demonstrated aperistalsis of the esophagus, despite no significant anatomic or mechanical obstructions seen during upper endoscopy. The patient underwent a subsequent revision to a RYGB, whereby the symptoms resolved. Calcineurin inhibitor levels remained stable. There were no episodes of graft rejection. At 3 months liver function tests remained stable. Excess weight loss averaged 55.5 % at 6 months.

Though data is limited it can be concluded that bariatric surgery is feasible in a post-liver transplant setting and can be considered as a treatment option in patients with morbid obesity post liver transplant and as a treatment of reccurent steatohepatitis when conservative measures fail.

18.7 Bariatric Surgery Before Heart Transplant in Advanced Heart Failure

The efficacy and safety of bariatric surgery in patients with advanced heart failure has only been reported in a small number of studies. Lim et al. reported seven patients with left ventricular ejection fraction (LVEF) ≤25 % who underwent laparoscopic bariatric surgery with no major perioperative complications. Postoperative LVEF improved to a median of 30 %. There was no mortality reported. Four patients met listing criteria of which two patients underwent successful cardiac transplantation. Three patients showed marked improvement of their LVEF and functional status removing the requirement for transplantation [27]. McCloskey et al. reported 14 patients with severe cardiomyopathy who underwent bariatric surgery (10 underwent laparoscopic LRYGB, 1 open RYGB, 2 SGs, and 1 laparoscopic AGB). The complications were pulmonary edema in 1, hypotension in 1, and transient renal insufficiency in 2. Mean excess weight loss at 6 months was 50.4. The mean left ventricular ejection fraction at 6 months had significantly improved from 23 to 32 %. Two patients underwent successful transplantation after weight loss [28]. Ramani et al. compared 12 morbidly obese patients with a mean LVEF of 22 % who underwent bariatric surgery and then compared outcomes with 10 matched controls. They noted a significant improvement in LVEF in 12 patients who underwent bariatric surgery, but not in the 10 controls. Also the bariatric surgery group had lower hospital readmission rates than controls. One bariatric surgery patient was successfully transplanted, and another listed for transplantation [29].

Bariatric surgery is an effective means of weight loss in patients with low LVEF, and is associated with low risk of complications in experienced equipped centers and many patients subsequently qualify for cardiac transplantation. Weight loss in these patients can improve cardiac function and in some may obviate the need for cardiac transplantation.

Recommendations

- Bariatric surgery can be safely performed in patients with CKD/ESRD with minimal morbidity. This helps in improving their candidacy for future renal transplantation.
- Bariatric surgery can also be safely performed in the post-renal transplant setting without any alteration in the dosages of the immunosuppressant drugs.
- A sleeve gastrectomy or a RYGB can be safely performed in patients with compensated cirrhosis without portal HT without fear of liver decompensation and mortality.
- Concomitant liver transplant with sleeve gastrectomy may be considered in a clinical trial setting.
- Bariatric surgery is feasible in a post-liver transplant setting as a treatment option of recurrent steatohepatitis when conservative measures fail.
- Bariatric surgery is feasible in patients with advanced heart failure in experienced equipped centers. This improves candidacy for cardiac transplantation and this weight loss may sometimes obviate the need for transplantation.

References

1. Bumgardner GL, Henry ML, Elkhammas E, Wilson GA, Tso P, Davies E, et al. Obesity as a risk factor after combined pancreas/kidney transplantation. Transplantation. 1995;60(12):1426–30.
2. Sawyer RG, Pelletier SJ, Pruett TL. Increased early morbidity and mortality with acceptable long-term function in severely obese patients undergoing liver transplantation. Clin Transplant. 1999;13(1 Pt 2):126–30.
3. Meier-Kriesche HU, Vaghela M, Thambuganipalle R, Friedman G, Jacobs M, Kaplan B. The effect of body mass index on long-term renal allograft survival. Transplantation. 1999;68(9):1294–7.
4. Braunfeld MY, Chan S, Pregler J, Neelakanta G, Sopher MJ, Busuttil RW, et al. Liver transplantation in the morbidly obese. J Clin Anesth. 1996;8(7):585–90.
5. Grady KL, White-Williams C, Naftel D, Costanzo MR, Pitts D, Rayburn B, et al. Are preoperative obesity and cachexia risk factors for post heart transplant morbidity and mortality: a

multi-institutional study of preoperative weight-height indices. Cardiac Transplant Research Database (CTRD) Group. J Heart Lung Transplant Off Publ Int Soc Heart Transplant. 1999;18(8):750–63.
6. Koshy AN, Coombes JS, Wilkinson S, Fassett RG. Laparoscopic Gastric Banding Surgery Performed in Obese Dialysis Patients Prior to Kidney Transplantation. Am J Kidney Dis. 2008;52(4):e15–7.
7. Newcombe V, Blanch A, Slater GH, Szold A, Fielding GA. Laparoscopic Adjustable Gastric Banding Prior to Renal Transplantation. Obes Surg. 2005;15(4):567–70.
8. Alexander JW, Goodman HR, Gersin K, Cardi M, Austin J, Goel S, et al. Gastric bypass in morbidly obese patients with chronic renal failure and kidney transplant. Transplantation. 2004;78(3):469–74.
9. Takata MC, Campos GM, Ciovica R, Rabl C, Rogers SJ, Cello JP, et al. Laparoscopic bariatric surgery improves candidacy in morbidly obese patients awaiting transplantation. Surg Obes Relat Dis Off J Am Soc Bariatr Surg. 2008;4(2):159–64; discussion 164–5.
10. Lin MYC, Tavakol MM, Sarin A, Amirkiai SM, Rogers SJ, Carter JT, et al. Laparoscopic sleeve gastrectomy is safe and efficacious for pretransplant candidates. Surg Obes Relat Dis. 2013;9(5):653–8.
11. Moore LW, Gaber AO. Patterns of early weight change after renal transplantation. J Ren Nutr. 1996;6(1):21–5.
12. Rogers CC, Alloway RR, Alexander JW, Cardi M, Trofe J, Vinks AA. Pharmacokinetics of mycophenolic acid, tacrolimus and sirolimus after gastric bypass surgery in end-stage renal disease and transplant patients: a pilot study. Clin Transplant. 2008;22(3):281–91.
13. Szomstein S, Rojas R, Rosenthal RJ. Outcomes of laparoscopic bariatric surgery after renal transplant. Obes Surg. 2010;20(3):383–5.
14. Keeffe EB, Gettys C, Esquivel CO. Liver transplantation in patients with severe obesity. Transplantation. 1994;57(2):309–11.
15. Shimizu H, Phuong V, Maia M, Kroh M, Chand B, Schauer PR, et al. Bariatric surgery in patients with liver cirrhosis. Surg Obes Relat Dis Off J Am Soc Bariatr Surg. 2013;9(1):1–6.
16. Shimizu H, Phuong V, Maia M, Kroh M, Chand B, Schauer PR, et al. Bariatric surgery in patients with liver cirrhosis. Surg Obes Relat Dis. 2013;9(1):1–6.
17. Dallal RM, Mattar SG, Lord JL, Watson AR, Cottam DR, Eid GM, et al. Results of laparoscopic gastric bypass in patients with cirrhosis. Obes Surg. 2004;14(1):47–53.
18. Campsen J, Zimmerman M, Shoen J, Wachs M, Bak T, Mandell MS, et al. Adjustable gastric banding in a morbidly obese patient during liver transplantation. Obes Surg. 2008;18(12): 1625–7.
19. Heimbach JK, Watt KDS, Poterucha JJ, Ziller NF, Cecco SD, Charlton MR, et al. Combined liver transplantation and gastric sleeve resection for patients with medically complicated obesity and end-stage liver disease. Am J Transplant Off J Am Soc Transplant Am Soc Transpl Surg. 2013;13(2):363–8.
20. Munoz SJ, Deems RO, Moritz MJ, Martin P, Jarrell BE, Maddrey WC. Hyperlipidemia and obesity after orthotopic liver transplantation. Transplant Proc. 1991;23(1 Pt 2):1480–3.
21. Palmer M, Schaffner F, Thung SN. Excessive weight gain after liver transplantation. Transplantation. 1991;51(4):797–800.
22. Malik SM, de Vera ME, Fontes P, Shaikh O, Sasatomi E, Ahmad J. Recurrent disease following liver transplantation for nonalcoholic steatohepatitis cirrhosis. Liver Transpl. 2009;15(12): 1843–51.
23. Duchini A, Brunson ME. Roux-en-Y gastric bypass for recurrent nonalcoholic steatohepatitis in liver transplant recipients with morbid obesity. Transplantation. 2001;72(1):156–9.
24. Tichansky DS, Madan AK. Laparoscopic Roux-en-Y gastric bypass is safe and feasible after orthotopic liver transplantation. Obes Surg. 2005;15(10):1481–6.
25. Butte JM, Devaud N, Jarufe NP, Boza C, Pérez G, Torres J, et al. Sleeve gastrectomy as treatment for severe obesity after orthotopic liver transplantation. Obes Surg. 2007;17(11): 1517–9.

26. Lin MYC, Tavakol MM, Sarin A, Amirkiai SM, Rogers SJ, Carter JT, et al. Safety and feasibility of sleeve gastrectomy in morbidly obese patients following liver transplantation. Surg Endosc. 2013;27(1):81–5.
27. Lim C-P, Fisher OM, Falkenback D, Boyd D, Hayward CS, Keogh A, et al. Bariatric Surgery Provides a "Bridge to Transplant" for Morbidly Obese Patients with Advanced Heart Failure and May Obviate the Need for Transplantation. Obes Surg. 2016;26(3):486–93.
28. McCloskey CA, Ramani GV, Mathier MA, Schauer PR, Eid GM, Mattar SG, et al. Bariatric surgery improves cardiac function in morbidly obese patients with severe cardiomyopathy. Surg Obes Relat Dis Off J Am Soc Bariatr Surg. 2007;3(5):503–7.
29. Ramani GV, McCloskey C, Ramanathan RC, Mathier MA. Safety and efficacy of bariatric surgery in morbidly obese patients with severe systolic heart failure. Clin Cardiol. 2008;31(11):516–20.

Part V

Postoperative Pathways

Perioperative Venous Thromboembolism Prophylaxis After Bariatric Surgery

19

Rachel Maria Gomes

19.1 Introduction

Obesity is both an independent and an additive risk factor for venous thromboembolism (VTE) [1, 2]. This is attributed to elevated levels of leptin, tissue factor, coagulation factors VII and VIII, thrombin, fibrinogen, von Willebrand factor, plasminogen activator inhibitor 1 that cause hypercoagulability [3]. Dyslipidemia, hyperglycemia, inflammation, oxidative stress and endothelial dysfunction associated with obesity may also be contributory [3]. Patients undergoing bariatric surgery for morbid obesity are at increased risk for VTE in the perioperative period [4]. A retrospective cohort study showed that bariatric patients had a mean of 3.4 risk factors (ranging from 2 to 7 factors) for the development of VTE [5]. Thus all patients are atleast at a moderate to high risk for VTE. The reported incidence of symptomatic VTE in bariatric surgery series is approximately 1–5.4 % for open surgery and <1 % for laparoscopic surgery. VTE is also a leading cause of mortality after bariatric surgery. In an autopsy study of 10 roux-en-Y gastric bypass (RYGB) patients by Melinek et al, 3 out of 10 postoperative mortalities were directly a result of pulmonary embolism (PE) and 8 out of 10 patients had microscopic evidence of PE at autopsy despite the use of prophylaxis [6].

In this chapter we aim to discuss the various deep venous thrombosis (DVT) prophylaxis strategies based on the existing literature, which could serve as a guide in surgical practice. We do not yet have any standard guidelines on the exact protocol that needs to be adhered to.

R.M. Gomes, MS, FMAS
Bariatric Division, Upper Gastrointestinal Surgery and Minimal Access Surgery Unit, GEM Hospital and Research Centre, Coimbatore, India
e-mail: dr.gomes@rediffmail.com

P.R. Palanivelu et al. (eds.), *Bariatric Surgical Practice Guide*,
DOI 10.1007/978-981-10-2705-5_19

19.2 VTE Prevention with Pharmacologic Strategies

In clinical practice a majority of bariatric surgeons routinely use pharmacologic agents in adjunct to mechanical methods for venous thromboembolism prophylaxis. There is no standard agent, dose, or timing or duration of these medications. The most commonly used agents include unfractionated heparin (UFH) and low-molecular-weight heparins (LMWHs) (most commonly enoxaparin).

It is important to note that unlike UFH, LMWH therapy cannot be monitored using the activated partial thromboplastin time (aPTT). Hence anti-factor Xa assay is used to monitor LMWH therapy. LMWHs inhibit the coagulation process by binding to antithrombin which subsequently inhibits activated factor Xa. The methodology of an anti-factor Xa assay is that patient's plasma is added to a known amount of excess factor Xa and excess antithrombin. If LMWH is present in the patient plasma, it will bind to antithrombin and form a complex with factor Xa, inhibiting it. The amount of residual factor Xa is inversely proportional to the amount of heparin/LMWH in the plasma detected by adding a chromogenic substrate. This same assay can also be used to monitor unfractionated heparin therapy based on the same principles.

19.2.1 Unfractionated Heparin

Several studies utilizing unfractionated heparin (UFH) for VTE prophylaxis have been performed in the bariatric surgical setting. Prophylactic dosing for UFH ranged from fixed dose 5,000 U subcutaneously two to three times daily (BID or TID) to higher dosing of 7,500 U TID [6, 7]. Some used anti-FXa adjusted or activated partial thromboplastin time (aPTT) of 1.5 times control adjusted-dose of UFH subcutaneously 12 hourly [8]. Overall DVT/PE incidence was 0.4–1.2 % and bleeding episodes were 1.8–2.4 %. However it is known that UFH is limited by unpredictable pharmacokinetic and pharmacodynamics properties when given subcutaneously in normal weight individuals which may further be exacerbated by obesity. Some investigators studied UFH used as an intravenous infusion. While one showed no clinically evident thromboembolic event or major bleeding another study showed 0.12 % clinically evident thromboembolic events with 1.3 % patients with bleeding needing transfusion and 5 % of patients needing termination of heparin therapy due to acute drop in hematocrit [9, 10].

However comparison data suggests that LMWH may be more effective than UFH for prevention of VTE among bariatric surgery patients. A study was conducted by the Michigan Bariatric Surgery Collaborative comparing VTE prophylaxis strategies. Three dominant prophylaxis strategies were used UFH preoperatively and postoperatively (UFH/UFH), UFH preoperatively and LMWH postoperatively (UFH/LMWH), and LMWH pre and postoperatively (LMWH/LMWH). Overall, adjusted rates of VTE were significantly lower for the LMWH/LMWH and UFH/LMWH compared with the UFH/UFH group. While UFH/LMWH and LMWH/LMWH were similarly effective in patients at low risk of VTE, LMWH/LMWH seemed more effective than UFH/LMWH for high-risk patients. There were no significant differences in rates of hemorrhage among the treatment strategies [11]. Also as LMWH has more consistent and predictable anticoagulant activity it has replaced UFH for most indications because of predictability and convenient dosing.

19.2.2 Low Molecular Weight Heparin

19.2.2.1 Enoxaparin

Enoxaparin is the most commonly used LMWH. Pharmacodynamic studies in obese and morbidly obese show that peak anti-FXa levels are often below recommended target anti-FXa levels for VTE prevention when standard doses of LMWH are used for VTE prophylaxis [11–13]. Higher doses of LMWH may be required in the morbidly obese patients. Several studies have looked at different dosing regimens and measured anti-FXa levels, in the bariatric surgical patient, to ensure appropriate prophylactic doses. Enoxaparin has been administered with doses ranging from 30 to 60 mg either as daily or twice daily frequency. In one retrospective review of Enoxaparin 30 mg 12 hourly versus 40 mg 12 hourly, a higher incidence of DVT (5.4 % vs 0.6 %) was seen in the 30 mg group with no differences in haemorrhage [14]. In another non-randomised study on comparison of Enoxaparin 30 mg 12 hourly with 40 mg 12 hourly studying levels of anti-Xa levels it was seen that after the first dose, 30.8 % of the patients receiving 40 mg were within an appropriate therapeutic range compared to 0 % in the group receiving 30 mg. After the third dose, only 41 % of patients in the 40 mg group and 9 % of patients in the 30 mg group were within therapeutic range. No patient had any bleeding complications. The authors concluded that 30 mg every 12 h may not be enough to achieve the desired anti-Xa levels and that 40 mg every 12 h shows only a slight improvement over the 30 mg regimen [15]. In one more non-randomised study on comparison of Enoxaparin 40 mg 12 hourly with 60 mg 12 hourly studying levels of anti-Xa levels it was seen that mean anti-Xa levels were higher in the 60 mg group but both groups achieved a therapeutic anti-Xa level [16].

In the multicenter retrospective study of the prophylaxis against VTE outcomes in bariatric surgery patients receiving enoxaparin (PROBE study), enoxaparin prophylaxis dosing in bariatric surgery patients were compared at 5 medical centers. One centre administered only 30 mg subcutaneous once preoperatively, one centre administered 30 mg subcutaneous every 24 h post discharge for 10 days, two centres administered 40 mg subcutaneous every 24 h postoperatively and one centre administered 40 mg subcutaneous every 12 h postoperatively. There were 6 PEs and 1 DVT recorded. 6 of the 7 episodes occurred after discontinuation of enoxaparin. One patient who developed a PE while on enoxaparin and 3 of the 7 episodes were found in the center that provided a dose of 30 mg subcutaneous every 24 h post discharge but not peri-operatively [17]. Thus it can be concluded that 0.4 mg 12 hourly may be the ideal prophylactic dose to be used in morbidly obese patients.

Borkgren-Okonek et al used enoxaparin dosing according to body mass index (BMI). Patients with a BMI less than or equal to 50 kg/m^2 were given 40 mg of enoxaparin subcutaneous every 12 h, while patients with BMI greater than 50 kg/m^2 were given

60 mg subcutaneous every 12 h. In the 40 mg group, none of the patients were supratherapeutic, whereas the 60 mg group showed similar numbers of patients with subtherapeutic and supratherapeutic levels. The authors concluded that using higher than standard dosing and stratifying patients by BMI was effective at preventing VTEs [18].

A recent study investigating the correlation between anti-Xa levels and the percentage of patients that reach the desired prophylactic range for anti-Xa levels with 0.4 mg fixed-dose enoxaparin twice daily after bariatric surgery demonstrated a strong negative correlation between body weight and peak anti-Xa levels. Thirty-eight percent of patients with excessive body weight (>150 kg) had subprophylactic anti-Xa levels with fixed-dose twice daily 0.4 mg enoxaparin while 35 % of patients with lower body weight (<110 kg) were above the advised prophylactic range. Thus a weight based dosing may be more appropriate [19]. A pragmatic approach as suggested by the HAT Committee of the UK Clinical Pharmacy Association in the NHS practice guidelines for doses of thromboprophylaxis at extremes of body weight may be followed. Non-obese patients receiving the efficacious enoxaparin 40 mg once daily using data from the MEDENOX trial, translates to a weight based dose of 0.4–0.8 mg/kg. If patients >100 kg receive 40 mg twice daily and patients >150 kg receive 60 mg twice daily they would be receiving a similar weight based dose to non-obese patients. Patients <100 kg can be treated with 0.4 mg once daily. This may be a simple practical option to address patients at extremes of weight.

Thus in summary, strongest data seem to support the use of 40 mg of enoxaparin SC every 12 h. The use of this dose was shown to decrease the risk of VTE in patients undergoing bariatric surgery compared to 0.3 mg 12 hourly and to bring more patients to a desired anti-Xa level with low frequency of sub-prophylactic doses when compared to 0.6 mg 12 hourly which had unlikely sub-prophylactic doses but higher frequency of supraprophylactic doses. However if sub-grouped according to weight, supra-prophylactic and sub-prophylactic are common at extremes of weight (<100 and >150 kg). Thus at weights less than 100 kg standard 0.4 mg once daily dose may be used and above 150 kg 0.6 mg 12 hourly may be used. BMI based dosing of 40 mg enoxaparin SC every 12 h in those <50 BMI and 60 mg of enoxaparin SC every 12 h in those >50 BMI may be considered based on a single well conducted study.

Although it appears that consideration could be made to use higher doses of LMWH to achieve proper therapeutic levels, the true clinical significance of this has yet to be proven. It is not well defined if this practice may lead to a decreased risk of VTE complications and/or if an increased rate of major bleeding complications will occur.

19.2.2.2 Other Low Molecular Weight Heparins

Very few studies have been conducted based on other low molecular weight heparins. In a randomized controlled trial a dose of 5,700 IU Nadroparin was as effective as 9,500 IU dose and with fewer bleeding complications [20]. In a multicenter, open-label, pilot study in bariatric surgical patients a parnaparin dose of 4,250 IU/day was equivalent to 6,400 IU/day for VTE prevention [21]. In a retrospective study it was concluded that 7,500 IU dalteparin dosage was appropriate for the majority of morbidly obese patients undergoing bariatric surgery [22].

19.2.3 Fondaparinux

In the recently published results of the EFFORT trial, a randomized double-blind pilot trial of enoxaparin versus fondaparinux for thromboprophylaxis in bariatric surgical patients, patients were randomized to receive either 40 mg enoxaparin twice daily or 5 mg fondaparinux sodium once daily. Adequate antifactor Xa levels were more common with fondaparinux (74.2 %) than with enoxaparin (32.4 %) [23]. The incidence of DVT was low and similar in both the groups. No major adverse events occurred in either arm. The authors concluded that Fondaparinux was much more likely to produce target prophylactic antifactor Xa levels than enoxaparin. Both regimens appear to be equally effective at reducing the risk of DVT. Further prospective studies are needed to determine the optimal DVT prophylaxis regimen in the bariatric surgical population. However because of the risk of bleeding without established reversal agent, Fondaparinux should be should be used with caution.

19.3 Duration of Venous Thromboprophylaxis'

In a study by Steele et al in 2011 it was demonstrated that the risk for VTE after bariatric surgery extends well beyond the initial hospitalization. The incidence of VTE during the index surgical hospitalization was 0.88 % [24]. This cumulative rate rose to 2.17 % at 1 month and 2.99 % by 6 months post-surgery. Over 74 % of VTE events occurred after discharge. Over one third of VTEs occurred 30 days post-bariatric surgery. This suggests that more aggressive extended prophylaxis should be considered in patients at higher risk for VTE but there are insufficient data to recommend specific duration of administration. Randomized controlled trials in other high-risk groups for VTE such as patients undergoing cancer surgery and orthopedic surgery suggest that 30 days of extended thromboprohylaxis can significantly reduce VTE events versus 1 week [25, 26]. These findings can be extrapolated to bariatric surgery patients and extended pharmacologic thromboprophylaxis for up to 4 weeks after discharge may be warranted in certain high risk patients undergoing bariatric surgery.

19.4 VTE Prevention with Mechanical Strategies

19.4.1 Mechanical Methods

Only few studies have examined the use of mechanical VTE prophylaxis alone in bariatric surgery patients. In a retrospective study comparing enoxaparin twice daily with patients who received sequential compression devices and early ambulation only (selective pharmacologic anticoagulation in high risk only) rates of DVT and PE rates were no different between the groups with higher bleeding complications in the LMWH group. The authors concluded that adequate VTE prophylaxis is achieved by only using sequential compression devices (SCDs), early ambulation, with adequate hydration, and shorter operating times in all but the high-risk population. Fewer bleeding complications occur without the use of anticoagulants [27].

In another study comparing a VTE prophylactic regimen of calf-length pneumatic compression devices placed before anesthesia induction and mandatory ambulation beginning on the day of operation with pharmacologic treatment for VTE prevention,DVT and PE rates were 0.31 % and 0.10 %, respectively, and a bleeding complication rate was 0.73 % for the latter. All patients had short operating times. The authors concluded that if patients have short operative times and were not high risk for VTE early ambulation and compliance with SCDs was sufficient for adequate VTE prophylaxis with low bleeding episodes [28].

Both these studies excluded patients who were at high risk for VTE. Also the limitations of poor compliance with mechanical prophylaxis is well known. At present, the existing evidence is not sufficient enough for recommendations on mechanical prophylaxis only and mechanical methods are often an accompaniment to some form of chemical thromboprophylaxis. It may be considered if a high bleeding risk precludes the use of pharmacologic prophylaxis in patients.

19.4.2 Inferior Vena Cava Filters

Reported VTE that occurs after bariatric surgery does so despite of pharmacologic prophylaxis which has led to the increased use of temporary inferior vena cava filters (IVCFs). Factors which make bariatric patients high risk have not been established, however most commonly considered factors are prior VTE, immobility, hypercoagulable conditions and body mass index >55 kg/m^2,obesity hypoventilation syndrome with associated elevated pulmonary artery pressure [29]. Some studies support a decreased rate of PE and death in high risk patients when prophylactic IVCF are used [30–33]. However in one study, more than half of the prophylactic IVCF patients had a fatal pulmonary embolism or complications directly related to the IVCF itself, including filter migration or thrombosis of the vena cava. Subgroup analysis couldn't identify improved outcomes for any particular group [34]. One study reported a longer length of hospital stay, higher incidence of DVT and had a higher mortality from PE and indeterminate causes [35]. Data from the Bariatric Outcomes Longitudinal Database also showed that IVCF resulted in a higher incidence of VTE [36]. A systematic review of 11 published studies of IVCF suggests that retrievable IVCF placement in bariatric surgery patients results in a low rate of complications and may reduce postoperative PE, particularly in high-risk bariatric surgery patients. None of the 11 studies included in the systematic review was a randomized trial, eight were case series and four were comparative studies of IVCF to no IVCF (two of these four cohort studies showed no significant difference in PE). Also complications of IVCF placement may not have been adequately considered [37]. In summary, the routine use of retrievable IVCF placement in bariatric surgery patients is not supported by the available evidence. It may reduce postoperative PE, particularly in high-risk bariatric surgery patients but insertion-related complications have been described and need to be considered.

Recommendations

- VTE is the leading cause of mortality after bariatric surgery hence venous thromboprophylaxis is of utmost importance.
- Ideal dosing regimen in morbidly obese patients is 40 mg of enoxaparin SC every 12 h with adjustments at extremes of weight (<100 and >150 kg).
- Mechanical methods is to be routinely combined with chemical thromboprophylaxis.
- Routine use of retrievable IVCF placement is not recommended but may used in selected high risk patients.
- Venous thromboprophylaxis needs to be started 12–36 h preoperatively and continued for a total of 8–10 days postoperatively.
- Extended pharmacologic thromboprophylaxis for up to 4 weeks after discharge may be warranted in high risk patients.

References

1. Stein PD, Beemath A, Olson RE. Obesity as a risk factor in venous thromboembolism. Am J Med. 2005;118(9):978–80.
2. Abdollahi M, Cushman M, Rosendaal FR. Obesity: risk of venous thrombosis and the interaction with coagulation factor levels and oral contraceptive use. Thromb Haemost. 2003;89(3): 493–8.
3. Allman-Farinelli MA. Obesity and venous thrombosis: a review. Semin Thromb Hemost. 2011;37(8):903–7.
4. Prystowsky JB, Morasch MD, Eskandari MK, Hungness ES, Nagle AP. Prospective analysis of the incidence of deep venous thrombosis in bariatric surgery patients. Surgery. 2005;138(4):759–63; discussion 763–5.
5. Cotter SA, Cantrell W, Fisher B, Shopnick R. Efficacy of venous thromboembolism prophylaxis in morbidly obese patients undergoing gastric bypass surgery. Obes Surg. 2005;15(9): 1316–20.
6. Melinek J, Livingston E, Cortina G, Fishbein MC. Autopsy findings following gastric bypass surgery for morbid obesity. Arch Pathol Lab Med. 2002;126(9):1091–5.
7. Miller MT, Rovito PF. An approach to venous thromboembolism prophylaxis in laparoscopic Roux-en-Y gastric bypass surgery. Obes Surg. 2004;14(6):731–7.
8. Shepherd MF, Rosborough TK, Schwartz ML. Heparin thromboprophylaxis in gastric bypass surgery. Obes Surg. 2003;13(2):249–53.
9. F Shepherd M, Rosborough TK, Schwartz ML. Unfractionated heparin infusion for thromboprophylaxis in highest risk gastric bypass surgery. Obes Surg. 2004;14(5):601–5.
10. Quebbemann B, Akhondzadeh M, Dallal R. Continuous intravenous heparin infusion prevents peri-operative thromboembolic events in bariatric surgery patients. Obes Surg. 2005;15(9): 1221–4.

11. Sanderink G-J, Le Liboux A, Jariwala N, Harding N, Ozoux M-L, Shukla U, et al. The pharmacokinetics and pharmacodynamics of enoxaparin in obese volunteers. Clin Pharmacol Ther. 2002;72(3):308–18.
12. Mayr AJ, Dünser M, Jochberger S, Fries D, Klingler A, Joannidis M, et al. Antifactor Xa activity in intensive care patients receiving thromboembolic prophylaxis with standard doses of enoxaparin. Thromb Res. 2002;105(3):201–4.
13. Frederiksen SG, Hedenbro JL, Norgren L. Enoxaparin effect depends on body-weight and current doses may be inadequate in obese patients. Br J Surg. 2003;90(5):547–8.
14. Scholten DJ, Hoedema RM, Scholten SE. A comparison of two different prophylactic dose regimens of low molecular weight heparin in bariatric surgery. Obes Surg. 2002;12(1):19–24.
15. Rowan BO, Kuhl DA, Lee MD, Tichansky DS, Madan AK. Anti-Xa levels in bariatric surgery patients receiving prophylactic enoxaparin. Obes Surg. 2008;18(2):162–6.
16. Simone EP, Madan AK, Tichansky DS, Kuhl DA, Lee MD. Comparison of two low-molecular-weight heparin dosing regimens for patients undergoing laparoscopic bariatric surgery. Surg Endosc. 2008;22(11):2392–5.
17. Hamad GG, Choban PS. Enoxaparin for thromboprophylaxis in morbidly obese patients undergoing bariatric surgery: findings of the prophylaxis against VTE outcomes in bariatric surgery patients receiving enoxaparin (PROBE) study. Obes Surg. 2005;15(10):1368–74.
18. Borkgren-Okonek MJ, Hart RW, Pantano JE, Rantis PC, Guske PJ, Kane JM, et al. Enoxaparin thromboprophylaxis in gastric bypass patients: extended duration, dose stratification, and antifactor Xa activity. Surg Obes Relat Dis Off J Am Soc Bariatr Surg. 2008;4(5):625–31.
19. Celik F, Huitema ADR, Hooijberg JH, van de Laar AWJM, Brandjes DPM, Gerdes VEA. Fixed-dose enoxaparin after bariatric surgery: the influence of body weight on peak anti-xa levels. Obes Surg. 2015;25(4):628–34.
20. Kalfarentzos F, Stavropoulou F, Yarmenitis S, Kehagias I, Karamesini M, Dimitrakopoulos A, et al. Prophylaxis of venous thromboembolism using two different doses of low-molecular-weight heparin (nadroparin) in bariatric surgery: a prospective randomized trial. Obes Surg. 2001;11(6):670–6.
21. Imberti D, Baldini E, Pierfranceschi MG, Nicolini A, Cartelli C, De Paoli M, et al. Prophylaxis of venous thromboembolism with low molecular weight heparin in bariatric surgery: a prospective, randomised pilot study evaluating two doses of parnaparin (BAFLUX Study). Obes Surg. 2014;24(2):284–91.
22. Simoneau M-D, Vachon A, Picard F. Effect of prophylactic dalteparin on anti-factor Xa levels in morbidly obese patients after bariatric surgery. Obes Surg. 2010;20(4):487–91.
23. Steele KE, Canner J, Prokopowicz G, Verde F, Beselman A, Wyse R, et al. The EFFORT trial: preoperative enoxaparin versus postoperative fondaparinux for thromboprophylaxis in bariatric surgical patients: a randomized double-blind pilot trial. Surg Obes Relat Dis Off J Am Soc Bariatr Surg. 2015;11(3):672–83.
24. Steele KE, Schweitzer MA, Prokopowicz G, Shore AD, Eaton LC, Lidor AO, Makary MA, Clark J, Magnuson TH. The long-term risk of venous thromboembolism following bariatric surgery. Obes Surg. 2011;21(9):1371–6.
25. Bergqvist D, Benoni G, Björgell O, Fredin H, Hedlundh U, Nicolas S, et al. Low-molecular-weight heparin (enoxaparin) as prophylaxis against venous thromboembolism after total hip replacement. N Engl J Med. 1996;335(10):696–700.
26. Bergqvist D, Agnelli G, Cohen AT, Eldor A, Nilsson PE, Le Moigne-Amrani A, et al. Duration of prophylaxis against venous thromboembolism with enoxaparin after surgery for cancer. N Engl J Med. 2002;346(13):975–80. 2011;21(9):1371–6.
27. Frantzides CT, Welle SN, Ruff TM, Frantzides AT. Routine anticoagulation for venous thromboembolism prevention following laparoscopic gastric bypass. JSLS. 2012;16(1):33–7.
28. Clements RH, Yellumahanthi K, Ballem N, Wesley M, Bland KI. Pharmacologic prophylaxis against venous thromboembolic complications is not mandatory for all laparoscopic Roux-en-Y gastric bypass procedures. J Am Coll Surg. 2009;208(5):917–21; discussion 921–3.
29. Vaziri K, Devin Watson J, Harper AP, Lee J, Brody FJ, Sarin S, et al. Prophylactic inferior vena cava filters in high-risk bariatric surgery. Obes Surg. 2011;21(10):1580–4.

30. Schuster R, Hagedorn JC, Curet MJ, Morton JM. Retrievable inferior vena cava filters may be safely applied in gastric bypass surgery. Surg Endosc. 2007;21(12):2277–9.
31. Keeling WB, Haines K, Stone PA, Armstrong PA, Murr MM, Shames ML. Current indications for preoperative inferior vena cava filter insertion in patients undergoing surgery for morbid obesity. Obes Surg. 2005;15(7):1009–12.
32. Obeid FN, Bowling WM, Fike JS, Durant JA. Efficacy of prophylactic inferior vena cava filter placement in bariatric surgery. Surg Obes Relat Dis Off J Am Soc Bariatr Surg. 2007;3(6):606–8; discussion 609–10.
33. Trigilio-Black CM, Ringley CD, McBride CL, Sorensen VJ, Thompson JS, Longo GM, et al. Inferior vena cava filter placement for pulmonary embolism risk reduction in super morbidly obese undergoing bariatric surgery. Surg Obes Relat Dis Off J Am Soc Bariatr Surg. 2007;3(4):461–4.
34. Birkmeyer NJO, Share D, Baser O, Carlin AM, Finks JF, Pesta CM, et al. Preoperative placement of inferior vena cava filters and outcomes after gastric bypass surgery. Ann Surg. 2010;252(2):313–8.
35. Li W, Gorecki P, Semaan E, Briggs W, Tortolani AJ, D'Ayala M. Concurrent prophylactic placement of inferior vena cava filter in gastric bypass and adjustable banding operations in the Bariatric Outcomes Longitudinal Database. J Vasc Surg. 2012;55(6):1690–5.
36. Winegar DA, Sherif B, Pate V, DeMaria EJ. Venous thromboembolism after bariatric surgery performed by Bariatric Surgery Center of Excellence Participants: analysis of the Bariatric Outcomes Longitudinal Database. Surg Obes Relat Dis. 2011;7(2):181–8.
37. Rajasekhar A, Crowther M. Inferior vena caval filter insertion prior to bariatric surgery: a systematic review of the literature. J Thromb Haemost. 2010;8(6):1266–70.

Perioperative Management of Medical Comorbidities After Bariatric Surgery

20

Praveen Raj Palanivelu, Mohammed Ismail, Padmakumar, and Deepak Subramaniam

20.1 Introduction

With evolution, we have moved away from the concept of 'bariatric surgery' towards 'metabolic surgery' where we look beyond just weight loss [1]. Recent evidences from literature clearly show that the surgical remission of type 2 diabetes mellitus (T2DM) is now possible in the long term without the need for medications [2, 3]. It has also been shown that the reduction in medications post bariatric surgery has a significant economic benefit with reduction of medication costs required for the treatment of diabetes, hypertension and dyslipidemia [4]. This surgical concept of treatment of diabetes has been endorsed by many diabetic associations including the International Diabetic Federation (IDF) [5].

In this chapter we intend to cover the principles of diabetes medication usage following bariatric surgery with an aim to define a post-operative treatment protocol.

P.R. Palanivelu, MS, DNB, DNB(SGE), FALS, FMAS (✉)
Bariatric Division, Upper Gastrointestinal Surgery and Minimal Access Surgery Unit, GEM Hospital and Research Centre, Coimbatore, India
e-mail: drraj@geminstitute.in

M. Ismail, MS, FICS, FMAS
Raihan Institute of Medical Science, Erattupetta, Moulana Hospital, Perinthalmannna, India
e-mail: mohameddr@msn.com

Padmakumar, DNB, MNAMS, DipALS, FAIS
Sunrise Hospital, Kochi, India
e-mail: drrpadmakumar@gmail.com

D. Subramaniam, MS, MRCS
Department of Surgery, Fortis Malar Hospital, Chennai, India
e-mail: deeps_msgs@yahoo.co.in

P.R. Palanivelu et al. (eds.), *Bariatric Surgical Practice Guide*,
DOI 10.1007/978-981-10-2705-5_20

20.2 Postoperative Management of Diabetes Mellitus

20.2.1 Challenges in Post-operative Diabetic Care

The principles of post-operative diabetic management has not been clearly defined. As the time taken for the remission to occur is variable, along with a subgroup of patients who will fail to achieve complete remission, defining a specific management protocol is important. But as outlined by Fenske et al. this has a lot of challenges [6].

1. Varied management strategies among various centers
2. The exact definition of remission/cure is still controversial
3. No validated treatment protocol currently exists for post bariatric patients

The recent ADA (American Diabetology Association) definition for complete remission of T2DM states return to normal glucose values (HbA1C <5.7 %, fasting capillary glucose (FCG) <5.6 mmol/L) for at least 1 year after bariatric surgery without glucose lowering medication [7].

Predicting the time scale for glycemic control to occur in the post-operative period is difficult and variable [8, 9]. Many centers tend to stop all hypoglycemic agents and insulin abruptly in anticipation of remission and to prevent the occurrence of hypoglycemia [8, 10–12]. However a healthy glucose environment is needed in the immediate post-operative period when the alteration of the incretin milieu could allow the pancreas to undergo regeneration. Hence glucotoxiticity should be avoided, which could hamper the beta cell glycemic memory [6]. For this a well-defined protocol of immediate T2DM management is needed to avoid both hypoglycemia and glucotoxicity.

The other factor to be considered is long-term management of T2DM after bariatric surgery. Many long term studies have pointed out the direct relationship between T2DM relapse and the time interval after surgery. The Swedish Obese subjects (SOS) study published a follow up report where the T2DM remission rates decreased from 72.3 % at 2 years to 30.4 % at 15 years [13]. No much literature exists for the clinical management of these post bariatric surgery patients with recurrence of diabetes.

20.2.2 Currently Used Anti-diabetic Medications and Use in Relationship to Bariatric Surgery (Kashyap et al.)

20.2.2.1 Biguanides

The most popular drug in this group is metformin, which increases insulin sensitivity by suppressing hepatic gluconeogenesis and opposition of glucagon action [14]. It has been quite popular with bariatric physicians for its ability to promote weight loss. It is important to know that the bioavailability is increased post bariatric surgery, the dosages need to be adjusted cautiously [15].

20.2.2.2 Thiazolidinediones

Also called the proliferator-activated receptor (PPAR) agonists or glitazones, this works primarily by increasing the insulin sensitivity. But since the mechanism of action is by reducing the visceral fat and increasing the subcutaneous fat, is known to promote weight gain. Hence could be used as a second line therapy to metformin for residual T2DM [16].

20.2.2.3 Sulfonyl Ureas

Unlike metformin and thiazolidinediones, sulfonyl ureas enhance insulin secretion by direct action on beta cells [17]. Hence it carries a higher risk of inducing hypoglycemia and weight regain [17, 18]. It has also been shown to carry higher risk of inducing hyperinsulinemic hypoglycemia and symptoms of dumping syndrome [18]. Hence it has to be used cautiously and can be considered as option for treatment of T2DM in the background of poor beta cell function and also to prevent further beta cell failure, along with an insulin sensitizing agent.

20.2.2.4 Insulin

In patients failing to respond adequately to insulin sensitizers or insulin secretogogues, treatment with insulin becomes important. In the immediate post-operative setting, this could be in the form of sliding scale short acting insulin or fixed dose long acting insulin. It has also been shown that a protocol based individualized insulin titration in combination with OHA s could offer better glycemic control [6].

20.2.2.5 GLP-1 Analogues/DPP4 Inhibitors

With increasing understanding on the role of incretins in T2DM remission following bariatric surgery, research has been focused in developing drugs mimicking the actions of these incretins. The most commonly studied incretin is the GLP-1 secreted in the L cells of the ileum, which is trophic to the beta cells and also improving insulin sensitivity. Native GLP-1 has a very short plasma half-life and novel methods have been developed to augment its half-life, so that its anti-hyperglycemic effects can be exploited. They analogues can be broadly classified as exendin-based therapies (exenatide, DPP-4-resistant analogues (lixisenatide, albiglutide), and analogues of human GLP-1 (liraglutide, taspoglutide) [19].

Research on obese rate models with T2DM has suggested that the use of these agents improves surgically induced weight loss [20]. Also a recent meta-analysis has demonstrated excellent glycemic control in T2DM patients [21]. Considering its role in both weight management and glycemic control, these drugs could find potential use in the post bariatric patient with inadequate remission or relapse of diabetes.

20.2.2.6 Others [16]

Sodium-glucose co-transporter 2 (SGLT-2) inhibitors or glifozins are agents that work by inhibiting glucose reabsorption in the renal tubules and increasing glucose excretion in the urine. Level 1 evidence shows the role for these agents in promoting weightloss, glycemic control and regulation of blood pressure.

Phentermine, a sympathomimetic amine which is an appetite suppressant is used along with Topiramate, a monosaccharide to increase satiety. CONQUER trial has shown that the combination when used with metformin demonstrated better weight loss and glycemic control when compared to metformin and placebo.

Orlistat is a gastric and pancreatic lipase inhibitor that works by reducing dietary fat absorption. Researchers have documented the role of this drug in producing weight loss and decreasing insulin resistance. The possible underlying mechanisms include improved insulin sensitivity, incomplete dietary fat digestion, GLP-1 release and reducing the visceral adiposity.

Lorcaserin is a selective serotonin 5-HT2C receptor agonist that decreases food intake and increases satiety. The BLOOM-DM trial has shown better weight loss and T2DM control when used along with metformin and sulfonylureas.

The four drugs mentioned above, with their potential role in weight loss and also improving glycemic control could possibly find role in the immediate and late management of type 2 diabetes following bariatric surgery. With no existing literature for the use of these drugs in post bariatric surgery patients, the exact role and the timing of initiation is still not clear.

20.2.3 Current Literature on Post-operative T2DM Management

Fenske et al. demonstrated that a protocol driven management compared to a non protocol management demonstrated a better glycemic control and more successful remission rates [6]. In the protocol based approach group, they discharged patients with 1 g of metformin twice daily along with glargine insulin based on the insulin requirements in the post-operative period. The patients were periodically contacted by SMS and insulin dosages were adjusted based on the fasting glucose values. Plasma glucose levels and HbA1C were measured before surgery and 3, 6 and 12 months after roux-en-Y gastric bypass (RYGB) surgery. Metformin was continued for 3 months and stopped only if the FCG levels reached normal values. In the non-protocol based approach group, the patients were managed and treated individually by the primary care physician or secondary care diabetologist by reduction and withdrawal or increase of glucose lowering medications, but not based on any protocol.

A recent retrospective review was published by Tritsch et al. of 88 sleeve gastrectomy patients operated at a single center, which assessed the medications used by their patients in the post-operative period. Patients receiving only one OHA in the pre-operative period did not require any medication at discharge [22]. Patients requiring more than one OHA were discharged on metformin only. Among insulin users, those with less than 30 units usage did not require any insulin at discharge and those with more than 30 units usage required 60 % less insulin use at discharge which persisted for a month. The patients were then regularly followed up for further adjustment and titration, with an average of five follow-up appointments at 6 months postoperatively.

The mean requirement of insulin in these patients dropped from 42 units in the pre-operative period to 16.1 units in the immediate post-operative period to 13.3 units at 6 months. Only 2 out of 9 patients requiring long term insulin discontinued insulin completely. They also observed that amongst the OHAs, the secretogogues followed by biguanides were frequently discontinued. Secretogogues have a well establised risk of hypoglycemia. They also observed an average 60% reduction in insulin in the immediate post-operative period with further decreases upto 6 months post-operatively.

A recent RCT which compared the use of once daily glargine versus the sliding scale insulin, the patients in the glargine group demonstrated better control of hyperglycemia along with fewer hypoglycemic events [23]. It is also surprising to note that even in patients with poor beta cell reserve indicated by low C peptide levels, following bariatric surgery there was a good number of patients going off insulin with remission and improvement [24].

20.2.4 Role of Weight Loss in T2DM Management

Although the exact links between obesity and T2DM is not very clear, positive energy balance, visceral adiposity and adipokine mediated inflammation are contributors to insulin resistance and altered insulin secretion [25–27]. The durability of T2DM remission has also been closely associated with durable weight loss and weight maintenance in the long-term [2, 28, 29]. Considering this close linkage of weight management to remission of T2DM, clinicians must be aware of the various factors that influence weight loss after surgery [16]. This same explanation would hold good for the differential rates of T2DM remission and relapse between restrictive and malabsorptive surgeries where the restrictive procedures have been associated with higher weight regain [3, 30, 31].

Since psychological and eating disorders have been closely linked to suboptimal weight loss, evaluation of the mental health and identifying eating disorders is of paramount importance for weight management and control of T2DM [32, 33]. It has also been shown that regular outpatient attendance and participation in support groups have better weight loss outcomes, such interventions may also contribute to better glycemic control [34, 35].

20.2.5 Management of Non-remission/Relapse

It is prudent to confirm T2DM as opposed to type 1 diabetes or latent-onset autoimmune diabetes (LADA), as obesity prevalence is increasing in all types of diabetes. Considering a possibility of a defect in β cell secretion as the underlying cause of non-remission or re-emergence, it is prudent to obtain indices of C-peptide and autoimmune status [16]. Long pre-operative T2DM duration, insulin use, poor glycemic control despite oral hypoglycemic agents, and microvascular complications are all additional indicators of inadequate β cell function [3].

No guidelines exist for the optimum management strategy for these patients. Khanna et al. has proposed management strategies for this group of patients depending upon the type of surgery performed. They also stress that for each type of surgery (restrictive vs malabsorptive) the management strategy should depend upon whether is patient has inadequate weight loss or weight regain or beta cell failure and stresses the need for better weight management strategies [16].

Hence weight management, both in the short and long term holds an important key in better glycemic control. The following pathway has been proposed by Khanna et al. for these subset of patients [16].

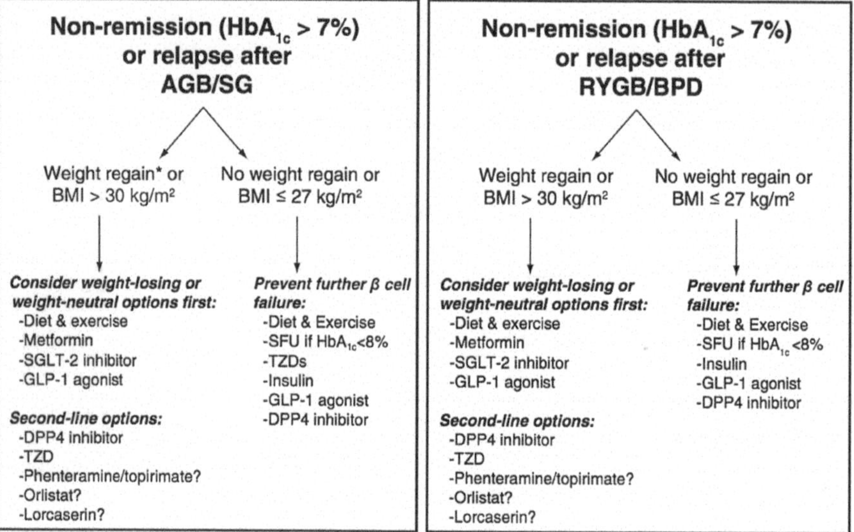

Based on the above discussion, the following protocol can be used in the post-operative period.

1. Monitor sugars in the immediate post-operative period and manage with sliding scale insulin/glargine insulin if needed.
2. If sugars are normal in the post-operative period then no OHA is needed
3. If sugars are high with minimal requirement of insulin only Metformin 1 g BD may be prescribed.
4. If the need for insulin is higher in the post-operative period discharge with 1 g Metformin BD and long acting insulin based on the requirement.
5. Monitor on a regular basis and titrate accordingly.
6. HbA1C to be done 3 months, 6 months and 1 year.

20.3 Postoperative Management of Hypertension

20.3.1 Obesity and Hypertension

Obesity is a major risk factor for hypertension and there is ample epidemiological evidence supporting the association between increased weight and increased blood pressure [36–38]. In addition, many studies have demonstrated that weight loss lowers blood pressure [39, 40]. After bariatric surgery, a decrease of 1 % in body weight leads to 1 mmHg decrease in systolic blood pressure and 2 mmHg decrease in diastolic blood pressure [41–43]. Buchwald and colleagues showed a significant reduction in hypertension in a systematic meta-analysis of 136 articles which included 22,094 patients and across all surgical procedures [8]. In particular, the percentages of patients in the total population whose hypertension resolved or improved were 61.7 % and 78.5 %, respectively.

According to a comparative study of Bariatric Surgery versus Intensive Medical Therapy in Obese Patients with Diabetes, conducted by Philip et al. on 150 patients there was a significant reduction in the number of hypertension medications after the two bariatric procedures [44]. Similarly we now have enough data on the positive effects of bariatric surgery in improvement/remission of hypertension [45–47]. Few data exist on factors associated with hypertension remission post-bariatric surgery. No information exists on factors that may actually predict hypertension relapse. Indeed, reviews of smaller surgical series have shown that normotensive or mildly hypertensive obese individuals do not achieve a significant reduction in blood pressure after gastric bypass compared with individuals with substantially elevated blood pressure [48].

20.3.2 Currently Used Antihypertensive Agents

A. *Diuretics:* bumetanide, furosemide, hydrochlorothiazide, spironolactone, triamterene
B. *Sympathoplegic agents:* methodopa, clonidine, guanfacine, thrimethaphan, guanethidine, propranolol, reserpine, methoprolol, nadolol, carteolol, pindolol, labetalol, prazosin
C. *Direct vasodilators:* hydralazine, minoxidil, sodium nitroprusside, diazoxide
D. *ACE inhibitors and angiotensin receptor antagonists:* captopril, enalapril, benazepril, quinapril, losartan, valsartan, saralasin

20.3.3 Current Literature on Post-operative Hypertension Management

As discussed above many studies have shown a drastic reduction in the use and number of antihypertensive drugs after bariatric surgery. But we have only limited data on the post-operative protocols on the usage of the different types of agents. In a recent retrospective review by Tritsch et al. on patients operated for sleeve gastrectomy at their center, the average hypertension medications reduced from 2.21 to 1.23, 1.21 and 1.18 at 1, 3 and 6 months respectively [22]. The most commonly stopped medications were thiazide diuretics. This was done to prevent volume depletion, hypotension and kidney injury. For patients with hypertension and T2DM together, a tendency to continue ACEi (Angiotensin converting enzyme inhibitors) and ARB (Angiotensin receptor blockers) was noted due to their renal protective effects. Beta blockers were continued for the benefit of perioperative beta blockade. Further changes when needed were done based on the 7th Report of the Joint National Committee on Prevention, Detection, Evaluation and Treatment of High blood pressure [49].

Though surgically induced, sustained weight loss does not seem to have a beneficial effect on blood pressure, it does lower pulse pressure which, is an independent predictor of coronary artery disease and cardiovascular mortality [50–52]. We hence need more data to help design post-operative hypertension management pathways. The above discussion may help design protocols and institution specific protocols have to be designed.

20.4 Postoperative Management of Dyslipidemia

20.4.1 Obesity and Dyslipidemia

Dyslipidemia is one of the comorbidities associated with obesity. After bariatric surgery, dyslipidemia management is much easier. Lipid parameters typically improve after bariatric surgery, but the effects have been inconsistent and may depend on the surgical procedure performed. The effects of various surgical procedures have been discussed in detail in the section on bariatric surgery in dyslipidemia in Chap. 3. If bariatric surgery consistently improves dyslipidemia, there may be associated cost savings in lipid-modifying medications.

20.4.2 Currently Used Dyslipidemic Agents

1. To lower LDL: Statin; second choice: bile acid binding resin or fenofibrate
2. To increase HDL: Fibrate (or nicotinic acid, with careful monitoring)
3. To lower Triglycerides: Fibrate (gemfibrozil, fenofibrate), high-dose statin (in hyper-triglyceridemic subjects with high LDL levels).
4. To treat combined hyperlipidemia: High-dose statin; second choice: statin + fibrate (gemfibrozil, fenofibrate); third choice: bile acid binding resin + fibrate (gemfibrozil or fenofibrate), or statin + nicotinic acid (with careful monitoring of glycemic control)

20.4.3 Current Literature on Post-operative Dyslipidemia Management

A comparative study, Bariatric Surgery versus Intensive Medical Therapy in Obese Patients with Diabetes, conducted on 150 patients showed that the levels of total and LDL cholesterol showed decrease and that there was a significant reduction in the number of medications needed to treat hyperlipidemia in the two surgical groups (gastric bypass and sleeve gastrectomy). Lipid-lowering drugs were required at baseline in 86 % and 78 % of patients assigned to undergo gastric bypass and sleeve gastrectomy, respectively, but use declined to 27 % and 39 % after 12 months [42].

Several series examining the effect of bariatric surgery on dyslipidemia have reported significant improvement in lipid profiles after bariatric surgery. There are marked reductions in LDL, increased HDL and decreased triglycerides [53]. In the Swedish Obesity Study significant improvements were observed in triglyceride and HDL levels at 2 and 10 years in the surgical versus the control group [54]. Although the total cholesterol was significantly different at 2 years, there was no significant difference at 10 years. However, the RYGB subgroup demonstrated significant improvements in total cholesterol, triglycerides and HDL at 10 years.

In the meta-analysis by Buchwald and colleagues, hyperlipidemia, hypercholesterolemia and hypertriglyceridemia were significantly improved across all surgical procedures at 2 year follow-up [8]. Segal et al. investigated the use of antilipemic drugs in 6235 bariatric surgery patients in a cohort study. The study reported that 59 % of the non-diabetic patients and 54 % of the diabetic patients showed a decrease in the need for the drug intake in the treatment of dyslipidemia 12 months after the surgery, thus indicating a substantial resolution of dyslipidemia after the surgical intervention [55]. Taken together, these studies suggest that bariatric surgery not only allows for sustained weight loss, but is a viable treatment option for correcting dyslipidemia in morbidly obese individuals.

Recommendations

- Glucotoxiticity can hamper beta cell glycemic recovery in the immediate post-operative period and should be avoided.
- A protocol driven T2DM management results in better glycemic control and more successful remission rates than a non protocol management.
- Based on sugars patients can be discharged without medications if sugars are normal. If sugars are high patients are discharged on Metformin with or without long acting insulin with close follow up for dosage adjustments.
- Long acting insulins are to be preferred to a sliding scale method of insulin usuage.
- Bariatric surgery results in improvement/remission of hypertension needing monitoring and reduction in the dose and number of antihypertensive drugs.
- Bariatric surgery consistently improves dyslipidemia and dyslipidemic agents need to be reduced postoperatively.

References

1. Hickey MS, Pories WJ, MacDonald KG, Cory KA, Dohm GL, Swanson MS, et al. A new paradigm for type 2 diabetes mellitus: could it be a disease of the foregut? Ann Surg. 1998;227(5):637–43; discussion 643–4.
2. Brethauer SA, Aminian A, Romero-Talamás H, Batayyah E, Mackey J, Kennedy L, et al. Can diabetes be surgically cured? Long-term metabolic effects of bariatric surgery in obese patients with type 2 diabetes mellitus. Ann Surg. 2013;258(4):628–36; discussion 636–7.
3. Lee W-J, Hur KY, Lakadawala M, Kasama K, Wong SKH, Lee Y-C. Gastrointestinal metabolic surgery for the treatment of diabetic patients: a multi-institutional international study. J Gastrointest Surg Off J Soc Surg Aliment Tract. 2012;16(1):45–51; discussion 51–2.
4. Nguyen NT, Varela JE, Sabio A, Naim J, Stamos M, Wilson SE. Reduction in prescription medication costs after laparoscopic gastric bypass. Am Surg. 2006;72(10):853–6.
5. Dixon JB, Zimmet P, Alberti KG, Rubino F. International diabetes federation taskforce on epidemiology and prevention. Bariatric surgery: an IDF statement for obese type 2 diabetes. Arq Bras Endocrinol Metabol. 2011;55(6):367–82.
6. Fenske WK, Pournaras DJ, Aasheim ET, Miras AD, Scopinaro N, Scholtz S, et al. Can a protocol for glycaemic control improve type 2 diabetes outcomes after gastric bypass? Obes Surg. 2012;22(1):90–6.
7. American Diabetes Association. Standards of medical care in diabetes – 2012. Diabetes Care. 2012;35 Suppl 1:S11–63.
8. Buchwald H, Avidor Y, Braunwald E, Jensen MD, Pories W, Fahrbach K, et al. Bariatric surgery: a systematic review and meta-analysis. JAMA. 2004;292(14):1724–37.
9. Hall TC, Pellen MGC, Sedman PC, Jain PK. Preoperative factors predicting remission of type 2 diabetes mellitus after Roux-en-Y gastric bypass surgery for obesity. Obes Surg. 2010;20(9):1245–50.
10. Buchwald H, Estok R, Fahrbach K, Banel D, Jensen MD, Pories WJ, et al. Weight and type 2 diabetes after bariatric surgery: systematic review and meta-analysis. Am J Med. 2009;122(3):248–56. e5.
11. Action to Control Cardiovascular Risk in Diabetes Study Group; Gerstein HC, Miller ME, Byington RP, Goff DC, Bigger JT, et al. Effects of intensive glucose lowering in type 2 diabetes. N Engl J Med. 2008;358(24):2545–59.
12. Duckworth W, Abraira C, Moritz T, Reda D, Emanuele N, Reaven PD, et al. Glucose control and vascular complications in veterans with type 2 diabetes. N Engl J Med. 2009;360(2):129–39.
13. Sjöström L, Peltonen M, Jacobson P, Ahlin S, Andersson-Assarsson J, Anveden Å, et al. Association of bariatric surgery with long-term remission of type 2 diabetes and with microvascular and macrovascular complications. JAMA. 2014;311(22):2297–304.
14. Pernicova I, Korbonits M. Metformin – mode of action and clinical implications for diabetes and cancer. Nat Rev Endocrinol. 2014;10(3):143–56.
15. Padwal RS, Gabr RQ, Sharma AM, Langkaas L-A, Birch DW, Karmali S, et al. Effect of gastric bypass surgery on the absorption and bioavailability of metformin. Diabetes Care. 2011;34(6):1295–300.
16. Khanna V, Kashyap SR. Clinical management of type 2 diabetes mellitus after bariatric surgery. Curr Atheroscler Rep. 2015;17(10):59.
17. Kahn SE, Cooper ME, Del Prato S. Pathophysiology and treatment of type 2 diabetes: perspectives on the past, present, and future. Lancet Lond Engl. 2014;383(9922):1068–83.
18. Bennett WL, Maruthur NM, Singh S, Segal JB, Wilson LM, Chatterjee R, et al. Comparative effectiveness and safety of medications for type 2 diabetes: an update including new drugs and 2-drug combinations. Ann Intern Med. 2011;154(9):602–13.
19. Gupta V. Glucagon-like peptide-1 analogues: an overview. Indian J Endocrinol Metab. 2013;17(3):413–21.
20. Habegger KM, Kirchner H, Yi C-X, Heppner KM, Sweeney D, Ottaway N, et al. GLP-1R agonism enhances adjustable gastric banding in diet-induced obese rats. Diabetes. 2013;62(9):3261–7.

21. Liu S-C, Tu Y-K, Chien M-N, Chien K-L. Effect of antidiabetic agents added to metformin on glycaemic control, hypoglycaemia and weight change in patients with type 2 diabetes: a network meta-analysis. Diabetes Obes Metab. 2012;14(9):810–20.
22. Tritsch AM, Bland CM, Hatzigeorgiou C, Sweeney LB, Phillips M. A retrospective review of the medical management of hypertension and diabetes mellitus following sleeve gastrectomy. Obes Surg. 2015;25(4):642–7.
23. Datta S, Qaadir A, Villanueva G, Baldwin D. Once-daily insulin glargine versus 6-hour sliding scale regular insulin for control of hyperglycemia after a bariatric surgical procedure: a randomized clinical trial. Endocr Pract Off J Am Coll Endocrinol Am Assoc Clin Endocrinol. 2007;13(3):225–31.
24. Aminian A, Brethauer SA, Daigle CR, Kirwan JP, Burguera B, Kashyap SR, et al. Outcomes of bariatric surgery in type 2 diabetic patients with diminished pancreatic secretory reserve. Acta Diabetol. 2014;51(6):1077–9.
25. Scheen AJ, Van Gaal LF. Combating the dual burden: therapeutic targeting of common pathways in obesity and type 2 diabetes. Lancet Diabetes Endocrinol. 2014;2(11):911–22.
26. Defronzo RA. Banting lecture. From the triumvirate to the ominous octet: a new paradigm for the treatment of type 2 diabetes mellitus. Diabetes. 2009;58(4):773–95.
27. Eckel RH, Kahn SE, Ferrannini E, Goldfine AB, Nathan DM, Schwartz MW, et al. Obesity and type 2 diabetes: what can be unified and what needs to be individualized? J Clin Endocrinol Metab. 2011;96(6):1654–63.
28. Chikunguwo SM, Wolfe LG, Dodson P, Meador JG, Baugh N, Clore JN, et al. Analysis of factors associated with durable remission of diabetes after Roux-en-Y gastric bypass. Surg Obes Relat Dis Off J Am Soc Bariatr Surg. 2010;6(3):254–9.
29. DiGiorgi M, Rosen DJ, Choi JJ, Milone L, Schrope B, Olivero-Rivera L, et al. Re-emergence of diabetes after gastric bypass in patients with mid- to long-term follow-up. Surg Obes Relat Dis Off J Am Soc Bariatr Surg. 2010;6(3):249–53.
30. Heber D, Greenway FL, Kaplan LM, Livingston E, Salvador J, Still C, et al. Endocrine and nutritional management of the post-bariatric surgery patient: an Endocrine Society Clinical Practice Guideline. J Clin Endocrinol Metab. 2010;95(11):4823–43.
31. Himpens J, Dobbeleir J, Peeters G. Long-term results of laparoscopic sleeve gastrectomy for obesity. Ann Surg. 2010;252(2):319–24.
32. Karmali S, Brar B, Shi X, Sharma AM, de Gara C, Birch DW. Weight recidivism post-bariatric surgery: a systematic review. Obes Surg. 2013;23(11):1922–33.
33. Odom J, Zalesin KC, Washington TL, Miller WW, Hakmeh B, Zaremba DL, et al. Behavioral predictors of weight regain after bariatric surgery. Obes Surg. 2010;20(3):349–56.
34. Martin DJ, Lee CMY, Rigas G, Tam CS. Predictors of weight loss 2 years after laparoscopic sleeve gastrectomy. Asian J Endosc Surg. 2015;8(3):328–32.
35. Robinson AH, Adler S, Stevens HB, Darcy AM, Morton JM, Safer DL. What variables are associated with successful weight loss outcomes for bariatric surgery after 1 year? Surg Obes Relat Dis Off J Am Soc Bariatr Surg. 2014;10(4):697–704.
36. National Cholesterol Education Program (NCEP) Expert Panel on Detection, Evaluation, and Treatment of High Blood Cholesterol in Adults (Adult Treatment Panel III). Third Report of the National Cholesterol Education Program (NCEP) Expert Panel on Detection, Evaluation, and Treatment of High Blood Cholesterol in Adults (Adult Treatment Panel III) final report. Circulation. 2002;106(25):3143–421.
37. Dyer AR, Elliott P, Shipley M. Body mass index versus height and weight in relation to blood pressure. Findings for the 10,079 persons in the INTERSALT study. Am J Epidemiol. 1990;131(4):589–96.
38. Hajjar I, Kotchen TA. Trends in prevalence, awareness, treatment, and control of hypertension in the United States, 1988–2000. JAMA. 2003;290(2):199–206.
39. Mokdad AH, Ford ES, Bowman BA, Dietz WH, Vinicor F, Bales VS, et al. Prevalence of obesity, diabetes, and obesity-related health risk factors, 2001. JAMA. 2003;289(1):76–9.
40. Gelber RP, Gaziano JM, Manson JE, Buring JE, Sesso HD. A prospective study of body mass index and the risk of developing hypertension in men. Am J Hypertens. 2007;20(4):370–7.

41. Aucott L, Poobalan A, Smith WCS, Avenell A, Jung R, Broom J. Effects of weight loss in overweight/obese individuals and long-term hypertension outcomes: a systematic review. Hypertension. 2005;45(6):1035–41.
42. Dornfeld LP, Maxwell MH, Waks AU, Schroth P, Tuck ML. Obesity and hypertension: long-term effects of weight reduction on blood pressure. Int J Obes. 1985;9(6):381–9.
43. The hypertension prevention trial: three-year effects of dietary changes on blood pressure. Hypertension Prevention Trial Research Group. Arch Intern Med. 1990;150(1):153–62.
44. Schauer PR, Kashyap SR, Wolski K, Brethauer SA, Kirwan JP, Pothier CE, et al. Bariatric surgery versus intensive medical therapy in obese patients with diabetes. N Engl J Med. 2012;366(17):1567–76.
45. Benaiges D, Sagué M, Flores-Le Roux JA, Pedro-Botet J, Ramón JM, Villatoro M, et al. Predictors of hypertension remission and recurrence after bariatric surgery. Am J Hypertens. 2016;29:653–9.
46. Alexander JK, Amad KH, Cole VW. Observations on some clinical features of extreme obesity, with particular reference to cardiorespiratory effects. Am J Med. 1962;32(4):512–24.
47. Ikramuddin S, Korner J, Lee W-J, Connett JE, Inabnet WB, Billington CJ, et al. Roux-en-Y gastric bypass vs intensive medical management for the control of type 2 diabetes, hypertension, and hyperlipidemia: the Diabetes Surgery Study randomized clinical trial. JAMA. 2013;309(21):2240–9.
48. Donadelli SP, Salgado W, Marchini JS, Schmidt A, Amato CAF, Ceneviva R, et al. Change in predicted 10-year cardiovascular risk following Roux-en-Y gastric bypass surgery: who benefits? Obes Surg. 2011;21(5):569–73.
49. Chobanian AV, Bakris GL, Black HR, Cushman WC, Green LA, Izzo JL, et al. The seventh report of the joint national committee on prevention, detection, evaluation, and treatment of high blood pressure: the JNC 7 report. JAMA. 2003;289(19):2560–72.
50. Franklin SS, Khan SA, Wong ND, Larson MG, Levy D. Is pulse pressure useful in predicting risk for coronary heart disease? The Framingham heart study. Circulation. 1999;100(4):354–60.
51. Benetos A, Rudnichi A, Safar M, Guize L. Pulse pressure and cardiovascular mortality in normotensive and hypertensive subjects. Hypertension. 1998;32(3):560–4.
52. Lee ML, Rosner BA, Weiss ST. Relationship of blood pressure to cardiovascular death: the effects of pulse pressure in the elderly. Ann Epidemiol. 1999;9(2):101–7.
53. Bouldin MJ, Ross LA, Sumrall CD, Loustalot FV, Low AK, Land KK. The effect of obesity surgery on obesity comorbidity. Am J Med Sci. 2006;331(4):183–93.
54. Sjöström CD, Peltonen M, Wedel H, Sjöström L. Differentiated long-term effects of intentional weight loss on diabetes and hypertension. Hypertension. 2000;36(1):20–5.
55. Segal JB, Clark JM, Shore AD, Dominici F, Magnuson T, Richards TM, et al. Prompt reduction in use of medications for comorbid conditions after bariatric surgery. Obes Surg. 2009;19(12):1646–56.

Perioperative Management of Obstructive Sleep Apnea After Bariatric Surgery

21

Rachel Maria Gomes

21.1 Introduction

Obstructive sleep apnea (OSA) is a disease characterized by episodes of cessation or decrease in respiratory airflow. Though this disease has multifactorial etiology, obesity is the most important risk factor. Other predisposing factors include age >50 years, male gender, neck circumference >40 cms, connective tissue disorders, hypothyroidism, tonsillar or adenoid hypertrophy, craniofacial abnormalities, retrognathia, macroglossia and lifestyle factors of smoking and alcohol consumption [1–6]. More than 90% of adult patients with OSA are obese and a minority have structural abnormalities or other risk factors of OSA.

The consequences of OSA are usually chronic with a negative long-term effect [6]. Its health impact includes premature deaths, sudden death from cardiac causes, nocturnal cardiac arrhythmias, hypertension (around 25% have associated OSA), ischaemic heart disease (OSA is an independent predictor of myocardial infarction& increased mortality) and stroke (OSA is an independent predictor of stroke) [7–10]. Its societal impact includes increased daytime sleepiness, increased road traffic accidents, decreased intellect, behavioral and personality changes, nocturnal enuresis and sexual dysfunction [11–13].

This disease is highly prevalent in the bariatric surgical population. Sleep studies performed during the preoperative assessment for bariatric surgery have suggested an overall prevalence of 50–90% [14, 15]. Though this condition is a chronic disease, in a perioperative bariatric surgery patient, anesthetic drugs and surgical stress exacerbate the baseline problem. Post-operatively there is increased risk of

R.M. Gomes, MS, FMAS
Bariatric Division, Upper Gastrointestinal Surgery and Minimal Access Surgery Unit, GEM Hospital and Research Centre, Coimbatore, India
e-mail: dr.gomes@rediffmail.com

P.R. Palanivelu et al. (eds.), *Bariatric Surgical Practice Guide*,
DOI 10.1007/978-981-10-2705-5_21

short–term morbidity which includes post-operative cardiac events, cardiac arrest, cardiac arrhythmias, desaturations, re-intubations, ICU transfers etc. These patients are also more likely to receive ventilatory support and ICU care with an overall increased hospital stay [16].

While OSA is characterized only by sleep-disordered breathing, a subset of morbidly obese patients may have an associated non-obstructive pulmonary condition, called obesity hypoventilation syndrome (OHS). OHS is an entity characterized by obesity with daytime hypoventilation with or without sleep-disordered breathing in the absence of an alternative neuromuscular, mechanical or metabolic explanation for hypoventilation. While patients with simple OSA have eucapnia during the daytime, those with OHS have persistent daytime hypercapnia and chronic respiratory acidosis. OHS on arterial blood analysis is characterized by hypoxemia ($PaO2 < 70$ mmHg) and hypercarbia ($PaCO2 > 45$ mmHg) while breathing room air in an awake, resting morbidly obese patient. This sub-population is at higher risk of developing pulmonary hypertension, right-sided cardiac failure and early mortality compared to eucapnic patients with OSA [17].

21.2 Pathophysiology of OSA

The nasopharynx and oropharynx form a passageway for air to the trachea. The tone of the nasopharyngeal and oropharyngeal musculature maintains the patency of the upper airway when awake. During sleep these relax resulting in relative obstruction of the airway. Although the mechanisms are still poorly understood, OSA in obesity is associated with deposition of fat around the tongue and soft tissues in the pharynx which decrease the upper airway passageway to the trachea which combined with decreased tone during sleep causing their collapse at this time thus obstructing the airway [18, 19]. Insulin resistance and inflammatory cytokines also possibly contribute to the pathological and somatic manifestations of OSA [20, 21].

The sequence of events that occur during sleep are as follows. With sleep onset, there is a loss of the upper airway reflex and pharyngeal dilator muscle activity decreases, the pharynx closes and the apnea begins. During the apnea, hypoxia and hypercapnia develop causing a decrease in both heart rate and blood pressure leading to increasing ventilatory effort. When this effort reaches a threshold level, the patient arouses with a reflex surge in sympathetic autonomic tone, with tachycardia and hypertension. Pharyngeal muscle activity is restored, and the airway opens. The patient then hyperventilates to correct the blood gas derangements, returns to sleep, and the cycle begins again. As a result, sleep can be severely disrupted by the repetitive arousals needed to end the apneas, and episodes of cyclic hypoxia and hypercapnia. Also as most apneic episodes are accompanied by hypoxemia, hypercapnia and surges in sympathetic autonomic tone these repeatedly stress the patient's cardiovascular system increasing the risk of several cardiovascular consequences.

OHS has a different pathophysiology from OSA. OHS is hypothesized to be caused by mechanical factors that include increased abdominal pressure raising the diaphragm, increased chest wall weight, fatty deposition within the diaphragm and intercostal muscles decreasing the strength of the respiratory muscles as well as lung circulatory abnormalities. However as this is common to all obese patients and since only a small subset of obese patients suffer from OHS it is suggested that the pathophysiology of OHS is contributed to by a combination of an impaired central drive to ventilate in response to both hypoxia and hypercapnia alongside impaired respiratory mechanics [22].

21.3 Diagnosis of OSA

Diagnosis is based on history and physical examination. Clinical symptoms include loud snoring, witnessed apnea, arousal with gasping and choking, disrupted sleep, restless sleep, daytime sleepiness and inappropriate falling asleep. Clinical signs include obesity, increased neck circumference >40 cm, retrognathia and increased mallampatti score. Several clinical screening tools for OSA have been developed, such as the Epworth Sleepiness Score, the Maintenance of Wakefulness Test, the Berlin Questionnaire and the STOP-BANG Questionnaire, with variable sensitivities and specificities [23–26]. The standard method of diagnosing OSA is via polysomnography (PSG). During each hour of sleep, the number of apneas, defined as complete cessation of airflow, and hypopneas, defined as a 50–90 % decrease in airflow and at least a 4 % drop in oxygen saturation for >10 s, are recorded. An "apnea hypopnea index" (AHI), or "respiratory disturbance index" (RDI) is used to quantitate these apneas and hypopneas. In general, an AHI of less than 5 is normal, 5–15 is mild sleep apnea, >15 is moderate sleep apnea and >30 severe sleep apnea. In addition to substantiating the diagnosis of OSA the role of a sleep study is to make recommendations for treatment (requirement and level of continuous positive airway pressure (CPAP) or bi-level positive airway pressure (Bi-PAP)).

21.4 Treatment of OSA

Treatment is indicated in moderate to severe OSA. Mild OSA does not warrant any specialized treatment. CPAP is highly effective in the treatment of OSA in adults [27]. Positive pressure ventilation functions as a pneumatic splint for the collapsing upper airway. It improves objective and subjective measures of OSA. However poor adherence to CPAP is widely recognized (~35 % drop-outs) as a significant limiting factor for OSA treatment, in addition to the cost [28, 29].

Several surgical procedures aimed at increasing airway patency do exist. Uvulopalatoplasty is the most widely performed pharyngeal surgical technique for OSA. It is mainly targeted at improving snoring. When assessed objectively by preoperative and postoperative PSG it has been shown that only around one-third of patients obtain a satisfactory response though significant improvements were noted in quality of life. It has also been shown to be not very effective in patients with a BMI >28 kg/m^2 [30].

Weight loss by any method is a well-documented treatment for OSA. Modest weight loss of 10–20% by lifestyle changes is associated with improvement of symptoms and greater than 26% reduction in AHI [31]. Bariatric surgery is associated with significant improvement of symptoms and greater than 50% reduction in AHI in the long term offering marked improvement [32, 33].

21.5 Screening, Evaluation and Optimization of OSA in a Bariatric Surgical Patient

Some studies in literature recommend routine screening for OSA prior to bariatric surgery reporting a high prevalence of OSA and a poor correlation with OSA based on clinical symptoms alone [14, 15]. Other studies looking into the outcomes of patients subjected to PSG suggest that only clinical screening with optimization of those detected does not increase postoperative pulmonary complications. Most institutions in clinical practice refer only patients with clinical symptoms of OSA for PSG and do not make this a routine preoperative test prior to bariatric surgery.

Of the several clinical screening tools available, the STOP-BANG questionnaire is most commonly used and was originally developed for the surgical population. It is useful in the preoperative setting to predict OSA severity and triage patients for further confirmatory testing [34]. The STOP-BANG scoring tool has been detailed in Table 21.1. Patients with STOP-BANG scores 0–2 may be considered low risk, 3–4 intermediate risk, and 5–8 high risk for OSA [26, 35].

There is evidence to show that OSA increases postoperative complications, especially oxygen desaturation [36]. Also OSA patients who did not use PAP devices prior to surgery but required PAP therapy after surgery had increased complication rates [36]. Peri-operative CPAP significantly reduces postoperative AHI and improves oxygen saturation in surgical patients with moderate and severe OSA [37]. There is also evidence to show that CPAP in addition to respiratory benefits may lead to an improvement in hypertension and other related co-morbidities especially for patients with moderate to severe OSA [38].

Table 21.1 STOP-BANG scoring tool

Do you **S**nore loudly? Yes/no
Do you often feel **T**ired, sleepy, or fatigued during the day? Yes/no
Has anyone **O**bserved you stop breathing? Yes/no
Have you been diagnosed with high blood **P**ressure? Yes/no
BMI > 35? Yes/no
Age > 50? Yes/no
Neck circumference > 17″ (male), 16″ (female)? Yes/no
Gender = male? Yes/no
Every 'Yes' answer is scored 1 point Patients with scores 0–2 may be considered low risk, 3–4 intermediate risk, and 5–8 high risk of OSA

STOP-BANG scores can be used for the eventual decision to evaluate a patient preoperatively with polysomnography. For patients with STOP-BANG score 5–8 (high risk of moderate to severe OSA) a polysomnography should be considered for diagnosis and treatment. This is especially important in patients with comorbid diseases (uncontrolled hypertension, heart failure, arrhythmias, pulmonary hypertension, cerebrovascular disease, and severe metabolic syndrome) wherein diagnosis and treatment will help for both respiratory optimization and co-morbidity stabilization. Patients with an intermediate risk of OSA based on STOP-BANG may represent false positives on screening, or may have less severe OSA and may proceed for surgery without further testing with perioperative OSA precautions. Patients deemed to be low risk on screening with score 0–2 on STOP-BANG are unlikely to have OSA. These patients may proceed for surgery with routine perioperative care.

No sufficient data exist in literature regarding the optimal time for pre-operative CPAP therapy in order to decrease the risk of perioperative complications. It has been shown that patients treated with therapeutic CPAP for 3 weeks showed significant reductions in the apnea-hypopnea index, decrease in fatigue, increase in vigor and decreased sleepiness [39]. It is reasonable to incorporate some time (~3 weeks) for adaptation to the device and benefits of CPAP in the preoperative period but whether this will translate into decreased complications postoperatively is still not known.

21.6 Perioperative Care of the Bariatric Patient with OSA

Patients with OSA who undergo bariatric surgery have an increased risk of perioperative complications [16]. The duration of this increased risk extends to around 1 week post-operatively of which the first 3 days after surgery pose the greatest risk for apnea from drug-induced sleep and the next 4 days pose a higher risk because of REM sleep rebound secondary to disturbed sleep architecture in the immediate post-operative period.

This increased risk peri-operatively mandates that certain 'OSA risk mitigation' strategies be followed in the preoperative, intraoperative and postoperative period [40].

OSA risk mitigation includes several steps.

- Preoperatively
  Sedative medications should be avoided.
- Intra-operatively
  Difficult mask ventilation/difficult intubation should be anticipated.
  CPAP pre-oxygenation and awake intubation should be considered.
  Proton pump inhibitors and rapid sequence induction should be followed as chances of as GERD (gastroesophageal reflux disease) is high.
  Short acting anesthetic agents should be used.
- Post-operatively

As there is an increased incidence of post-extubation obstruction it is essential that full reversal of neuromuscular blockade is verified.

Extubation should be done only when fully active and conscious.

Semi-upright position should be used for extubation and recovery.

An oral or nasal airway should be used to maintain airway.

- For postoperative care

Multimodal analgesia techniques should be preferred.

Avoid opiods whenever possible and use non steroidal anti-inflammatory agents (NSAIDs).

Clonidine or Dexmedetomidine can be used as pain adjuvant or as opiod sparing agents.

If needed IV bolus narcotics can be used and basal infusion can be avoided.

- For postoperative monitoring

Continuous pulse oximetry monitoring should be used with ready access to medical intervention.

Select higher risk patients such as those with severe OSA, multiple comorbidities, superobesity, or advanced age may be monitored in an ICU setting at the discretion of the surgeon/intensivist.

Monitoring can be stopped once oxygen saturation of >90 % is maintained in room air and during sleep, with no hypoxemia/airway obstruction.

21.7 Use of CPAP in the Postoperative Period

There exist no clear guidelines on the usage of CPAP in the post-operative period. Perioperative CPAP significantly reduces postoperative AHI and improves oxygen saturation in surgical patients with moderate and severe OSA [37]. However studies have also shown that postoperative CPAP and Bi-PAP can be safely omitted if patients are observed in a monitored setting and their pulmonary status is optimized by aggressive incentive spirometry and early ambulation [41, 42]. It should also be noted that there is no increase in overall or pulmonary complications despite non-routine use of CPAP [41, 42]. However it may still be required in select patients with worsening pulmonary status postoperatively. Importantly postoperative use of CPAP should not be viewed as potentially adverse to outcomes following bariatric surgery. Evidence in literature shows that the risk of anastomotic complications is not increased [43].

Thus in patients with diagnosed OSA who undergo bariatric surgery and who were using CPAP may be required to use CPAP in the post-operative period occasionally. It is often best if the patient brings their own CPAP mask, with or without their machine, with them to the hospital. This ensures the equipment fits the patient well and is readily available for use in the postoperative period.

It has been shown that >62 % of patients have significant residual disease after bariatric surgery in the long term, with an AHI of more than 15 [32]. Though there is significant subjective improvement in most patients absence of clinical symptoms does not necessarily correlate with normalization of AHI and/or severity of sleep apnea. The severity of preoperative OSA often influences the degree to which OSA improves or resolves after bariatric surgery. Many patients may still need treatment of OSA based on their AHI. Institutions differ in their practice regarding the use of CPAP in the long term post bariatric surgery. While some discontinue use others re-titrate the settings and continue to use postoperatively. However as long term effects of OSA is of concern and as continuing weight loss will have a continuing improvement of OSA, surgeons can consider repeat PSG testing after significant weight loss and restart CPAP accordingly. Currently no consensus or recommendation exists regarding indications or timing for repeat PSG either in the general population or after bariatric surgery.

Recommendations

- Weight loss by any method is a well-documented treatment for OSA.
- The standard method of diagnosing OSA is via polysomnography (PSG) which can be selectively used based on preoperative symptoms by clinical screening tools.
- Patients with moderate to severe OSA should be optimized preoperatively with continuous positive airway pressure (CPAP) for a minimum period of 3 weeks
- Postoperative CPAP and Bi-PAP can be safely omitted if patients are observed in a monitored setting and optimized by aggressive incentive spirometry and early ambulation.
- Postoperative CPAP and Bi-PAP can be used in select patients with worsening pulmonary status postoperatively without the risk of anastomotic complications.
- The need for continuing CPAP in the postoperative period may be based on clinical findings.

References

1. Wilhelm CP, de Shazo RD, Tamanna S, Ullah MI, Skipworth LB. The nose, upper airway, and obstructive sleep apnea. Ann Allergy Asthma Immunol Off Publ Am Coll Allergy Asthma Immunol. 2015;115(2):96–102.
2. Tan H-L, Kheirandish-Gozal L, Abel F, Gozal D. Craniofacial syndromes and sleep-related breathing disorders. Sleep Med Rev. 2015;27:74–88.
3. Davies RJ, Ali NJ, Stradling JR. Neck circumference and other clinical features in the diagnosis of the obstructive sleep apnoea syndrome. Thorax. 1992;47(2):101–5.
4. Ryan CM, Pillar G. Adolescent obesity, adenotonsillar hypertrophy, and obstructive sleep apnea. Am J Respir Crit Care Med. 2015;191(11):1220–2.
5. Simsek G, Karacayli C, Ozel A, Arslan B, Muluk NB, Kilic R. Blood parameters as indicators of upper airway obstruction in children with adenoid or adenotonsillar hypertrophy. J Craniofac Surg. 2015;26(3):e213–6.

6. Strobel RJ, Rosen RC. Obesity and weight loss in obstructive sleep apnea: a critical review. Sleep. 1996;19(2):104–15.
7. Floras JS. Hypertension and sleep apnea. Can J Cardiol. 2015;31(7):889–97.
8. Torres G, Sánchez-de-la-Torre M, Barbé F. Relationship between OSA and hypertension. Chest. 2015;148(3):824–32.
9. Lyons OD, Bradley TD. Heart failure and sleep apnea. Can J Cardiol. 2015;31(7):898–908.
10. Lyons OD, Ryan CM. Sleep apnea and stroke. Can J Cardiol. 2015;31(7):918–27.
11. Bhattacharyya N. Sleep and health implications of snoring: a populational analysis. Laryngoscope. 2015;125(10):2413–6.
12. Husnu T, Ersoz A, Bulent E, Tacettin O, Remzi A, Bulent A, et al. Obstructive sleep apnea syndrome and erectile dysfunction: does long term continuous positive airway pressure therapy improve erections? Afr Health Sci. 2015;15(1):171–9.
13. Osorio RS, Gumb T, Pirraglia E, Varga AW, Lu S-E, Lim J, et al. Sleep-disordered breathing advances cognitive decline in the elderly. Neurology. 2015;84(19):1964–71.
14. O'Keeffe T, Patterson EJ. Evidence supporting routine polysomnography before bariatric surgery. Obes Surg. 2004;14(1):23–6.
15. Frey WC, Pilcher J. Obstructive sleep-related breathing disorders in patients evaluated for bariatric surgery. Obes Surg. 2003;13(5):676–83.
16. Liao P, Yegneswaran B, Vairavanathan S, Zilberman P, Chung F. Postoperative complications in patients with obstructive sleep apnea: a retrospective matched cohort study. Can J Anesth Can Anesth. 2009;56(11):819–28.
17. Castro-Añón O, de Llano LA P, De la Fuente Sánchez S, Golpe R, Méndez Marote L, Castro-Castro J, et al. Obesity-hypoventilation syndrome: increased risk of death over sleep apnea syndrome. PLoS One. 2015;10(2):e0117808.
18. Westbrook PR. Sleep disorders and upper airway obstruction in adults. Otolaryngol Clin North Am. 1990;23(4):727–43.
19. Shelton KE, Woodson H, Gay S, Suratt PM. Pharyngeal fat in obstructive sleep apnea. Am Rev Respir Dis. 1993;148(2):462–6.
20. Vgontzas AN, Papanicolaou DA, Bixler EO, Kales A, Tyson K, Chrousos GP. Elevation of plasma cytokines in disorders of excessive daytime sleepiness: role of sleep disturbance and obesity. J Clin Endocrinol Metab. 1997;82(5):1313–6.
21. Vgontzas AN, Papanicolaou DA, Bixler EO, Hopper K, Lotsikas A, Lin HM, et al. Sleep apnea and daytime sleepiness and fatigue: relation to visceral obesity, insulin resistance, and hypercytokinemia. J Clin Endocrinol Metab. 2000;85(3):1151–8.
22. Shahi B, Praglowski B, Deitel M. Sleep-related disorders in the obese. Obes Surg. 1992;2(2):157–68.
23. Banks S, Barnes M, Tarquinio N, Pierce RJ, Lack LC, McEvoy RD. Factors associated with maintenance of wakefulness test mean sleep latency in patients with mild to moderate obstructive sleep apnoea and normal subjects. J Sleep Res. 2004;13(1):71–8.
24. Chung F, Yegneswaran B, Liao P, Chung SA, Vairavanathan S, Islam S, et al. Validation of the Berlin questionnaire and American Society of Anesthesiologists checklist as screening tools for obstructive sleep apnea in surgical patients. Anesthesiology. 2008;108(5):822–30.
25. Serafini FM, MacDowell Anderson W, Rosemurgy AS, Strait T, Murr MM. Clinical predictors of sleep apnea in patients undergoing bariatric surgery. Obes Surg. 2001;11(1):28–31.
26. Chung F, Abdullah HR, Liao P. STOP-bang questionnaire: a practical approach to screen for obstructive sleep apnea. Chest. 2016;149(3):631–8.
27. Giles TL, Lasserson TJ, Smith BJ, White J, Wright J, Cates CJ. Continuous positive airways pressure for obstructive sleep apnoea in adults. Cochrane Database Syst Rev. 2006;1:CD001106.
28. Campos-Rodriguez F, Martinez-Alonso M, Sanchez-de-la-Torre M, Barbe F; Spanish Sleep Network. Long-term adherence to continuous positive airway pressure therapy in non-sleepy sleep apnea patients. Sleep Med. 2016;17:1–6.
29. Guralnick AS, Pant M, Minhaj M, Sweitzer BJ, Mokhlesi B. CPAP adherence in patients with newly diagnosed obstructive sleep apnea prior to elective surgery. J Clin Sleep Med JCSM Off Publ Am Acad Sleep Med. 2012;8(5):501–6.

30. Rollheim J, Miljeteig H, Osnes T. Body mass index less than 28 kg/m2 is a predictor of subjective improvement after laser-assisted uvulopalatoplasty for snoring. Laryngoscope. 1999; 109(3):411–4.
31. Peppard PE, Young T, Palta M, Dempsey J, Skatrud J. Longitudinal study of moderate weight change and sleep-disordered breathing. JAMA. 2000;284(23):3015–21.
32. Greenburg DL, Lettieri CJ, Eliasson AH. Effects of surgical weight loss on measures of obstructive sleep apnea: a meta-analysis. Am J Med. 2009;122(6):535–42.
33. Ashrafian H, Toma T, Rowland SP, Harling L, Tan A, Efthimiou E, et al. Bariatric surgery or Non-surgical weight loss for obstructive sleep apnoea? a systematic review and comparison of meta-analyses. Obes Surg. 2015;25(7):1239–50.
34. Seet E, Chua M, Liaw CM. High STOP-BANG questionnaire scores predict intraoperative and early postoperative adverse events. Singapore Med J. 2015;56(4):212–6.
35. Chung F, Yang Y, Liao P. Predictive performance of the STOP-Bang score for identifying obstructive sleep apnea in obese patients. Obes Surg. 2013;23(12):2050–7.
36. Liao P, Yegneswaran B, Vairavanathan S, Zilberman P, Chung F. Postoperative complications in patients with obstructive sleep apnea: a retrospective matched cohort study. Can J Anaesth J Can Anesthésie. 2009;56(11):819–28.
37. Liao P, Luo Q, Elsaid H, Kang W, Shapiro CM, Chung F. Perioperative auto-titrated continuous positive airway pressure treatment in surgical patients with obstructive sleep apnea: a randomized controlled trial. Anesthesiology. 2013;119(4):837–47.
38. O'Connor GT, Caffo B, Newman AB, Quan SF, Rapoport DM, Redline S, et al. Prospective study of sleep-disordered breathing and hypertension. Am J Respir Crit Care Med. 2009;179(12):1159–64.
39. Tomfohr LM, Ancoli-Israel S, Loredo JS, Dimsdale JE. Effects of continuous positive airway pressure on fatigue and sleepiness in patients with obstructive sleep apnea: data from a randomized controlled trial. Sleep. 2011;34(1):121–6.
40. Chung F. Obstructive sleep apnea and anesthesia– what an anesthesiologist should know? 2014. Available from: http://www.stopbang.ca/pdf/refresher.pdf.
41. Grover BT, Priem DM, Mathiason MA, Kallies KJ, Thompson GP, Kothari SN. Intensive care unit stay not required for patients with obstructive sleep apnea after laparoscopic Roux-en-Y gastric bypass. Surg Obes Relat Dis Off J Am Soc Bariatr Surg. 2010;6(2):165–70.
42. Jensen C, Tejirian T, Lewis C, Yadegar J, Dutson E, Mehran A. Postoperative CPAP and BiPAP use can be safely omitted after laparoscopic Roux-en-Y gastric bypass. Surg Obes Relat Dis Off J Am Soc Bariatr Surg. 2008;4(4):512–4.
43. Ramirez A, Lalor PF, Szomstein S, Rosenthal RJ. Continuous positive airway pressure in immediate postoperative period after laparoscopic Roux-en-Y gastric bypass: is it safe? Surg Obes Relat Dis Off J Am Soc Bariatr Surg. 2009;5(5):544–6.

Enhanced Recovery After Bariatric Surgery

22

Faruq Badiuddin

22.1 Introduction

Enhanced recovery after surgery (ERAS) protocols are multimodal perioperative care pathways designed to achieve early recovery after surgical procedures by maintaining preoperative organ function and reducing the profound stress response following surgery. The key elements of ERAS protocols include preoperative counseling, optimization of nutrition, standardized analgesic and anesthetic regimens and early mobilization. Despite the significant body of evidence indicating that ERAS protocols lead to improved outcomes, they challenge traditional surgical doctrine, and as a result their implementation has been slow [1]. Also referred to as Fast Track Surgery (FTS) these protocols have been successfully practiced in colorectal surgery over many years [2]. The body of evidence is quite compelling, but so far their adoption in bariatric surgery has been rather sporadic and patchy.

Traditionally bariatric surgery has been perceived as being a 'high risk' surgery partly due to the difficulties with anesthesia of the obese patient and the existence of multiple co-morbidities in these patients. In part, the perceptions which were derived from the days of open bariatric surgery, where post-operative complications used to be high, are still active with the practitioners of bariatric surgery. With the widespread adoption of the laparoscopic approach in bariatric surgery, peri-operative morbidity has fallen dramatically. Recent evidence fromthe Longitudinal Assessment of Bariatric Surgery (LABS) group has shown us that the peri-operative mortality and morbidity of bariatric surgery is as low as that of laparoscopic cholecystectomy [3]. There are sporadic reports of some centers successfully adopting ERAS programs [4–8]. A wider adoption of such protocols has the potential to alter the perceptions that Bariatric Surgery is not so dangerous or complicated, leading to greater acceptance of bariatric surgery by patients and referring physicians.

F. Badiuddin, MS, FRCS (England)
Department of General, Bariatric and Upper GI Surgery, Mediclinic Dubai Mall, Dubai, UAE
e-mail: faruq1@gmail.com

P.R. Palanivelu et al. (eds.), *Bariatric Surgical Practice Guide*,
DOI 10.1007/978-981-10-2705-5_22

22.2 Principles of ERAS

ERAS Programs require the adoption of the philosophy of early recovery by all members of the team involved in the care of the obese patient, similar to the processes and protocols laid out in a Day Surgery Unit.

The key elements of an ERAS Program incorporate the following

1. Pre-operative information to the patient
2. Pre-operative optimization of organ function
3. Stress reduction in the operating room
4. Effective pain relief and prophylaxis for nausea and vomiting
5. Modification of the post-operative care with the aim of early mobilization and early enteral feeding

The expected outcomes of an ERAS program are

1. Reduction in morbidity
2. Enhanced recovery
3. Early discharge
4. Patient satisfaction
5. Cost savings

22.3 Designing an ERAS Program

The design and implementation of an ERAS Program involves the creation of procedure specific care plans, staff training on the principles of ERAS, and multi-disciplinary collaboration between the pre-operative team, the surgeon, the endocrinologist/physician, the anesthetic team and the post-operative nursing professionals, and most importantly the involvement of the patient who is fully informed of the post-operative journey. In a larger organization it may be desirable to appoint designated personnel who should be part of the "ERAS Bariatric Team" and who receive appropriate training into the ERAS protocols.

Clear guidelines for the pre-operative care pathways, intraoperative protocols and post- operative care plans should be developed and all personnel receive rigorous training in the implementation of these pathways.

22.3.1 Pre-operative Pathways

22.3.1.1 Pre-operative Investigations and Treatments

- Investigation for H. Pylori infection and eradication therapy
- Investigation of vitamin deficiencies and correction
- Investigation for anemia and appropriate treatment

- Investigation of metabolic disease and optimization of metabolic status including the recommendations on post-operative management of diabetes in the immediate post-operative period
- Investigation for cardio-respiratory function and appropriate treatment including the recommendations on post-operative management of hypertension and heart disease.
- Upper GI endoscopy is increasingly being adopted as an essential pre –op evaluation modality routinely. However, in a patient who gives a history of GERD or other suspicious upper GI symptoms, this should be a mandatory step.

22.3.1.2 Pre-operative Optimization Diet

- Fat Free Diet
- Vitamin Supplements
- Protein Supplements

The purpose of this diet is to build a reserve of essential nutrients in anticipation of a low nutrition catabolic post-operative state, when the patient receives only a liquid diet until 2 weeks. The second objective is to reduce the hepatic steatosis to make the surgery safer by slimming down the liver so it can be easily lifted off the stomach and does not get traumatized and bleed during surgery.

22.3.1.3 Patient Counseling on the Recovery Process

- Early Enteral Nutrition
- Early Mobilization
- Incentive Spirometry

These measures should be clearly discussed and demonstrated to the patient during the pre-operative visit. This is a critical requirement as patient's active participation in the implementation of the postoperative care pathways is essential to ensure predictable outcomes.

22.3.2 Intra Operative Protocols

Several intra-operative measures have an impact on the post-operative recovery process. The objective is to reduce the inflammatory response to surgical trauma, to prevent post-operative nausea and vomiting, reduce pain enabling early mobilization and commencing early enteral nutrition. Several of the measures described below are designed to get the patient upright immediately after surgery and spend as little time as possible in bed.

22.3.2.1 Minimally Invasive Techniques

The migration from open to laparoscopic surgery was a game changer in the widespread adoption of bariatric surgery and the reduction in the morbidities and the mortality associated with bariatric surgery. The most common complications related to bariatric surgery prior to the introduction of laparoscopic surgery were related to the state of recumbency i.e. DVT and PE as well as basal pneumonias. The advantages of laparoscopic surgery are well known, but become especially important in the context of bariatric surgery where a shorter operating time and reduction in the surgical trauma making this otherwise major surgery as safe as a laparoscopic cholecystectomy. An efficient and co-ordinated operating team familiar with the procedure and surgeon to reduce the total operating time to less than 120 min further reduces the incidence of complications including DVT [9].

22.3.2.2 Ultra Short Acting Volatile Anesthetic Agents and Muscle Relaxants

It is important to have the patient breathe spontaneously as soon as possible immediately after surgery, so that assisted ventilation and oxygenation can be discontinued. The longer the patient remains under the influence of muscle relaxants the longer it takes to have the patient mobilizing.

Neuromuscular blockade (NMB) achieved with the continuous infusion of a combination of Propofol and Remefentanil seems to achieve this objective of shortening the anesthetic time and avoids the hangover effect of the drugs in the immediate post op period. Opioids to be avoided or only used in small doses during anesthesia. Remefentanil has been also known to reduce the surgical stress response. The technique of "intravenous anesthesia" and not using anesthetic gases helps recover the patient rapidly after the procedure. Use of long acting local anesthetics intraperitoneally and at the port sites also has the beneficial effects of reduction in the stress response

22.3.2.3 Intraoperative Prophylaxis for Nausea and Vomiting

One of the most important measures especially in gastric surgery with stapling or anastomosis is the prevention of retching and vomiting in the immediate post-operative period. These symptoms could be a consequence of the side effects of the anesthetic and narcotic agents often used during anesthesia as well as the effect of the surgery on the stomach. Arguably these measures would prevent potential bleeds (intra or extra luminal) and any strain and weakening of the staple lines. Therefore prophylaxis started early in the intraoperative period would prevent these actions in the recovery room as well as post operatively in the ward thereafter. 5HT3 receptor antagonists (Ondansetron) and Dexamethasone 4 mg to be given at the start of the operation and the Ondansetron to be continued for 24 h thereafter [10].

22.3.2.4 Intraoperative Dexamethasone

Dexamethasone 4 mg given at the start of surgery has been shown to effectively suppress the post-operative inflammatory response associated with the surgical trauma, reduce the incidence of nausea and vomiting, and reduce the requirement of strong analgesic agents. We believe that corticosteroids also reduce the edema around the staple lines and anastomoses thus allowing effective enteral feeding in the immediate aftermath of surgery [11].

22.3.2.5 Intraoperative Intermittent Calf Compression

It is well established that use of intermittent calf compression devices reduces the incidence of deep venous thrombosis (DVT) and pulmonary embolism (PE). In bariatric surgery, the sitting position used promotes pooling of blood in the legs and using sequential compression device prevents pooling and clotting thereby reducing the incidence of clots that may later progress to DVT [9].

22.3.2.6 Prevention of Hypothermia

Hypothermia leads to hypoxia; shivering and muscle stiffness with consequent diaphragmatic splinting lowers oxygen saturation, increasing patient discomfort and pain. This is also known to lowering platelet count and increasing the chances of bleeding.

Preventing hypothermia in the operating room (OR) with the use of body warmers, warmed IV fluids and warmed oxygen are several measures used to prevent hypothermia and accelerate the recovery process

22.3.2.7 Sparing Use of IV Fluids

Excessive IV fluids especially when not warmed lead to patient discomfort and increase in fluid retention. This also might increase pulmonary edema and reduce spontaneous oxygenation. Keeping the patient dry in the immediate post-operative period may also benefit in the wake of the reduction in the renal output from the post inflammatory response.

22.3.2.8 No NG Tubes, Catheters, Epidurals, Drains or Oxygen Tubes

Having an unencumbered patient allows for early mobilization. We have found that using drains and catheters as well as other similar equipment, unless it is a clinical necessity, is the key to early mobilization and fast tracking the patient to early ambulation and feeding. In our series we have only sparingly used these modalities for a specific indication and not as routine practice.

22.3.2.9 Peritoneal and Gastric Washout

A thorough peritoneal washout until the saline "returns clear" to remove blood and clots reduces peritoneal irritation and the consequent pain and therefore the necessity of using strong narcotics.

We wash the stomach with 250 ml of normal saline soon after the methylene blue leak test before removing the gastric tube. This is done with pressure (Gastric stress test) that ensures the clearance of residual methylene blue as well as blood and clots from the stomach. In addition, when done under vision of the laparoscope, the surgeon is able to evaluate clearance of the saline from the stomach tube and know that there are no rotational deformities or clot obstructions that might lead to post-operative vomiting.

22.3.3 Post-operative Pathway

22.3.3.1 Non-narcotic Analgesia

We have effectively used intra-peritoneal Bupivacaine to reduce the incidence of pain from the peritoneal irritation from residual $CO^2$and blood in the peritoneal cavity and reduce the dose of analgesics. It is common practice to use a combination of Paracetamol and non steroidal anti-inflammatory agents (NSAIDs) post laparoscopic surgery for analgesia. Bariatric surgery is no different. As long as the trauma to the abdominal wall is minimized by using muscle splitting trocars, and ensuring minimal residual blood in the peritoneal cavity, narcotic analgesia is rarely required. In fact narcotics delay recovery by making the patients drowsy, encourages them to stay in bed, and induces nausea and vomiting, impedes breathing and spontaneous oxygenation; discourages enteral feeding and the use of respirometer. In addition they do not reduce the inflammatory response as NSAIDs do.

In our practice, there is an express instruction to inform the surgeon if the resident doctor feels obliged to administer a narcotic analgesia. The premise is if the patient pain score is significant enough to require a narcotic analgesic, then it might be a circumstance to review the patient for a complication that might require an early exploration. Anti-spasmodics are also routinely administered to prevent gastric spasm, another potent cause for visceral pain and nausea.

22.3.3.2 Incentive Spirometry

Starting 2 hours after return to ward the patient starts using the respirometer. Preventing basal collapse and allowing the lungs to expand minimizes the risk of developing pulmonary complications. The key is making the patient believe they can do it. We allow the patient to use the respirometer in the clinic at the immediate pre-operative visit to get them to understand how to use this device and the target of reaching the flow to 1200 ml/min. They are also given to understand that this is an essential act to prevent complications that might prolong their hospital stay or necessitate readmission. This modality requires the active participation of patient and requires effective pre-operative counseling and demonstration to be effective in the post-operative period. Despite this, compliance may be a problem and active encouragement from the post operative ward personnel in combination with effective pain relief ensures a better compliance rate. Not using narcotics and allowing the patient to sit while using the device gives better results.

22.3.3.3 Early Mobilization

Obese patients are best nursed in the sitting position. Pre-operative counseling to sit in preference to sleeping and to walk atleast twice on the day of surgery, and active efforts by the ward staff to ensure compliance ensures early mobilization. In addition, effective non-narcotic analgesia keeps the patient alert and willing to mobilize out of bed early.

22.3.3.4 Routine Anti-emetics

We prescribe anti-emetics to be administered at 6 hourly intervals regularly instead of "as required". Anticipating nausea and vomiting and administering anti emetics routinely helps keeping the patient nausea free and ensures adequate oral intake of liquids.

22.3.3.5 Early Nutrition

Early liquid intake is a critical step in giving confidence to patients that they can manage themselves at home soon after discharge. The premise is, if the operated stomach is not considered waterproof right after surgery then one should rethink their stapling technique. As long as one has ensured a negative leak test and stress test, administration of water immediate post operatively is safe. The patient is advised to drink continuously at 10–15 min intervals, and to take gulps instead of sips. Once the patients have demonstrated satisfactory warm water intake by day two, they would be allowed all clear liquids. Warm liquids are tolerated better than cold ones.

22.3.3.6 Early Discharge from Hospital

Patients are ready to be discharged by day two (1st post op day) after they have demonstrated adequate fluid intake, vitals are stable, pain is under control and there is no nausea or vomiting.

They are prescribed liquid paracetamol, diclofenac suppositories, DVT prophylaxis, as well as a proton pump inhibitor.

They are told to ensure a minimum of 2000–2500 ml of clear liquids per day for 1 week.

22.3.3.7 24 Hour Helpline to the Specialist Bariatric Nurse or Resident Doctor

One of the essential components of an ERAS program is to ensure easy access to the surgeons practice in case of an adverse situation. A 24 h access to a member of the ERAS team should be available to the patient or the relative. This can prevent unnecessary readmissions and guarantee appropriate early care in case of a genuine emergency.

22.4 Advantages of ERAS Programs

The major positive outcomes of ERAS programs are

1. Minimizing complications associated with recumbency such as deep venous thrombosis, pulmonary embolism, and basal Pneumonia
2. Minimizing the risks associated with prolonged hospital stay such as hospital acquired infections.
3. Reducing the cost of hospitalization
4. Patient satisfaction

These outcomes translates into surgeries no longer being considered as high risk as previously considered and thereby greater acceptance of these procedures.

22.5 Limitations of ERAS Programs

Elderly patients who have other co-morbidities which would require medical supervision for their cardiovascular disease or pulmonary disease may be unsuitable for early discharge. Patients who live alone and may not have a responsible adult supervising them at home may also be unsuitable candidates for early discharge. Patients whose pain control is inadequate or those who continue to have nausea preventing adequate liquid intake may need longer hospital stay until satisfactory hydration status could be ensured.

Conclusions

- Fast track surgery programs have been successfully implemented in Colorectal Surgeries [2]. There have been very few reports of FTS or ERAS programs within the Bariatric Surgery literature.
- Results from centers which have adopted such protocols show that the same Fast Track principles can be applied to Bariatric Surgery too quite safely without any additional morbidity or mortality. In fact the incidence of complications is reduced through the FTS Program due to the shorter hospital stay [1, 4, 12, 13].
- Significant cost savings from shorter hospital stay [12].
- A multidisciplinary approach is essential.
- Helps achieve higher patient satisfaction

Recommendations

- The success of a ERAS program depends on the collabaration of a a committed and trained multi-disciplinary team.
- Preoperative pathways in ERAS protocols should include optimization of comorbidities and nutrition and patient counseling on the recovery process.
- Intraoperative protocols should include use of ultra short acting volatile anesthetic agents and muscle relaxants:, prophylaxis for nausea and vomiting, prevention of hypothermia, peritoneal and gastric washout, avoiding use of tubes, and sparing use of iv fluids.
- Postoperative pathways should include effective pain relief, early mobilization, spirometry, routine prophylaxis for nausea and vomiting, early discharge with post-discharge easy access in case of adverse events.

References

1. Dogan K, Kraaij L, Aarts EO, Koehestanie P, Hammink E, van Laarhoven CJHM, et al. Fast-track bariatric surgery improves perioperative care and logistics compared to conventional care. Obes Surg. 2015;25(1):28–35.
2. Sosada K, Wiewiora M, Piecuch J, Zurawiński W. Fast track in large intestine surgery - review of randomized clinical trials. Wideochir Inne Tech Małoinwazyjne. 2013;8(1):1–7.

3. Flum DR, Belle SH, King WC, et al. Peri-operative safety in the longitudinal assessment of bariatric surgery. N Engl J Med. 2009;361(5):445–54.
4. Geubbels N, Bruin SC, Acherman YIZ, van de Laar AWJM, Hoen MB, de Brauw LM. Fast track care for gastric bypass patients decreases length of stay without increasing complications in an unselected patient cohort. Obes Surg. 2014;24(3):390–6.
5. Elliott JA, Patel VM, Kirresh A, Ashrafian H, Le Roux CW, Olbers T, et al. Fast-track laparoscopic bariatric surgery: a systematic review. Updates Surg. 2013;65(2):85–94.
6. Lemanu DP, Srinivasa S, Singh PP, Johannsen S, MacCormick AD, Hill AG. Optimizing perioperative care in bariatric surgery patients. Obes Surg. 2012;22(6):979–90.
7. Bamgbade OA, Adeogun BO, Abbas K. Fast-track laparoscopic gastric bypass surgery: outcomes and lessons from a bariatric surgery service in the United Kingdom. Obes Surg. 2012;22(3):398–402.
8. Bergland A, Gislason H, Raeder J. Fast-track surgery for bariatric laparoscopic gastric bypass with focus on anaesthesia and peri-operative care. Experience with 500 cases. Acta Anaesthesiol Scand. 2008;52(10):1394–9.
9. Kim JYS, Khavanin N, Rambachan A, McCarthy RJ, Mlodinow AS, De Oliveria GS, et al. Surgical duration and risk of venous thromboembolism. JAMA Surg. 2015;150(2):110–7.
10. Gan TJ, Meyer T, Apfel CC, Chung F, Davis PJ, Eubanks S, et al. Consensus guidelines for managing postoperative nausea and vomiting. Anesth Analg. 2003;97(1):62–71, table of contents.
11. De Oliveira GS, Castro-Alves LJS, Ahmad S, Kendall MC, McCarthy RJ. Dexamethasone to prevent postoperative nausea and vomiting: an updated meta-analysis of randomized controlled trials. Anesth Analg. 2013;116(1):58–74.
12. Jacobsen HJ, Bergland A, Raeder J, Gislason HG. High-volume bariatric surgery in a single center: safety, quality, cost-efficacy and teaching aspects in 2,000 consecutive cases. Obes Surg. 2012;22(1):158–66.
13. Sommer T, Larsen JF, Raundahl U. Eliminating learning curve-related morbidity in fast track laparoscopic Roux-en-Y gastric bypass. J Laparoendosc Adv Surg Tech A. 2011;21(4):307–12.

Part VI

Surgical Complications After Bariatric Surgery

Management of Leaks After Sleeve Gastrectomy

23

Rachel Maria Gomes, Rajkumar Palaniappan, Aparna Bhasker, Shivram Naik, and Sumeet Shah

23.1 Introduction

Laparoscopic sleeve gastrectomy (LSG) is the most commonly performed 'stand-alone' bariatric procedure in India. Staple line gastric leaks occur infrequently but cause significant and prolonged morbidity [1]. A constructed LSG results in high intra-gastric pressure in comparison to a normal stomach [2]. This high intra-gastric pressure is quoted as a reason why LSG has a higher leak rate and sleeve leaks tend to be more prolonged than anastomotic techniques like gastric bypass etc.

R.M. Gomes, MS, FMAS (✉)
Bariatric Division, Upper Gastrointestinal Surgery and Minimal Access Surgery unit, GEM Hospital and Research Centre, Coimbatore, India
e-mail: dr.gomes@rediffmail.com

R. Palaniappan, MS, MMAS, FUCS, DMAS, FMAS, FALS
Institute of Bariatrics, Apollo Hosptals, Chennai, India
e-mail: raj@doctor.com

A. Bhasker, MS
Department of Bariatric Surgery, Saifee Hospital, Mumbai, India
e-mail: aparna@codsindia.com

S. Naik, MS, FAIS, FICS, FRCS(Glasgow)
Aster CMI Hospital, Bangalore, India
e-mail: hvshivaram@gmail.com

S. Shah, MS, DNB, MNAMS, FIAGES, FMAS
Bariatric and Metabolic Surgical Services, Rockland Group of Hospitals, New Delhi, India
e-mail: sumeetshah01@gmail.com

P.R. Palanivelu et al. (eds.), *Bariatric Surgical Practice Guide*,
DOI 10.1007/978-981-10-2705-5_23

23.2 Diagnosis of Sleeve Leaks

Clinical suspicion and contrast enhanced CT (CECT) scan constitute the mainstay for the diagnosis of sleeve leaks. Clinically systemic inflammation and peritonitis are usually the main signs for early-onset sleeve leak, whereas intra-abdominal abscesses and pulmonary symptoms reveal delayed-onset leaks like gastro-bronchial fistulas and gastrocolic fistulas [3]. Tachycardia, tachypnea, fever and vomiting along with a low urine output must alert the surgeons and warrant further investigations. A high white blood cell count or a raised creatinine level must raise the suspicions of a leak. Gastrograffin swallow tests performed in patients with a clinically suspected leak are commonly false negative [3]. A high clinical suspicion for a gastric leak should be immediately followed up with a CECT scan. Ultrasound imaging cannot detect abnormalities because of obesity and small size walled off collections with a sub-diaphragmatic location [1]. A CECT will differentiate localized leaks from diffuse spread and identify abscesses or fistulous tracts. A leak of contrast material at CECT may or may not be identified. However in the morbidly obese patients there may be instances when it may not be technically possible for these patients to fit on CT consoles due to high body weight and diagnostic laparoscopy may be the final choice of intervention [4]. Endoscopy if done early can identify the position of the fistula and any associated stenosis [5]. At the time of surgical re-exploration an obvious fistulous opening may be identified. However intraoperative identification and localization of the site of leak may not be possible in some cases [6].

23.3 Classification of Sleeve Leaks

23.3.1 Clinical Classification

Csendes et al. and Burgos et al. proposed a clinical classification based on time of appearance after surgery, clinical severity, and location of leaks as follows [7, 8].

Based on clinical presentation gastric leaks were classified as follows:

1. Type I (Subclinical): Presence of leakage without early septic complications corresponding to drainage through a fistulous track and/or without generalised dissemination to the pleural or abdominal cavity with or without appearance of contrast medium in any of the abdominal drains.
2. Type II (Clinical): Presence of leakage with early septic complications corresponding to drainage by an irregular pathway (no well-formed fistulous tract) and a more generalised dissemination into the pleural or abdominal cavity with or without appearance of contrast medium in any of the abdominal drains.

Based on the time when the leaks presented, they were classified as follows:

1. Early (leaks appearing 1–3 days after surgery),
2. Intermediate (leaks appearing 4–7 days after surgery), and
3. Late (leaks appearing ≥8 days after surgery).

Rosenthal et al. proposed a clinical classification in the International Sleeve Gastrectomy Expert Panel Consensus Statement as follows [9].

Type	Presentation
Acute	Within 7 days
Early	Within 1–6 weeks
Late	Within 6–12 weeks
Chronic	>12 weeks from surgery

23.3.2 Radiological Classification

Nedelcu et al. proposed a radiological classification based on CT findings as follows [4].

Type of leak	Collection on radiology	Leak visualization	Staple line region
I	<5 cm in LUQ	a – No leak b – Positive leak	S – Superior part M – Middle part I – Inferior part
II	>5 cm in LUQ		
III	Diffuse abdominal collection		
IV	Thoracic collection		

23.3.3 Endoscopic Classification

Galvao Neto et al. proposed an endoscopic classification as follows [5].

Type	Region of leak
High	Upper 1/3 of stapler line
Middle	Middle 1/3 of stapler line
Low	Lower 1/3 of stapler line

23.4 Management Options

Considering the variability of presentation and the complexity of management no clear guidelines exist regarding the optimal management options for sleeve leak. The treatment options for postoperative leaks after bariatric surgery mainly depend on the timing of leaks at presentation. The main principles of management of sleeve leak include adequate drainage, closure of leak and nutrition.

This chapter aims to review the existing literature for better understanding of the management processes after a sleeve gastrectomy leak.

23.4.1 Management of Early or Intermediate Leaks

Clinically systemic inflammation and peritonitis are the main signs for early-onset sleeve leaks. Hence surgery is almost always performed for early-onset sleeve leaks. The re-intervention can be a laparoscopic or open washout and drainage. If the site of leak is not identifiable simple drainage alone may be performed by placing a drain next to the staple line. An alternative approach to control the leak site is placement of a T-tube directly into the defect or laparoscopic endoscopic tube drainage through healthy distal antrum as described by some authors [6, 10, 11]. T-tube drainage technique consists of placing the T part of the drain directly into the defect. The drain is then exteriorized connecting to a bag drainage. The T-tube is left in place for 4–6 weeks and is slowly withdrawn over time (1–2 in per week) [12]. However, as access and identification of the perforation at the time of surgical exploration is not always easy and manipulations through this ischemic esophagogastric region may not be advisable, a modification in the form of a 'laparo-endoscopic gastrostomy' decompression has been recently described. Here a gastrostomy is placed through a healthy area of the distal antrum with intact vascularity draining the entire gastric tube from the esophagogastric junction to the antrum [13].

Re-suturing of a detected sleeve leak at the time of drainage is controversial as these closures tend to break down due to unhealthy tissue at the leak site. However studies have shown that early re-suturing within the first three days can result in successful closure versus re-suturing leaks after the third day [1, 7, 8] Hence this is considered as a 'favourable' window period and attempt at early surgical closure of the defect may be performed when re-exploration is early and tissues are healthy. If possible re-sleeve of the fistula site by stapling can be done with suture reinforcement [1]. Generalized peritonitis with hemodynamic instability is uncommon, but if present an immediate surgical repair of the fistula site may be deferred for later.

23.4.2 Management of Late Leaks

Adequate drainage and maintenance of nutrition form the mainstay of treatment when leaks are detected late. Drainage can be performed by percutaneous drainage or by surgical intervention. Surgery for drainage is considered mainly in patients with signs of peritonitis or hemodynamic instability. Definitive treatment options include endoscopic stenting, endobiliary drainage, roux-en-Y gastric bypass, total gastrectomy and fistulojujenostomy.

23.4.2.1 Endoscopic Exclusion of the Fistula

Over the last decade, there has been increasing use of self-expanding metal stents (SEMS) for the treatment of sleeve leaks. The objective of stenting has been to divert gastric contents from the fistula site and to bypass the distal stenotic portion if present. Casella and colleagues reported the use of endoscopic stents for sleeve leaks in three patients with 100 % success [14]. Oshiro and colleagues reported 100 % success in 2 patients of sleeve leak with covered endoscopic stents. [15]. Nyugen et al. reported 100 % success in three cases treated with endoscopic stenting [16]. Southwell et al. reported 95 % success with endoscopic stenting but significant stent migration in 19 % of primary stents [17]. Serra and colleagues reported on the use of coated self-expanding stents for management of leaks after laparoscopic sleeve gastrectomy (LSG) or duodenal switch in six patients with control of leaks in 83 % of cases [18]. Simon et al. reported 78 % success in patients with gastric staple line leaks after LSG treated with covered stents [19]. Eubanks et al. reported a success rate of 84 % with covered endoscopic stents with a success rate of 84 % for closure of sleeve leaks [20]. Tan et al. reported a success rate of 50 % in 8 cases of sleeve leaks with covered stents, with four patients requiring premature removal of the stent due to migration, hematemesis, and obstruction from kinking at the proximal aspect of the stent [6]. Fukumoto and colleagues reported a single case of endoscopic stent for leak after sleeve gastrectomy without success that required operative closure of the fistula [21].

Thus endoscopic stenting for gastric leaks has a variable success rate which is dependent on medical expertise available. The main advantages in using a stent include bridging the fistula resulting in source control and allowing for early oral nutrition. There exists a wide variation in practice with regards to the type of stent, the length and the diameter of the stent to be used and the number of stenting sessions required. However, it is clear from these series that stent placement is limited by a high rate of migration of around 30–60 %. In majority, the migration is within the stomach but in some cases even small bowel migration needing operative removal has been reported [20]. Thus multiple sessions of stenting could be required in many patients adding to the cost. Various maneuvers have been described to reduce migration with limited success. These include fixing the stent to the sleeve by suturing or using transnasally externalised threads, use of wider stents, use of partially covered stents (Ultraflex Boston Scientific, USA), use of stents with double layer anti-migratory cuffs [Beta stent (Taewoong Medical, Korea)] and use of stents with both a wider diameter and a long body (TaewoongNiti-S™ Megastent) [17]. The Taewoong Niti-S™ Megastent is a recently developed promising stent whose length and wide diameter limits migration. Its length provides effective drainage of the entire sleeve and wide diameter also helps to keep open stenotic areas [22]. Its length however results in its wide distal flare resting at the duodenum which can cause significant mucosal ulceration (decubitus ulcers). It is also not tolerated as well as the other stents. Other less commonly reported complications of stenting include mucosal overgrowth with retrieval problems and persistent vomiting with inability to tolerate the stent [18]. Other endoscopic therapies such as metal clips, over the scope clips (OTSC) and glue injection have been described and can be used as complementary therapy on a case to case basis [23–25].

In summary, endoscopic stent placement has a definite role in the management of sleeve leaks. But this management strategy needs special expertise, multiple sessions, has recognized complications with added costs. Although reasonable success rates have been reported, it still cannot be recommended as a standalone treatment option.

23.4.2.2 Endobiliary Drainage with Enteral Nutrition

Donatelli et al. recently described the use of endoscopically placed endobiliary catheters with enteral nutrition (EDEN) as an alternative to stenting [26]. These stents are placed through the fistula tract into the collection providing drainage. With time there is a reduction of the cavity size with closure. The author reported closure in 20 out of 21 patients without metallic stents. Though Donatelli et al. reported success with use in varied sized fistulous openings Nedeleu et al. recommended selected use in freely draining fistulae smaller than 10 mm and for leaks larger than 10 mm or of any size in the presence of sleeve stenosis to be managed with SEMS [27].

23.4.2.3 Definitive Surgical Options

More definitive surgical options include conversion of the LSG to a regular Roux-Y gastric bypass (RYGB), anastomosis of the jejunal Roux limb to the fistula and total gastrectomy.

Conversion of the sleeve to a RYGB is recommended as a surgical option for sleeve leak. The short distance from the esophagogastric junction to the fistula may not allow pouch construction above the leak in most cases. However the fistulous opening may not necessarily be excluded at the time of the procedure. Praveenraj et al. demonstrated that laparoscopic suturing of the fistulous opening in the remnant pouch with a RYGB leading to closure of the fistula [28, 29]. The authors suggested that converting a sleeve to a RYGB leads to decompression of the high intragastric pressure within the sleeve to a low pressure system. Also a Roux limb allows for better drainage than a sleeve, which can have functional disorders or stenotic areas. Conversion of the LSG to a RYGB may not be advisable in the presence of significant peritonitis.

Another definitive surgical option may be a fistula roux gastro-jejunostomy wherein the edges of the gastric opening are freshened and widened and a side-to side anastomosis is performed. Anastomosis of the jejunal Roux limb to the fistula was first described by Baltasar et al. in three patients who performed the procedure through laparotomy [30, 31]. Recently, van de Vrande et al. reported laparoscopic Roux limb placement in 11 patients with good results [32]. A side to side anastomosis is preferred as rotation of the Roux-en-Y loop will be less likely. A fistula loop jujenostomy is not recommended as it doesn't divert the bile flow and can make the fistula complex.

Total gastrectomy is a final option for persistent leak. Baltasar et al. reported total gastrectomy in nine patients performed by laparotomy for complications of LSG [33]. Moszkowicz et al. reported seven patients who required total gastrectomy for devastating complications, all performed by open approach [34]. Yaacov et al. reported a series of four patients with chronic fistulae, who failed conservative treatment and required total gastrectomy [35].

23.5 Complex Sleeve Fistulae

Gastro-bronchial fistulae (GBF) are an uncommon presentation of a chronic leak. Due to the high intra-gastric pressure a chronic leak tends to erode into the bronchus leading to a fistulization. Some surgeons prefer an invasive surgical procedure whereas others have preferred endoscopic stenting [36]. When surgical management was opted some only addressed the gastric fistula component whereas others in addition to tackling the gastric fistula variably combined thoracotomy with/without lung resection, with/without diaphragmatic resection and reconstruction [28, 37]. Thus it is difficult to come up with a recommended approach. GBF may be treated on the same lines as a simple sleeve leak fistula. Need for thoracotomy with/without lung resection with/without diaphragmatic resection and reconstruction can be decided on a case to case basis.

23.5.1 Gastro-colic Fistulae

This sequel may follow a long-standing chronic sleeve leak. Unlike GBF which may be treated initially on the same lines as simple sleeve leak fistulae, gastro-colic fistulae fail a more conservative approach and need operative intervention.. The treatment of choice described for benign gastro-colic fistulae is en bloc surgical resection of the fistula tract with a margin of adjacent tissue with closure of the defect at the sleeve and the colon. Laparoscopic resection of the fistula en-bloc from the stomach as well as the colonic side by longitudinally re-sleeving the stomach has been described in gastro-colic fistulae following sleeve leaks [38].

Recommendations

- Management of an early leak is by laparoscopic resuturing and drainage
- Decompression of the stomach is an intergral part of intermediate to late leak management. This can be in the form of endoscopic stenting or surgical diversion procedures.
- Multiple attempts of endoscopic stenting can be tried.
- Definitive surgery includes laparoscopic roux-en Y gastric bypass or total gastrectomy or fistulojejunostomy.

References

1. Praveenraj P, Gomes RM, Kumar S, Senthilnathan P, Parthasarathi R, Rajapandian S, et al. Management of gastric leaks after laparoscopic sleeve gastrectomy for morbid obesity- a tertiary care experience and design of a managment algorithm. J Min Access Surg. 2016;12(4):342–9.

2. Yehoshua RT, Eidelman LA, Stein M, Fichman S, Mazor A, Chen J, et al. Laparoscopic sleeve gastrectomy--volume and pressure assessment. Obes Surg. 2008;18(9):1083–8.
3. Bekheit M, Katri KM, Nabil W, Sharaan MA, El Kayal ESA. Earliest signs and management of leakage after bariatric surgeries: Single institute experience. Alex J Med. 2013;49(1):29–33.
4. Nedelcu M, Skalli M, Delhom E, Fabre JM, Nocca D. New CT scan classification of leak after sleeve gastrectomy. Obes Surg. 2013;23(8):1341–3.
5. GalvãoNeto M, Marins Campos J. Therapeutic flexible endoscopy after bariatric surgery: a solution for complex clinical scenarios. Cir Esp. 2015;93(1):1–3.
6. Tan JT, Kariyawasam S, Wijeratne T, Chandraratna HS. Diagnosis and management of gastric leaks after laparoscopic sleeve gastrectomy for morbid obesity. Obes Surg. 2010;20(4):403–9.
7. Csendes A, Braghetto I, León P, Burgos AM. Management of leaks after laparoscopic sleeve gastrectomy in patients with obesity. J Gastrointest Surg Off J Soc Surg Aliment Tract. 2010;14(9):1343–8.
8. Burgos AM, Braghetto I, Csendes A, Maluenda F, Korn O, Yarmuch J, et al. Gastric Leak After Laparoscopic-Sleeve Gastrectomy for Obesity. Obes Surg. 2009;19(12):1672–7.
9. Rosenthal RJ. International Sleeve Gastrectomy Expert Panel, Diaz AA, Arvidsson D, Baker RS, Basso N, et al. International Sleeve Gastrectomy Expert Panel Consensus Statement: best practice guidelines based on experience of >12,000 cases. Surg Obes Relat Dis Off J Am Soc Bariatr Surg. 2012;8(1):8–19.
10. Court I, Wilson A, Benotti P, Szomstein S, Rosenthal RJ. T-tube gastrostomy as a novel approach for distal staple line disruption after sleeve gastrectomy for morbid obesity: case report and review of the literature. Obes Surg. 2010;20(4):519–22.
11. El Hassan E, Mohamed A, Ibrahim M, Margarita M, Al Hadad M, Nimeri AA. Single-stage operative management of laparoscopic sleeve gastrectomy leaks without endoscopic stent placement. Obes Surg. 2013;23(5):722–6.
12. Nguyen NT, Armstrong C. Management of Gastrointestinal Leaks and Fistula. In: Nguyen NT, Blackstone RP, Morton JM, Ponce J, Rosenthal RJ, editors. The ASMBS Textbook of Bariatric Surgery. New York: Springer; 2015. p. 221–7.
13. Zachariah PJ, Lee W-J, Ser K-H, Chen J-C, Tsou J-J. Laparo-Endoscopic Gastrostomy (LEG) Decompression: a Novel One-Time Method of Management of Gastric Leaks Following Sleeve Gastrectomy. Obes Surg. 2015;25(11):2213–8.
14. Casella G, Soricelli E, Rizzello M, Trentino P, Fiocca F, Fantini A, et al. Nonsurgical treatment of staple line leaks after laparoscopic sleeve gastrectomy. Obes Surg. 2009;19(7):821–6.
15. Oshiro T, Kasama K, Umezawa A, Kanehira E, Kurokawa Y. Successful management of refractory staple line leakage at the esophagogastric junction after a sleeve gastrectomy using the HANAROSTENT. Obes Surg. 2010;20(4):530–4.
16. Nguyen NT, Nguyen X-MT, Dholakia C. The use of endoscopic stent in management of leaks after sleeve gastrectomy. Obes Surg. 2010;20(9):1289–92.
17. Southwell T, Lim TH, Ogra R. Endoscopic Therapy for Treatment of Staple Line Leaks Post-Laparoscopic Sleeve Gastrectomy (LSG): Experience from a Large Bariatric Surgery Centre in New Zealand. Obes Surg. 2015;26:1155–62.
18. Serra C, Baltasar A, Andreo L, Pérez N, Bou R, Bengochea M, et al. Treatment of gastric leaks with coated self-expanding stents after sleeve gastrectomy. Obes Surg. 2007;17(7):866–72.
19. Simon F, Siciliano I, Gillet A, Castel B, Coffin B, Msika S. Gastric leak after laparoscopic sleeve gastrectomy: early covered self-expandable stent reduces healing time. Obes Surg. 2013;23(5):687–92.
20. Eubanks S, Edwards CA, Fearing NM, Ramaswamy A, de la Torre RA, Thaler KJ, et al. Use of endoscopic stents to treat anastomotic complications after bariatric surgery. J Am Coll Surg. 2008;206(5):935–8; discussion 938–9.
21. Fukumoto R, Orlina J, McGinty J, Teixeira J. Use of Polyflex stents in treatment of acute esophageal and gastric leaks after bariatric surgery. Surg Obes Relat Dis Off J Am Soc Bariatr Surg. 2007;3(1):68–71; discussion 71–2.

22. Basha J, Appasani S, Sinha SK, Siddappa P, Dhaliwal HS, Verma GR, et al. Mega stents: a new option for management of leaks following laparoscopic sleeve gastrectomy. Endoscopy. 2014;46(Suppl 1 UCTN):E49–50.
23. Keren D, Eyal O, Sroka G, Rainis T, Raziel A, Sakran N, et al. Over-the-Scope Clip (OTSC) System for Sleeve Gastrectomy Leaks. Obes Surg. 2014;25(8):1358–63.
24. Vilallonga R, Himpens J, Bosch B, van de Vrande S, Bafort J. Role of Percutaneous Glue Treatment After Persisting Leak After Laparoscopic Sleeve Gastrectomy. Obes Surg. 2015;16:1–6.
25. Campos JM, Pereira EF, Evangelista LF, Siqueira L, Neto MG, Dib V, et al. Gastrobronchial fistula after sleeve gastrectomy and gastric bypass: endoscopic management and prevention. Obes Surg. 2011;21(10):1520–9.
26. Donatelli G, Ferretti S, Vergeau BM, Dhumane P, Dumont J-L, Derhy S, et al. Endoscopic Internal Drainage with Enteral Nutrition (EDEN) for treatment of leaks following sleeve gastrectomy. Obes Surg. 2014;24(8):1400–7.
27. Nedelcu M, Manos T, Cotirlet A, Noel P, Gagner M. Outcome of leaks after sleeve gastrectomy based on a new algorithm adressing leak size and gastric stenosis. Obes Surg. 2015;25(3):559–63.
28. Praveenraj P, Gomes RM, Kumar S, Senthilnathan P, Parthasarathi R, Rajapandian S, et al. Management of Type 1 Late Sleeve Leak with Gastrobronchial Fistula by Laparoscopic Suturing and Conversion to Roux-en-Y Gastric Bypass: Video Report. Obes Surg. 2015;25:2462.
29. Praveenraj P, Gomes RM, Kumar S, Senthilnathan P, Parthasarathi R, Rajapandian S, et al. Management of Type 2 Late Sleeve Leak by Laparoscopic Suturing and Conversion to Roux-en-Y Gastric Bypass: Video Report. Obes Surg. 2015;25(10):1984.
30. Baltasar A, Serra C, Bengochea M, Bou R, Andreo L. Use of Roux limb as remedial surgery for sleeve gastrectomy fistulas. Surg Obes Relat Dis Off J Am Soc Bariatr Surg. 2008;4(6):759–63.
31. Baltasar A, Bou R, Bengochea M, Serra C, Cipagauta L. Use of a Roux limb to correct esophagogastric junction fistulas after sleeve gastrectomy. Obes Surg. 2007;17(10):1408–10.
32. Van de Vrande S, Himpens J, El Mourad H, Debaerdemaeker R, Leman G. Management of chronic proximal fistulas after sleeve gastrectomy by laparoscopic Roux-limb placement. Surg Obes Relat Dis Off J Am Soc Bariatr Surg. 2013;9(6):856–61.
33. Serra C, Baltasar A, Pérez N, Bou R, Bengochea M. Total gastrectomy for complications of the duodenal switch, with reversal. Obes Surg. 2006;16(8):1082–6.
34. Moszkowicz D, Arienzo R, Khettab I, Rahmi G, Zinzindohoué F, Berger A, et al. Sleeve gastrectomy severe complications: is it always a reasonable surgical option? Obes Surg. 2013;23(5):676–86.
35. Ben Yaacov A, Sadot E, Ben David M, Wasserberg N, Keidar A. Laparoscopic total gastrectomy with Roux-y esophagojejunostomy for chronic gastric fistula after laparoscopic sleeve gastrectomy. Obes Surg. 2014;24(3):425–9.
36. Campos JM, Pereira EF, Evangelista LF, Siqueira L, Neto MG, Dib V, et al. Gastrobronchial fistula after sleeve gastrectomy and gastric bypass: endoscopic management and prevention. Obes Surg. 2011;21(10):1520–9.
37. Silva LB, Moon RC, Teixeira AF, Jawad MA, Ferraz ÁAB, Neto MG, et al. Gastrobronchial Fistula in Sleeve Gastrectomy and Roux-en-Y Gastric Bypass—A Systematic Review. Obes Surg. 2015;25(10):1959–65.
38. Bhasker AG, Khalifa H, Sood A, Lakdawala M. Management of gastro-colic fistula after laparoscopic sleeve gastrectomy. Asian J Endosc Surg. 2014;7(4):314–6.

24 Detection and Management of Internal Hernias

Praveen Raj Palanivelu

24.1 Introduction

Small bowel obstruction (SBO) after roux en Y gastric bypass (RYGB) is not uncommon and can be secondary to adhesions, anastomotic strictures, volvulus and internal hernias. However internal hernias (IH) are the most common cause in the laparoscopic era [1–3]. In fact IH is the most common and most frequently missed complication after LRYGB and can be even life-threatening if it results in bowel ischaemia or obstruction [4, 5]. Petersen W was the first surgeon to report an internal hernia after gastrojejunostomy [6]. Later in 1972 Petersen H described the Treitz hernia [7].

With an antecolic and antegastric technique, the potential defects are the mesenteric opening at the level of the jejunojejunostomy and the Petersen's space(The space between the Roux limb and the transverse colon). In the retrocolic technique, an additional potential site for the internal herniation is the window in the transverse colon created to bring up the loop. With the mesocolic defect being the commonest IH in retrocolic approach, the incidence of Petersen hernia seems to be increased with the antecolic approach [8]. Overall, the incidence of IH have been reported to be between 0.5 and 9 % [2, 9, 10].

24.2 Diagnosis

The presentation can be widely varied from severe acute abdominal pain requiring an emergency management to chronic intermittent abdominal pain requiring a conservative approach and semi elective laparoscopic exploration when

P.R. Palanivelu, MS, DNB, DNB(SGE), FALS, FMAS
Bariatric Division, Upper Gastrointestinal Surgery and Minimal Access Surgery Unit, GEM Hospital and Research Centre, Coimbatore, India
e-mail: drraj@geminstitute.in

P.R. Palanivelu et al. (eds.), *Bariatric Surgical Practice Guide*,
DOI 10.1007/978-981-10-2705-5_24

needed [8]. Patients with Petersen's hernia may have pain that could sometimes be ameliorated by adopting the hand and knee positions [11]. Considering the variability in the symptoms, the role of imaging assumes prime importance, especially in patients without any obvious signs of severe intestinal obstruction or peritonitis [8].

X-ray can identify intestinal obstruction, but most patients with internal hernias (IH) do not have evident signs of small bowel obstruction on plain films making contrast studies or CT necessary [11]. A CT scan can help make the diagnosis of an IH, especially when a mesenteric swirl sign is present, which is defined as a twisting pattern of mesenteric vessels indicating midgut volvulus. The other CT findings that can be seen are mushroom sign, hurricane eye, small bowel obstruction, clustered loops in the left hypochondrium, small bowel behind the superior mesenteric artery(SMA), right sided location of J-J anastomosis, dilated remnant stomach etc [12].

The sensitivity of the swirl sign varies between 60 and 100% and specificity between 63 and 94% [12–14]. The sensitivity and specificity of the other signs has a larger inter-observer variability and also lacks sensitivity. This variability could be related to the experience of the radiologist, as shown by Al-Mansour et al where a retrospective review by a board certified radiologist showed positive findings in a few CT films which were earlier reported normal [8]. This stresses the need for an experienced radiologist and also the need for surgeons to be familiar with the cross sectional imaging of these patients.

Marchini et al noticed two signs specific to Petersen's hernia with small bowel obstruction [15]. A sac like cluster of small bowel loops displaced towards the left mid-abdominal wall, coming from behind the Roux limb and in front of the angle of Treitz, and a horizontal course of engorged superior mesenteric vessels towards the left abdominal wall.

24.3 Mesenteric Closure and Relationship to Internal Hernia

The issue of mesenteric defect closure has been discussed in detail earlier in chapter 10 on the technique of RYGB. Petersen's hernia has been more commonly encountered in patients with mesenteric closure only. While the incidence of overall IH did not change with Petersens defect closure, the rates of Petersens hernia has actually reduced from 84 to 33% [8]. Rodriguez et al reported that with experience and change of technique, the incidence of IH can be reduced significantly [11]. From not closing the Petersens defect and dividing the mesentery until the base with closure of the defect with small bites to routine closure of the Petersens defect and avoiding the mesenteric division and thick interrupted bites on the mesentry reduced the IH incidence from 15.5 to 1.1%. This highlights the importance of good mesenteric closure in preventing internal hernias.

The data is divergent about the incidence of Petersens and mesenteric hernias. Koppmann et al depicted a higher rate of Petersen hernia(56 %) while Ianelli et al believes mesenteric hernias to be more prone with gravity facilitating the intestine projection into the space with lower position [16, 17]. Karcz et al had noted no significant difference in the incidence of both the types of hernias [18]. It was also noted that biliopancreatic limb was the most common to herniate and in the direction of left-right. In cases of alimentary limb or the common channel the direction was opposite. It was also interesting to note that following BPD-DS, the hernias were seen only at the Petersens and not the mesenteric defect. A classification system called SDL(Space-Direction-Limb) classification system has been proposed to help in clinical understanding and communication of information and possible evaluation of severity [18]. Al-Mansour et a reported 3 cases of bowel gangrene with Petersens hernia. This was in patients in whom only the JJ defect was closed and not the Petersens [8].

24.4 Management of Patients with Suspected/Proven IH

As discussed above, with the variability of clinical presentation and with CT scans prone to having false negative reports, a high index of suspicion is most important. And as suggested by Goudsmedt et al, from a surgical perspective, the CT sensitivity is more important than specificity and the clinical consequences of missing an IH is far more serious than performing an unnecessary diagnostic laparoscopy [12]. Hence the decision to go for surgery will be more dependent on clinical examination than on radiological findings. In their series of 131 diagnostic laparoscopy, only 73 patients had an IH and the remaining either had no IH or had bowel adhesions.

Management of the obstructive episodes requires reduction of the herniated bowel and closure of the defects which can done successfully by laparoscopy in most cases [16, 19–21]. Mansour et al had reported laparoscopic closure of IH in all cases except cases of gangrene and two other patients [8]. Rodriguez et al also showed that with experience they were successfully able to close all IH laparoscopically [11]. Hence laparoscopy is an excellent diagnostic and therapeutic tool to treat IH.

The first step is to explore the Petersens space by lifting the mesocolon on the right side of the alimentary limb. The bowel protruding from the posterior aspect of the alimentary limb towards the right side of the abdomen would suggest a Petersen hernia. The IC junction can then be identified and traced proximally and any herniation at this point can be identified and reduced appropriately. This has to be done carefully to avoid further twisting of the bowel. It is better to close any open defects even without any hernia to prevent subsequent hernias [11].

Recommendations

- The closure of intermesenteric defects has huge impact on the incidence of internal hernias and the complications associated with it.
- Closure of the Petersens hernia is controversial and although decreased the incidence of Petersens hernia, the overall incidence has not been reduced.
- The better the closure the better the outcome.
- With an experienced radiologist CT scan is usually diagnostic. The mesenteric swirl sign is highly sensitive and specific.
- High index of suspicion is required and even if imaging is not confirmatory, there needs to be a low threshold for diagnostic laparoscopy.
- Management of obstructed hernias requires reduction of the herniated bowel and closure of the defects and can be done successfully by laparoscopy. Other open defects even if not having any hernia should be closed and this reduces recurrence of hernia.

References

1. DeMaria EJ, Sugerman HJ, Kellum JM, Meador JG, Wolfe LG. Results of 281 consecutive total laparoscopic Roux-en-Y gastric bypasses to treat morbid obesity. Ann Surg. 2002;235(5):640–5; discussion 645–7.
2. Podnos YD, Jimenez JC, Wilson SE, Stevens CM, Nguyen NT. Complications after laparoscopic gastric bypass: a review of 3464 cases. Arch Surg Chic Ill 1960. 2003;138(9):957–61.
3. Capella RF, Iannace VA, Capella JF. Bowel obstruction after open and laparoscopic gastric bypass surgery for morbid obesity. J Am Coll Surg. 2006;203(3):328–35.
4. Gunabushanam G, Shankar S, Czerniach DR, Kelly JJ, Perugini RA. Small-bowel obstruction after laparoscopic Roux-en-Y gastric bypass surgery. J Comput Assist Tomogr. 2009;33(3):369–75.
5. Husain S, Ahmed AR, Johnson J, Boss T, O'Malley W. Small-bowel obstruction after laparoscopic Roux-en-Y gastric bypass: etiology, diagnosis, and management. Arch Surg Chic Ill 1960. 2007;142(10):988–93.
6. Petersen W. Ueber darmverschlingung nach der gastroenterostomie. Arch Klin Chir. 1900;62:94–114.
7. Petersen H. Treitz's hernia with total incarceration of the small intestine. Zentralblatt Für Chir. 1972;97(31):1112–5.
8. Al-Mansour MR, Mundy R, Canoy JM, Dulaimy K, Kuhn JN, Romanelli J. Internal hernia after laparoscopic antecolic Roux-en-Y gastric bypass. Obes Surg. 2015;25(11):2106–11.
9. Steele KE, Prokopowicz GP, Magnuson T, Lidor A, Schweitzer M. Laparoscopic antecolic Roux-en-Y gastric bypass with closure of internal defects leads to fewer internal hernias than the retrocolic approach. Surg Endosc. 2008;22(9):2056–61.
10. Mickevicius A, Sufi P, Heath D. Factors predicting the occurrence of a gastrojejunal anastomosis leak following gastric bypass. Wideochir Inne Tech Małoinwazyjne. 2014;9(3):436–40.
11. Rodríguez A, Mosti M, Sierra M, Pérez-Johnson R, Flores S, Dominguez G, et al. Small bowel obstruction after antecolic and antegastric laparoscopic Roux-en-Y gastric bypass: could the incidence be reduced? Obes Surg. 2010;20(10):1380–4.
12. Goudsmedt F, Deylgat B, Coenegrachts K, Van De Moortele K, Dillemans B. Internal hernia after laparoscopic Roux-en-Y gastric bypass: a correlation between radiological and operative findings. Obes Surg. 2015;25(4):622–7.

13. Iannuccilli JD, Grand D, Murphy BL, Evangelista P, Roye GD, Mayo-Smith W. Sensitivity and specificity of eight CT signs in the preoperative diagnosis of internal mesenteric hernia following Roux-en-Y gastric bypass surgery. Clin Radiol. 2009;64(4):373–80.
14. Lockhart ME, Tessler FN, Canon CL, Smith JK, Larrison MC, Fineberg NS, et al. Internal hernia after gastric bypass: sensitivity and specificity of seven CT signs with surgical correlation and controls. AJR Am J Roentgenol. 2007;188(3):745–50.
15. Kawkabani Marchini A, Denys A, Paroz A, Romy S, Suter M, Desmartines N, et al. The four different types of internal hernia occurring after laparascopic Roux-en-Y gastric bypass performed for morbid obesity: are there any multidetector computed tomography (MDCT) features permitting their distinction? Obes Surg. 2011;21(4):506–16.
16. Koppman JS, Li C, Gandsas A. Small bowel obstruction after laparoscopic Roux-en-Y gastric bypass: a review of 9,527 patients. J Am Coll Surg. 2008;206(3):571–84.
17. Iannelli A, Facchiano E, Gugenheim J. Internal hernia after laparoscopic Roux-en-Y gastric bypass for morbid obesity. Obes Surg. 2006;16(10):1265–71.
18. Karcz WK, Zhou C, Daoud M, Gong Z, Blazejczyk K, Keck T, et al. Modification of internal hernia classification system after laparoscopic Roux-en-Y bariatric surgery. Wideochir Inne Tech Małoinwazyjne. 2015;10(2):197–204.
19. Dresel A, Kuhn JA, Westmoreland MV, Talaasen LJ, McCarty TM. Establishing a laparoscopic gastric bypass program. Am J Surg. 2002;184(6):617–20; discussion 620.
20. Nguyen NT, Huerta S, Gelfand D, Stevens CM, Jim J. Bowel obstruction after laparoscopic Roux-en-Y gastric bypass. Obes Surg. 2004;14(2):190–6.
21. Papasavas PK, Caushaj PF, McCormick JT, Quinlin RF, Hayetian FD, Maurer J, et al. Laparoscopic management of complications following laparoscopic Roux-en-Y gastric bypass for morbid obesity. Surg Endosc. 2003;17(4):610–4.

Prevention and Management of Marginal Ulcers

25

Praveen Raj Palanivelu

Marginal ulcer (MU), is defined as "a peptic ulcer produced at the jejunal mucosa just distal to the gastro-jejunal anastomosis after partial gastrectomy for benign diseases, such as gastric or duodenal ulcer or after surgery for morbid obesity". It can be sub-divided into early (<12 months) and late (>12 months) based on the time of presentation for which both the underlying etiology and treatment may differ.

Due to more sufficient follow-up and increasing performance of gastric bypass procedures, a higher number of marginal ulcers are now being identified [1]. The incidence of marginal ulcers has been quite variable and has been reported to vary between 0.6 and 16% [2–4]. A recent review of literature had shown an overall incidence of 4.6% [5].

The severity of presentation has also been quite variable from being completely asymptomatic to more severe lethal presentation like bleeding, perforation etc. [6–12]. Most studies have reported that majority of MU are early, occurring within 12 months, starting as early as 1 month post-surgery. Late ulcers are relatively rare and have been reported upto 20 years post-surgery [2, 10, 13–15]. Asymptomatic ulcers have been reported in 7.6% of patients at 2 months and the mean time of symptom development is 4.3 months [4, 16]. A recent systematic review had reported that patients with early MU present with vague upper abdominal symptoms and that 57% of patients experience epigastric pain and 5.1% of patients present with bleeding [5]. On the contrary, patients with MU may not always be symptomatic with a significant number of patients with symptoms having normal endoscopic findings [17]. Hence, the positive predictive value of any individual symptom is low (40%) and a poor predictor of endoscopic pathology [4, 18]. This variability could be related to inflammation of the remnant stomach [17].

P.R. Palanivelu, MS, DNB, DNB(SGE), FALS, FMAS
Bariatric Division, Upper Gastrointestinal Surgery and Minimal Access Surgery Unit, GEM Hospital and Research Centre, Coimbatore, India
e-mail: drraj@geminstitute.in

P.R. Palanivelu et al. (eds.), *Bariatric Surgical Practice Guide*,
DOI 10.1007/978-981-10-2705-5_25

25.1 Pathogenesis and Risk Factors

Numerous mechanisms have been considered in the pathogenesis of MU which can be divided into surgical and non-surgical factors.

25.1.1 Surgical Factors

Amongst the surgical risk factors, small-vessel ischaemia and anastomotic tension are considered the most important factors [19]. The other important factors are discussed below.

Persistent acidity in a large gastric pouch in the absence of alkaline fluid from the duodenum exposing the jejunal mucosa to the undiluted gastric juice are contributing factors [20, 21]. Patients with a large, less proximal pouch are prone to higher risk of MU similar to patients with biliopancreatic diversion who have large gastric pouches, where the incidence of MU's are higher. This is probably related to higher parietal cell mass contributing to hyperacidity. A smaller standardized proximal pouch, limited to the cardia has been shown to reduce the occurrence of MU [20, 22, 23].

The three techniques of creation of gastrojejunostomy (linear stapled, circular stapled and hand sewn) does not have any significant impact in MU development [24]. The use of non-absorbable sutures in the course of anastomosis has also been suggested as a contributing factor [25, 26]. In a study by Rasmussen et al. it was seen that 32 % of the ulcer beds had remnants of suture material [16]. However, this was visible in 44 % vs 20 % in absorbable. He had also noted that the handsewn closure after linear stapled anastomosis, though short, is the possible site of the ulcer when non-absorbable sutures were used. Similar incidences have also been noted when non-absorbable sutures were used to reinforce a circular stapled anastamosis. It has also been shown that endoscopic removal of this suture material augmented ulcer healing [27]. The change of non-absorbable sutures to absorbable has reduced the incidence of MU [26, 28]. A recent report had shown that ante-colic creation of gastrojejunostomy (GJ) had higher marginal ulcer rates compared to retro-colic reconstruction [29].

25.1.2 Non-surgical Risk Factors

25.1.2.1 Smoking

Smoking is an independent and an important factor for development of MU. Wilson et al. had reported that the use of tobacco is an independent risk factor for developing MU [14]. In the review by Coblijin et al, it was also noted that a mean 35.8 % patients smoked while developing MU [5]. Additionally smoking increases the chances of recurrent ulcers and ulcers presenting with perforation. El-Hayek had suggested that smoking cessation is as important as proton pump inhibitor (PPI) therapy in ulcer healing [15]. It was also noted that the success of ulcer healing along with the time taken for the healing to happen is longer in smoking related MU.

25.1.2.2 NSAID Usage

Non steroidal anti-inflammatory drugs (NSAIDs) use may cause mucosal disruption due to inhibition of cyclo-oxygenase, causing decreased PGE2 levels and disruption of mucosal barrier [30, 31]. The use of NSAIDs increases the incidence of MU significantly [32, 33]. Similarly, it has also been noted to be an independent predicting factor for development of MU after LRYGB. Protection against MU was possible when PPI s were used simultaneously with NSAIDs [14]. The use of NSAIDs is not only related to the formation of MU, but also in inhibiting the healing of ulcer [34]. NSAID s were found to be risk factors for increasing the incidence of perforation similar to smoking [9, 35]. Sasse et al. had noted that with a zero tolerance policy to NSAID usage, the incidence of perforations had significantly reduced [36].

25.1.2.3 Helicobacter Pylori Infection

The incidence of infection with H. Pylori has been noted to be between 22 and 67 % [5]. Although most surgeons would prefer eradicating H. pylori prior to RYGB on the basis of inaccessibility to the gastric remnant, the role of H. pylori in the pathogenesis of MU is still inconclusive [37]. A few studies have shown a positive association of H. pylori to MU [16, 38, 39]. But a recent study from Rawlins et al. did not show any difference in the rate of complications between patients with and without H.pylori [40]. Similar results have been shown by many other authors [17, 41, 42]. It was also noted that H. pylori infection was associated with higher incidence of foregut symptoms and eradication of this had resolved these symptoms in most patients [43]. This is probably related to the bacteria related inflammation [44].

25.1.2.4 Other Factors

Hypertension was shown to be risk factor for development of MU in one study [30]. With regard to presence of DM, although one study showed an association, most others did not [7, 10, 16, 26, 36, 42]. No study has shown an association between alcohol and MU [15]. In one study it was noted that patients with history of gastroesophageal reflux disease (GERD) before surgery had a higher incidence of MU's compared to patients without GERD [45].

25.2 Prophylactic PPI Use

It has now become a routine by surgeons to prescribe PPI routinely following RYGB. The same was also shown by an international survey where 88 % of surgeons routinely preferred prophylactic PPI usage [37]. But whether this usage really impacts the outcome of MU and when used, the exact duration of usage has not been outlined.

In literature, the duration of postoperative PPI usage has been reported to be between 30 days to 2 years, a few have suggested lifelong usage too. But with the understanding that the gastric acidity has a big role in the pathophysiology of MU, PPIs continue to be widely used. Gumbs et al. had the rate of MU falling to zero with prophylactic PPI therapy compared to no PPI therapy, but the sample size was small [46]. A recent report also showed that prophylactic PPI usage had an impact in preventing MU [47]. D'Hondt et al. found no statistical difference in the incidence of MU with/without PPI prophylaxis in patients without H.pylori infection [42]. But what was interesting to note was that in pre-operatively H.pylori positive patients with eradication, PPI had a beneficial effect in protecting against MU. They hypothesised that pre-operative H.pylori infection could lead to gastritis leading to increased ulcer risk, which was reduced by PPI usage. Currently no Level 1 evidence exist on the actual impact of this usage.

Also based on the understanding of pathophysiology, it is also now clear that the first 12 months is when most MU's are seen. Hence it is more logical to continue PPI therapy for atleast for 1 year. The risks of continuing PPI for longer periods needs special consideration. Carr RJ has recently analyzed the existing literature to propose a management algorithm for MU [48]. For prophylaxis PPIs were recommended for 6–12 months along with risk factor modification for low risk patients with longer duration to be considered for higher risk patients e.g. patients with NSAID usage, smoking etc. Long term PPI therapy can cause calcium malabsorption with increasing risk of osteoporosis and hip fracture, iron and B12 deficiency and hence is to be used with caution [49–51].

25.3 Treatment of Primary MU

Diagnosis of MU requires a high index of suspicion and a low threshold for endoscopic evaluation. For patients with MUs, the treatment involves modification of patient risk factors and inhibition of gastric acid secretion which is successful in treating 68 to 100 % of MU s with relapse rates of 8 % [48]. Medical treatment consists of PPIs, H2 antagonists, Sucralfate, or a combination of these. The International survey by Steinemann et al. had shown that 68 % surgeons preferred PPI alone and 32 % preferred in combination with Sucralfate [37]. H2 blockers alone or in combination with sucralfate was less frequently used. High dose PPI monotherapy is highly successful in the treatment of MU's with healing rates varying between 2 and 7 months as documented by endoscopy [46, 52]. Dallal and Bailey had used a combination regimen of PPI and sucralfate with a step down management regime involving a month of high dose PPI and sucralfate which were weaned on a monthly basis [53]. They also claimed that sucralfate offers better treatment than PPI monotherapy. Hence we believe that sucralfate could be used for patients who develop MU during PPI prophylaxis. However, Azagury et al. [10],noted no difference in healing rates comparing PPI monotherapy to PPI and sucralfate.

The duration of PPI that needs to be continued after ulcer healing has also not been studied by any clinical trial. The international survey showed that more than 50 % of surgeons would continue medical therapy for a median of 6 months to prevent recurrence, most of them preferring PPI monotherapy [37]. Carr et al. in his review had suggested a lifelong PPI in patients with MU s after the healing of the ulcer [48]. But for this to be validated we need more long term and level 1 data.

25.4 Treatment of Refractory/Recurrent MU

Refractory MU is defined as persistence of an ulcer after initial conservative treatment. Evaluation is important at this juncture to find out anatomic abnormalities which could be the potential contributing factor for the refractory nature. This should include identification of a dilated gastric pouch, gastro-gastric fistulae and foreign body in the ulcer. If any of the above factors are identified, the treatment should be directed at appropriate correction of the same. This can be done using a combination of endoscopic and surgical techniques [10, 19, 22, 42, 54]. Although the majority of data has been for the open approach which is known to have greater complication rates and mortality, the recent data on laparoscopic revisions have proven safer and also effective [19, 36, 55–60].

The controversy is in patients without any identifiable abnormalities. The international survey showed that 56 % of surgeons preferred to continue with conservative treatment and would consider surgery only when complications arise. Forty one percent of surgeons preferred to revise the gastrojejunostomy with 18 % of those preferring to add a vagotomy. What was interesting to note in this survey was that the choice of approach was related to experience, with more than 50 % of surgeons with more than 200 surgeries experience, preferring a surgical approach compared to less experienced surgeons [37]. Although data on the right approach is lacking, surgical revision of the GJ can be considered in the event of failure of medical management, but the exact duration for failure needs further research. Some authors also advocate a vagotomy in an attempt to reduce the secretion of gastric acid [7, 10, 22, 61]. Even thoracoscopic vagotomy has been reported in one series, but with very high complication rates [62]. El-Hayek et al. suggested smoking as a major risk factor for development of MU and recommended urinary nicotine testing, reserving surgical intervention only for patients with negative tests [15]. Similar principles would hold good for recurrent MU's too, with importance being given to identification of the risk factor and lifelong PPI therapy.

25.5 Treatment of MU Perforation

The incidence of perforated MU after LRYGB is around 1–2 % of the general population, which means about 20 % of the patients with MU present with a perforation [5]. It is important to note that 70 % of the patients with perforation after MU have some identifiable risk factor like smoking, use of NSAIDS, steroids etc. Twenty percent of patients may not have any warning signs prior to perforation [9]. Based on the understanding of the treatment of perforated duodenal ulcer, laparoscopic approaches can reduce morbidity, post-operative pain, hospital stay and early return to work [63–65]. The same principle could be applied to perforated MU as well, where majority of the ulcers occur on the jejunal side of the GJ anastomosis on the antimesenteric border suitable for laparoscopic repair and patch closure. Laparoscopic patch repair has been shown to be an optimum solution [59, 66–68]. Although surgical revision with refashioning of the GJ is also possible, it is better avoided in an emergency which has higher blood loss, operating time and length of stay [35].

Recommendations

- Prophylactic PPI usage prevents marginal ulcer and should be continued for atleast 1 year.
- Long term PPI usage should be given to patients on NSAIDs and smokers.
- Medical treatment of marginal ulcers consists of PPIs with or without sucralfate along with risk factor modification.
- Refractory marginal ulcer in presence of a dilated gastric pouch, gastro-gastric fistulae or foreign body in the ulcer should be directed towards treatment of the identified abnormality.
- Refractory marginal ulcer without any identified abnormality need to undergo revision of the gastrojejunostomy with/without vagotomy.
- Marginal ulcer perforation can be treated with laparoscopic patch repair

References

1. Schneider BE, Villegas L, Blackburn GL, et al. Laparoscopic gastric bypass surgery: outcomes. J Laparoendosc Adv Surg Tech A. 2003;13(4):247–55.
2. Csendes A, Burgos A, Altuve J, et al. Incidence of marginal ulcer 1 month and 1 to 2 years after gastric bypass: a prospective consecutive endoscopic evaluation in 442 patients with morbid obesity. Obes Surg. 2009;19:135–8.
3. Hutter MM, Schirmer BD, Jones DB, et al. First report from the American College of Surgeons Bariatric Surgery Center Network: laparoscopic sleeve gastrectomy has morbidity and effectiveness positioned between the band and the bypass. Ann Surg. 2011;254(3):410–20; discussion 20–2.
4. Garrido Jr AB, Rossi M, Lima Jr SE, et al. Early marginal ulcer following Roux-en-Y gastric bypass under proton pump inhibitor treatment: prospective multicentric study. Arq Gastroenterol. 2010;47(2):130–4.
5. Coblijn UK, Goucham AB, Lagarde SM, et al. Development of ulcer disease after Roux-en-Y gastric bypass, incidence, risk factors, and patient presentation: a systematic review. Obes Surg. 2013;24:299–309.
6. MacLean LD, Rhode BM, Nohr C, et al. Stomal ulcer after gastric bypass. J Am Coll Surg. 1997;185(1):1–7.
7. Sapala JA, Wood MH, Sapala MA, et al. Marginal ulcer after gastric bypass: a prospective 3-year study of 173 patients. Obes Surg. 1998;8(5):505–16.
8. Howard L, Malone M, Michalek A, et al. Gastric bypass and vertical banded gastroplasty—a prospective randomized comparison and 5-year follow-up. Obes Surg. 1995;5(1):55–60.
9. Felix EL, Kettelle J, Mobley E, et al. Perforated marginal ulcers after laparoscopic gastric bypass. Surg Endosc. 2008;22(10):2128–32.
10. Azagury DE, Abu Dayyeh BK, Greenwalt IT, et al. Marginal ulceration after Roux-en-Y gastric bypass surgery: characteristics, risk factors, treatment, and outcomes. Endoscopy. 2011;43(11):950–4.
11. Caruana JA, McCabe MN, Smith AD, et al. Risk of massive upper gastrointestinal bleeding in gastric bypass patients taking clopidogrel. Surg Obes Relat Dis. 2007;3(4):443–5.
12. Higa KD, Boone KB, Ho T. Complications of the laparoscopic Roux- en-Y gastric bypass: 1,040 patients—what have we learned? Obes Surg. 2000;10(6):509–13.
13. Sanyal AJ, Sugerman HJ, Kellum JM, et al. Stomal complications of gastric bypass: incidence and outcome of therapy. Am J Gastroenterol. 1992;87:1165–9.

14. Wilson JA, Romagnuolo J, Byrne TK, Morgan K, Wilson FA. Predictors of endoscopic findings after Roux-en-Y gastric bypass. Am J Gastroenterol. 2006;101(10):2194–9.
15. El-Hayek K, Timratana P, Shimizu H, et al. Marginal ulcer after Roux-en-Y gastric bypass: what have we really learned? Surg Endosc. 2012;26(10):2789–96.
16. Rasmussen JJ, Fuller W, Ali MR. Marginal ulceration after laparoscopic gastric bypass: an analysis of predisposing factors in 260 patients. Surg Endosc. 2007;21(7):1090–4.
17. Marano BJ. Endoscopy after Roux-en-Y gastric bypass: a community hospital experience. Obes Surg. 2005;15(3):342–5.
18. Huang CS, Forse RA, Jacobson BC, et al. Endoscopic findings and their clinical correlations in patients with symptoms after gastric bypass surgery. Gastrointest Endosc. 2003;58:859–66. PMID: 14652553.
19. Patel RA, Brolin RE, Gandhi A. Revisional operations for marginal ulcer after Roux-en-Y gastric bypass. Surg Obes Relat Dis. 2009;5(3):317–22.
20. Siilin H, Wanders A, Gustavsson S, et al. The proximal gastric pouch invariably contains acid-producing parietal cells in Roux-en-Y gastric bypass. Obes Surg. 2005;15(6):771–7.
21. Mason EE, Munns JR, Kealey GP, et al. Effect of gastric bypass on gastric secretion. Am J Surg. 1976;131(2):162–8.
22. Printen KJ, Scott D, Mason EE. Stomal ulcers after gastric bypass. Arch Surg. 1980;115(4):525–7.
23. Sapala JA, Wood MH, Sapala MA, et al. The micropouch gastric bypass: technical considerations in primary and revisionary operations. Obes Surg. 2001;11(1):3–17.
24. Bendewald FP, Choi JN, Blythe LS, et al. Comparison of hand-sewn, linear-stapled, and circular-stapled gastrojejunostomy in laparoscopic Roux-en-Y gastric bypass. Obes Surg. 2011;21(11):1671–5.
25. Vasquez JC, Wayne Overby D, Farrell TM. Fewer gastrojejunostomy strictures and marginal ulcers with absorbable suture. Surg Endosc. 2009;23(9):2011–5.
26. Sacks BC, Mattar SG, Qureshi FG, et al. Incidence of marginal ulcers and the use of absorbable anastomotic sutures in laparoscopic Roux- en-Y gastric bypass. Surg Obes Relat Dis. 2006;2(1):11–6.
27. Frezza EE, Herbert H, Ford R, et al. Endoscopic suture removal at gastrojejunal anastomosis after Roux-en-Y gastric bypass to prevent marginal ulceration. Surg Obes Relat Dis. 2007;3(6):619–22.
28. Capella JF, Capella RF. Gastro-gastric fistulas and marginal ulcers in gastric bypass procedures for weight reduction. Obes Surg. 1999;9(1):22–7; discussion.
29. Ribeiro-Parenti L, Arapis K, Chosidow D, et al. Comparison of marginal ulcer rates between antecolic and retrocolic laparoscopic Roux-en-Y gastric bypass. Obes Surg. 2015;25(2):215–21.
30. Bhayani N, Oyetunji T. Predictors of marginal ulcers after laparoscopic Roux-en-Y gastric bypass. J Surg Res. 2012;203(1):24–9.
31. Soll A, Weinstein W, Kurata J, et al. Nonsteroidal anti-inflammatory drugs and peptic ulcer disease. Ann Intern Med. 1991;114(4):307–19.
32. Huang JQ, Sridhar S, Hunt RH. Role of Helicobacter pylori infection and non-steroidal anti-inflammatory drugs in peptic-ulcer disease: a meta-analysis. Lancet. 2002;359(9300):14–22.
33. Tytgat GN. Etiopathogenetic principles and peptic ulcer disease classification. Dig Dis. 2011;29(5):454–8.
34. Konturek SJ, Konturek PC, Brzozowski T. Prostaglandins and ulcer healing. J Physiol Pharmacol. 2005;56 Suppl 5:5–31.
35. Wendling MR, Linn JG, Keplinger KM, et al. Omental patch repair effectively treats perforated marginal ulcer following Roux-en-Y gastric bypass. Surg Endosc. 2013;27(2):384–9.
36. Sasse K, Ganser J, Kozar M, et al. Seven cases of gastric perforation in Roux-en-Y gastric bypass patients: what lessons can we learn? Obes Surg. 2008;18:530–4.
37. Steinemann DC, Bueter M, Schiesser M, et al. Management of anastamotic ulcers after Roux en Y gastric bypass: results of an international survey. Obes Surg. 2014;24:741–6.
38. Hartin Jr CW, ReMine DS, Lucktong TA. Preoperative bariatric screening and treatment of Helicobacter pylori. Surg Endosc. 2009;23(11):2531–4.

39. Schirmer B, Erenoglu C, Miller A. Flexible endoscopy in the management of patients undergoing Roux-en-Y gastric bypass. Obes Surg. 2002;12(5):634–8.
40. Rawlins L, Rawlins MP, Brown CC, Schumacher DL. Effect of Helicobacter pylori on marginal ulcer and stomal stenosis after Roux-en-Y gastric bypass. Surg Obes Relat Dis. 2012;9(5):760–4.
41. Suggs WJ, Kouli W, Lupovici M, et al. Complications at gastrojejunostomy after laparoscopic Roux-en-Y gastric bypass: comparison between 21- and 25-mm circular staplers. Surg Obes Relat Dis. 2007;3(5):508–14.
42. D'Hondt MA, Pottel H, Devriendt D, et al. Can a short course of prophylactic low-dose proton pump inhibitor therapy prevent stomal ulceration after laparoscopic Roux-en-Y gastric bypass? Obes Surg. 2010;20(5):595–9.
43. Ramaswamy A, Lin E. Early effects of Helicobacter pylori infection in patients undergoing bariatirc surgery. Arch Surg. 2004;139(September 2001):1094–6.
44. Papasavas P, Gagne D, Donnelly P. Prevalence of Helicobacter pylori infection and value of preoperative testing and treatment in patients undergoing laparoscopic Roux-en-Y gastric bypass. Surg Obes Relat Dis. 2008;4:383–8.
45. Gilmore MM, Kallies KJ, Mathiason MA, Kothari SN. Varying marginal ulcer rates in patients undergoing laparoscopic Roux-en-Y gastric bypass for morbid obesity versus gastroesophageal reflux disease: is the acid pocket to blame? Surg Obes Relat Dis. 2013;9(6):862–6.
46. Gumbs A, Duffy A, Bell R. Incidence and management of marginal ulceration after laparoscopic Roux-Y gastric bypass. Surg Obes Relat Dis. 2006;2:460–3.
47. Coblijn UK, Lagarde SM, de Castro SM, et al. The influence of prophylactic proton pump inhibitor treatment on the development of symptomatic marginal ulceration in Roux-en-Y gastric bypass patients: a historic cohort study. Surg Obes Relat Dis. 2015;12:246–52. pii: S1550-7289(15)00141-0.
48. Carr WR, Mahawar KK, Balupuri S. An evidence-based algorithm for the management of marginal ulcers following Roux-en-Y gastric bypass. Obes Surg. 2014;24(9):1520–7.
49. Insogna KL. The effect of proton pump-inhibiting drugs on mineral metabolism. Am J Gastroenterol. 2009;104(Suppl (March)):S2–4.
50. Yang C-S, Lee W-J, Wang H-H, et al. The influence of Helicobacter pylori infection on the development of gastric ulcer in symptomatic patients after bariatric surgery. Obes Surg. 2006;16(6):735–9.
51. Vestergaard P, Rejnmark L, Mosekilde L. Proton pump inhibitors, histamine H2 receptor antagonists, and other antacid medications and the risk of fracture. Calcif Tissue Int. 2006;79:76–83.
52. Csendes A, Torres J, Burgos AM. Late marginal ulcers after gastric bypass for morbid obesity. Clinical and endoscopic findings and response to treatment. Obes Surg. 2011;21(9):1319–22.
53. Dallal R, Bailey L. Ulcer disease after gastric bypass surgery. Surg Obes Relat Dis. 2006;2:455–9.
54. Jordan JH, Hocking MP, Rout WR, et al. Marginal ulcer following gastric bypass for morbid obesity. Am Surg. 1991;57(5):286–8.
55. Madan AK, DeArmond G, Ternovits CA, et al. Laparoscopic revision of the gastrojejunostomy for recurrent bleeding ulcers after past open revision gastric bypass. Obes Surg. 2006;16(12):1662–8.
56. Brolin RE, Cody RP. Impact of technological advances on complications of revisional bariatric operations. J Am Coll Surg. 2008;206(3):1137–44.
57. Kolkman JJ, Meuwissen SG. A review on treatment of bleeding peptic ulcer: a collaborative task of gastroenterologist and surgeon. Scand J Gastroenterol Suppl. 1996;218:16–25.
58. Nguyen NT, Hinojosa MW, Gray J, et al. Reoperation for marginal ulceration. Surg Endosc. 2007;21(11):1919–21.
59. St Jean MR, Dunkle-Blatter SE, Petrick AT. Laparoscopic management of perforated marginal ulcer after laparoscopic Roux-en-Y gastric bypass. Surg Obes Relat Dis. 2006;2(6):668.
60. Racu C, Dutson EP, Mehran A. Laparoscopic gastrojejunostomy revision: a novel approach to intractable marginal ulcer management. Surg Obes Relat Dis. 2010;6(5):557–8.

61. Hedberg J, Hedenstrom H, Nilsson S, et al. Role of gastric acid in stomal ulcer after gastric bypass. Obes Surg. 2005;15(10):1375–8.
62. Hunter J, Stahl RD, Kakade M, et al. Effectiveness of thoracoscopic truncal vagotomy in the treatment of marginal ulcers after laparoscopic Roux-en-Y gastric bypass. Am Surg. 2012;78(6):663–8.
63. Siu WT, Leong HT, Law BKB, et al. Laparoscopic repair for perforated peptic ulcer: a randomized controlled trial. Ann Surg. 2002;235:313–9.
64. Lunevicius R, Morkevicius M. Management strategies, early results, benefits, and risk factors of laparoscopic repair of perforated peptic ulcer. World J Surg. 2005;29:1299–310.
65. Bertleff MJOE, Lange JF. Laparoscopic correction of perforated peptic ulcer: first choice? A review of literature. Surg Endosc. 2010;24:1231–9.
66. Lublin M, McCoy M, Waldrep DJ. Perforating marginal ulcers after laparoscopic gastric bypass. Surg Endosc. 2006;20(1):51–4.
67. Wheeler AA, de le Torre R, Fearing N. Laparoscopic repair of perforated marginal ulcer following Roux-en-Y gastric bypass: a case series. J Laparoendosc Adv Surg Tech A. 2011;21(1):57–60.
68. Binenbaum SJ, Dressner RM, Borao FJ. Laparoscopic repair of a free perforation of a marginal ulcer after Roux-en-Y gastric bypass: a safe alternative to open exploration. JSLS. 2007;11:383–8.

Prevention and Management of Gastro-Jejunostomy Anastomotic Strictures

26

Jakkapan Wittaya, Narong Boonyakard, Suthep Udomsawaengsup, and Praveen Raj Palanivelu

26.1 Introduction

A stricture of the gastrojejunal(GJ) anastomosis is one the most common complication after laparoscopic roux-en-Y gastric bypass(LRYGB), ranging from 2.9 to 23 % across numerous studies [1, 2]. An anastomotic stricture has to be suspected if the patient has frequent nausea, emesis and/or dysphagia with liquids or meal. A stricture can be confirmed by the inability to pass the gastroscope (10-mm) through the gastrojejunal anastomosis. It usually occurs 1 month after the surgery and can be classified as early or late (within or longer than 30 days after operation, respectively [3]. In this chapter we aim to discuss the different predisposing factors for stricture formation and also the management options.

26.2 Predisposing Factors

The risk factors based on existing literature include gastroesophageal reflux disease (GERD), younger age, antecolic construction of GJ, usage of fibrin glue around the anastomosis and usage of 21 mm circular stapler for creation of GJ [4–9].

Blackstone et al. found that young age and GERD were both independent risk factors for development of GJ stricture and that the odds of developing a GJ stricture decreased with increasing age [7]. However, other studies have not confirmed this association [1, 8]. Riberio-Parenti L et al. had shown that the incidence of stricture

J. Wittaya • N. Boonyakard • S. Udomsawaengsup, MD, FACS, FRCST (✉)
Chula Minimally Invasive Surgery Center, Chulalongkorn University, Bangkok, Thailand
e-mail: suthep.u@gmail.com

P.R. Palanivelu, MS, DNB, DNB(SGE), FALS, FMAS
Bariatric Division, Upper Gastrointestinal Surgery and Minimal Access Surgery Unit, GEM Hospital and Research Centre, Coimbatore, India
e-mail: drraj@geminstitute.in

P.R. Palanivelu et al. (eds.), *Bariatric Surgical Practice Guide*,
DOI 10.1007/978-981-10-2705-5_26

was more common with antecolic construction of GJ compared to a retrocolic method [9]. This could probably be related to the increased anastomotic tension at the site of GJ. The relationship of the various anastomotic to stricture formations is discussed below.

26.2.1 Linear Stapled(LSA) Versus Circular Stapled Anastamosis (CSA)

Marta Penna et al. had performed a meta-analysis comparing linear-stapled versus circular-stapled laparoscopic gastrojejunal anastomosis in morbid obesity, in which nine trials were included comprising 9374 patients (2946 linear vs. 6428 circular) [10]. Primary outcome analysis revealed a statistically significant increase in the rate of GJ stricture associated with CSA with a significantly reduced rate of wound infection, bleeding, and operative time associated with LSA hence recommending the preferential use of the linear stapling technique over circular stapling.

LSA requires closure of the enterotomy site using hand-sewn anastomosis, which can be either longitudinal or transverse closure. Mueller et al. compared these two techniques retrospectively and noticed that the rate of GJ stricture was 16.5 % with longitudinal closure compared to 0 % in the transverse technique [11].

26.2.2 Hand-Sewn Anastomosis Versus Circular-Stapler Anastomosis

Lois AW et al. retrospectively reviewed 190 patients for GJA complication after LRYGB, performed by two surgeons comparing hand-sewn anastomosis (HSA) versus CSA [12]. The CSA technique had significantly higher rate of non-life threatening anastomotic complications compared to the HSA technique. Operative times were also significantly longer for HSA, with the length of hospital stay and long-term weight loss being no different. A recent RCT by Abellan et al. had shown no differences in the incidence of stricture or other complications between the two groups [13].

26.2.3 Hand-Sewn Versus Linear-Stapler Versus Circular-Stapler

The rates of stricture formation have been 3–8 % with HSA, 0–6 % with LSA and 5–31 % with CSA. But majority of the strictures with the circular stapled technique have been with the 21 mm stapler [1, 5–7, 14–18]. Qureshi et al. reported a case-series, of 860 consecutive patients undergoing LRYGB using HSA, LSA, and CSA techniques at a single institution, with three different surgeons [19]. Each surgeon used only one of the three primary LRYGB technique already passing the learning curve, with experience of more than 100 cases. It was concluded that the CSA as the best overall GJA technique with lower rate of strictures.

Lee S et al. had shown that there was no difference in the three different techniques, with the linear technique having the lowest requirement for dilatation [20]. The comparison of all the three techniques by Bendewald FP et al. did not show any difference amongst the techniques [21]. A meta-analysis by Giordano et al. showed that the use of linear stapler compared to circular stapler was associated with a reduced risk of anastomotic stricture [22].

26.2.4 What sized Circular-Stapler Is Better?

Leyba JL et al. conducted a randomized control trial to compared 21-mm circular-stapler and linear-stapler GJA. A significantly higher rate of stricture was noted in the 21-mm CSA group [5]. The operating time and hospital stay were comparable in both groups with the percentage excess weight loss at 1 year following surgery being no different. Similar results were shown by Gould JC et al. where the stricture rate was higher with the 21-mm CSA comparing to the 25-mm CSA [6].

Hence, most surgeons prefer to use a 25 mm circular stapler because of the higher incidence of stricture with the use of 21 mm stapler [1, 5, 7, 14–17]. But it has been recently shown that with technical modification of using the anvil transorally and at the level of the stapler line, the ischaemia can be reduced with lower stricture rates [23]. And with no differences in weight loss outcomes between usage of 21 and 25 mm stapler, it is reasonable to use 25 mm stapler when circular staplers are preferred [16, 18, 24].

Since the results amongst the various techniques being conflicting, no technique can be considered superior to the other except that 21 mm circular stapling technique having a higher stricture rate, the choice of the technique should be based on individual surgeon's preference.

26.2.5 Treatment of GJA Stricture

Endoscopic dilatation has become the primary treatment modality for the treatment of GJ stricture following RYGB, due to the reproducibility and low morbidity associated with the procedure. However there are no well-designed studies indicating this to be the best treatment method and no consensus exist on the safety of this. A review of literature of 23 studies containing 760 patients with GJ stricture showed a 98 % success rate with endoscopic interventions [25]. No guidelines exist on whether the Savary-Gillard bougie or the through the scope (TTS) balloon is better. But most studies have reported the use of TTS with S-G dilators being rarely used. The smallest diameter of the balloon used was 6 mm and the largest being 25 mm. An initial size of 12 mm seems to be the best option [25]. Huang et al. proposes a size of 15 mm to be optimal to prevent recurrences also keeping the chances of perforations lower [26, 27]. Even 15 mm is not without risks as perforations have been reported with this approach too [28]. The procedures were most commonly performed as an out-patient procedure under conscious sedation. There exists no recommendation for the duration of dilatation to be used. Most authors used dilatation from 1 min upto 3 min. The mean number of dilatations required was 1.7/ patient. But most patients had a clinical resolution after a single procedure [25]. Contrast studies can be used selectively if patients showed any sign of possible perforation. The gastroscope has to be passed through the gastrojejunal anastomosis in all patients after dilation.

As seen in this review and from the reports of other authors, its now clear that endoscopic dilatation is safe & effective and is the first therapy for any GJ stricture [29, 30]. But it should also be noted that the outcomes of dilatation is better for early strictures compared to late strictures [29].

26.2.6 Perforation Following Dilatation

Perforation was the most commonest complication reported with an incidence of 1.82 %. The other complications noted were esophageal hematoma, Mallory-Weiss tear, severe abdominal pain, nausea and vomiting. Ukleja et al. reported three patients with radiologic evidence of perforation which were explored surgically, did not reveal any site of leak and were treated conservatively, with satisfactory outcomes [31]. Patients presenting with recurrent strictures after two successful dilatations can be treated with stenostomy, using a needle knife to make incisions in two to four quadrants of the stricture (Lee JK et al) or by revising the GJ surgically [32]. Self-expanding metallic stents have also been attempted in patients with refractory stricture, but these stents are not designed for this purpose the chances of migration is high.

Recommendations

- There is no difference in the incidence of stricture between the three techniques of anastomosis (circular vs linear vs hand sewn),except that with the circular stapled technique using 21 mm had higher rates of stricture.
- With no difference in weight loss outcomes between 25 and 21 mm, 25 mm is preferred if circular staplers are to be used.
- Endoscopic dilatation has become the primary treatment modality for the treatment of GJ stricture
- Considering the risks and benefits dilatation to a size of 15 mm is ideal.
- Perforations are the commonest complications after dilatations, hence a post dilatation imaging may be of benefit.
- Patients with recurrent strictures after two successful dilatations may be treated by a stenostomy using a needle knife.
- Failure of dilatations may require surgical revision of the GJ

References

1. Alasfar F, Sabnis AA, Liu RC, Chand B. Stricture rate after laparoscopic Roux-en-Y Gastric Bypass with a 21-mm circular stapler: the Cleveland Clinic experience. Med Princ Pract Int J Kuwait Univ Health Sci Cent. 2009;18(5):364–7.
2. Mathew A, Veliuona MA, DePalma FJ, Cooney RN. Gastrojejunal stricture after gastric bypass and efficacy of endoscopic intervention. Dig Dis Sci. 2009;54(9):1971–8.
3. Fernández-Esparrach G, Bordas JM, Llach J, Lacy A, Delgado S, Vidal J, et al. Endoscopic dilation with Savary-Gilliard bougies of stomal strictures after laparoscopic gastric bypass in morbidly obese patients. Obes Surg. 2008;18(2):155–61.
4. Ibele AR, Bendewald FP, Mattar SG, McKenna DT. Incidence of gastrojejunostomy stricture in laparoscopic Roux-en-Y gastric bypass using an autologous fibrin sealant. Obes Surg. 2014;24(7):1052–6.
5. Leyba JL, Llopis SN, Isaac J, Aulestia SN, Bravo C, Obregon F. Laparoscopic gastric bypass for morbid obesity-a randomized controlled trial comparing two gastrojejunal anastomosis techniques. J Soc Laparoendosc Surg. 2008;12(4):385–8.
6. Gould JC, Garren M, Boll V, Starling J. The impact of circular stapler diameter on the incidence of gastrojejunostomy stenosis and weight loss following laparoscopic Roux-en-Y gastric bypass. Surg Endosc. 2006;20(7):1017–20.
7. Blackstone RP, Rivera LA. Predicting stricture in morbidly obese patients undergoing laparoscopic Roux-en-Y gastric bypass: a logistic regression analysis. J Gastrointest Surg Off J Soc Surg Aliment Tract. 2007;11(4):403–9.
8. Takata MC, Ciovica R, Cello JP, Posselt AM, Rogers SJ, Campos GM. Predictors, treatment, and outcomes of gastrojejunostomy stricture after gastric bypass for morbid obesity. Obes Surg. 2007;17(7):878–84.
9. Ribeiro-Parenti L, Arapis K, Chosidow D, Dumont J-L, Demetriou M, Marmuse J-P. Gastrojejunostomy stricture rate: comparison between antecolic and retrocolic laparoscopic Roux-en-Y gastric bypass. Surg Obes Relat Dis Off J Am Soc Bariatr Surg. 2015;11(5):1076–84.
10. Penna M, Markar SR, Venkat-Raman V, Karthikesalingam A, Hashemi M. Linear-stapled versus circular-stapled laparoscopic gastrojejunal anastomosis in morbid obesity: meta-analysis. Surg Laparosc Endosc Percutan Tech. 2012;22(2):95–101.
11. Mueller CL, Jackson TD, Swanson T, Pitzul K, Daigle C, Penner T, et al. Linear-stapled gastrojejunostomy with transverse hand-sewn enterotomy closure significantly reduces strictures for laparoscopic Roux-en-Y gastric bypass. Obes Surg. 2013;23(8):1302–8.
12. Lois AW, Frelich MJ, Goldblatt MI, Wallace JR, Gould JC. Gastrojejunostomy technique and anastomotic complications in laparoscopic gastric bypass. Surg Obes Relat Dis Off J Am Soc Bariatr Surg. 2015;11(4):808–13.
13. Abellán I, López V, Lujan J, Abrisqueta J, Hernández Q, Frutos MD, et al. Stapling Versus Hand Suture for Gastroenteric Anastomosis in Roux-en-Y Gastric Bypass: a Randomized Clinical Trial. Obes Surg. 2015;25(10):1796–801.
14. Gonzalez R, Lin E, Venkatesh KR, Bowers SP, Smith CD. Gastrojejunostomy during laparoscopic gastric bypass: analysis of 3 techniques. Arch Surg Chic Ill 1960. 2003;138(2):181–4.
15. Rondan A, Nijhawan S, Majid S, Martinez T, Wittgrove AC. Low anastomotic stricture rate after Roux-en-Y gastric bypass using a 21-mm circular stapling device. Obes Surg. 2012;22(9):1491–5.
16. Nguyen NT, Stevens CM, Wolfe BM. Incidence and outcome of anastomotic stricture after laparoscopic gastric bypass. J Gastrointest Surg Off J Soc Surg Aliment Tract. 2003;7(8):997–1003; discussion 1003.
17. Dolce CJ, Dunnican WJ, Kushnir L, Bendana E, Ata A, Singh TP. Gastrojejunal strictures after Roux-en-Y gastric bypass with a 21-MM circular stapler. J Soc Laparoendosc Surg Soc Laparoendosc Surg. 2009;13(3):306–11.

18. Fisher BL, Atkinson JD, Cottam D. Incidence of gastroenterostomy stenosis in laparoscopic Roux-en-Y gastric bypass using 21- or 25-mm circular stapler: a randomized prospective blinded study. Surg Obes Relat Dis Off J Am Soc Bariatr Surg. 2007;3(2):176–9.
19. Qureshi A, Podolsky D, Cumella L, Abbas M, Choi J, Vemulapalli P, et al. Comparison of stricture rates using three different gastrojejunostomy anastomotic techniques in laparoscopic Roux-en-Y gastric bypass. Surg Endosc. 2015;29(7):1737–40.
20. Lee S, Davies AR, Bahal S, Cocker DM, Bonanomi G, Thompson J, et al. Comparison of gastrojejunal anastomosis techniques in laparoscopic Roux-en-Y gastric bypass: gastrojejunal stricture rate and effect on subsequent weight loss. Obes Surg. 2014;24(9):1425–9.
21. Bendewald FP, Choi JN, Blythe LS, Selzer DJ, Ditslear JH, Mattar SG. Comparison of hand-sewn, linear-stapled, and circular-stapled gastrojejunostomy in laparoscopic Roux-en-Y gastric bypass. Obes Surg. 2011;21(11):1671–5.
22. Giordano S, Salminen P, Biancari F, Victorzon M. Linear stapler technique may be safer than circular in gastrojejunal anastomosis for laparoscopic Roux-en-Y gastric bypass: a meta-analysis of comparative studies. Obes Surg. 2011;21(12):1958–64.
23. Khoraki J, Funk LM, Greenberg JA, Leverson G, Campos GM. The Effect of Route of Anvil Insertion on Stricture Rates with Circular Stapled Gastrojejunostomy During Laparoscopic Gastric Bypass. Obes Surg. 2016;26(3):517–24.
24. Owens ML, Sczepaniak JP. Size really does matter-role of gastrojejunostomy in postoperative weight loss. Surg Obes Relat Dis Off J Am Soc Bariatr Surg. 2009;5(3):357–61.
25. Campos JM, de FST M, Ferraz AAB, de JN B, Nassif PAN, Galvão-Neto Mdos P. Endoscopic dilation of gastrojejunal anastomosis after gastric bypass. Arq Bras Cir Dig ABCD Braz Arch Dig Surg. 2012;25(4):283–9.
26. Huang CS, Forse RA, Jacobson BC, Farraye FA. Endoscopic findings and their clinical correlations in patients with symptoms after gastric bypass surgery. Gastrointest Endosc. 2003;58(6):859–66.
27. Huang CS, Farraye FA. Endoscopy in the bariatric surgical patient. Gastroenterol Clin North Am. 2005;34(1):151–66.
28. Vance PL, de Lange EE, Shaffer HA, Schirmer B. Gastric outlet obstruction following surgery for morbid obesity: efficacy of fluoroscopically guided balloon dilation. Radiology. 2002;222(1):70–2.
29. Yimcharoen P, Heneghan H, Chand B, Talarico JA, Tariq N, Kroh M, et al. Successful management of gastrojejunal strictures after gastric bypass: is timing important? Surg Obes Relat Dis Off J Am Soc Bariatr Surg. 2012;8(2):151–7.
30. Carrodeguas L, Szomstein S, Zundel N, Lo Menzo E, Rosenthal R. Gastrojejunal anastomotic strictures following laparoscopic Roux-en-Y gastric bypass surgery: analysis of 1291 patients. Surg Obes Relat Dis Off J Am Soc Bariatr Surg. 2006;2(2):92–7.
31. Ukleja A, Afonso BB, Pimentel R, Szomstein S, Rosenthal R. Outcome of endoscopic balloon dilation of strictures after laparoscopic gastric bypass. Surg Endosc. 2008;22(8):1746–50.
32. Lee JK, Van Dam J, Morton JM, Curet M, Banerjee S. Endoscopy is accurate, safe, and effective in the assessment and management of complications following gastric bypass surgery. Am J Gastroenterol. 2009;104(3):575–82; quiz 583.

Management of Leaks After Gastric Bypass

27

Praveen Raj Palanivelu and Saravana Kumar

27.1 Introduction

The incidence of leaks after roux en Y gastric bypass (RYGB) is not uncommon and has been reported to be between 0 and 5.6 % with a mean of 2.6 % [1]. Although not so commonly debated like a sleeve leak, it still represents a major and serious bariatric surgical complication with high mortality rates [2]. Leak related mortality rates of 37.5–50 % has been reported and along with pulmonary embolism is an important cause of mortality [3–5].

27.2 Classification of Leaks

The presence of leak after any kind of gastric bypass can be classified based on three parameters as suggested by Csendes et al. [6–8].

27.2.1 Time of Appearance After Surgery

Early –1–4 days
Intermediate-5–9 days
Late-10 or more days.

Jacobsen et al. proposes an alternate classification with those within 5 days as early and more than 5 days as late leaks, as those leaks within 5 days are usually related to technical aspects of the surgery and anything after with a more complex etiology [9].

P.R. Palanivelu, MS, DNB, DNB(SGE), FALS, FMAS (✉)
S. Kumar, DNB (Gen. Surgery), MS, FMAS
Bariatric Division, Upper Gastrointestinal Surgery and Minimal Access Surgery Unit, GEM Hospital and Research Centre, Coimbatore, India
e-mail: drraj@geminstitute.in; drsakubariatric@gmail.com

P.R. Palanivelu et al. (eds.), *Bariatric Surgical Practice Guide*,
DOI 10.1007/978-981-10-2705-5_27

27.2.2 Severity of Leak

Based on the severity, leaks can be classified as,

Type I-localized
Type II-clinically significant leak

27.2.3 Location

Based on the site of leak, they can be classifies as follows:

Type 1-Gastric pouch
Type 2-Gastrojejunal (GJ) anastamosis
Type 3-Jejunal stump
Type 4-Jejunojejunal (JJ) anastomosis
Type 5-Excluded stomach
Type 6-Duodenal stump in resectional bypass
Type 7-Blind end jejunal limb

27.3 Risk Factors

Risk factors for leaks can be subdivided as surgical and non-surgical factors. The common surgical factors include anastomotic tension and ischaemia [10]. Anastomotic tension may result in stress that exceeds the disruptive forces of a stapled or sutured anastomosis contributing to a leak [3]. The position of the alimentary limb (antecolic vs retrocolic) has also been debated but no conclusive evidence exist [11–14]. Non surgical risk factors include advanced age, super-obesity, male sex, presence of multiple co-morbidities and previous bariatric operations [4, 5, 10, 15–18].

27.4 Diagnosis

A large number of patients do not present with the typical features of peritonitis and routine post-operative oral contrast studies fail to identify a significant proportion of leaks, which can delay diagnosis and treatment [13, 18–20]. Hence a high index of suspicion is important based on the clinical parameters. Mickevicius A et al reported that a pulse rate of >90 on day 1 had a sensitivity of 100% and specificity of 87% [21]. The same has been reported by others as well, that unexplained tachycardia as an early indicator of leak [22, 23]. Significant differences in temperature on day 2 and higher pain scores on day 3 are additional factors. Serum C-reactive protein (CRP) concentrations were also significantly high on day 2 and 3 in patients with leaks [21] In fact Jacobsen et al suggested that in patients with tachycardia exceeding 120/min, used more pain medication than expected and/or unable to be mobilized within 2 h after surgery were considered to have a bleeding or leak and was an indication for surgical exploration in the first 24 h [9].

Some surgeons prefer to perform a routine upper GI series (UGS) in the postoperative period as a routine when early leaks can be identified [3]. But it should be noted that the sensitivity of this routine UGI series has a low sensitivity and hence not routinely followed in may centers [3, 13]. If routinely followed, it is suggested that small localized leaks can be better diagnosed with barium sulfate, and not with liquid contrast medium like Gastrograffin or Hypaque [7].

Considering the morbidity associated with a missed leak being quite significant, CT scanning can be performed. Findings suggestive of an anastomotic leak include contrast extravasation from the gastrojejunostomy or the jejunojejunostomy, collections adjacent to the gastric pouch, diffuse abdominal fluid and the presence of free intraperitoneal gas. However, the sensitivity and specificity of both UGS and CT are directly dependent on the radiologist experience with post-operative anatomical changes after roux en Y gastric bypass (RYGB) [3].

27.5 Management of Leak

With the diagnosis of leak after RYGB, the choice is between conservative approach which is usually a combination of endoscopic/radiologic interventions or surgery(open/laparoscopy). Hamilton et al performed open re-exploration in all cases of leaks, at which time the abdomen was irrigated, leak repaired with placement of gastric feeding tubes and closed suction drains [13]. But it is interesting to note that in Ballesta's series that the hospital stay was prolonged in patients managed operatively with a mortality of 8.5 % [3]. This could be because of the more severe nature of the leak on whom surgery was performed with the hemodynamically stable patients being managed conservatively. Gonzalez et al reported that 12 % of patients had unsuccessful non-operative treatment and required subsequent operation because of systemic toxicity or poor clinical outcome [18].

But with better risk stratification and classification of leak based on severity, a significant numbers of patients could be conservatively managed especially for patients presenting late with hemodynamic stability with leak at the level of gastric pouch or gastrojejunal anastomosis [3]. Jacobsen et al reported that patients with Clavien-Dindo grade II or IIIA complications were treated conservatively and by surgery for IIIB and above [9]. The principles of conservative treatment includes nasojejunal tube placement guided under fluoroscopy and commencing enteral nutrition when possible (or parenteral nutrition), leaving behind the drains if present. If not, to place a 12 F drain by percutaneous approach. Medications like antibiotics as necessary. The patients have to be evaluated for the leak closure and hemodynamic stability on a regular basis [6–8]. Patients with hemodynamic instability, complicated leaks or presence of signs of sepsis should preferably be operated. Csendes e al suggested that leaks presenting early, type 2 and located at the GJ or the JJ, prompt surgical repair is preferred [24]. Schiesser et al reported successful closure of GJ leaks with a sequential approach of stenting, OTC(over the scope clips) and placement of percutaneous drains [25]. Endoscopic fibrin glue applications has also been attempted successfully [25] Patients delay in reporting signs and symptoms and delay in intervention were both associated with adverse outcomes [9].

Recommendations

- High index of suspicion based on clinical parameters like tachycardia, unusual pain and fever should prompt further evaluation
- Routine UGI series may pick up early leaks but has a high false negative rate.
- CT scans can be confirmatory but related to the experience of the radiologist.
- Haemodynamically stable patients can be managed by endoscopic/radiological means with good success
- Haemodynamically unstable patients needs surgical intervention and the overall mortality and hospital stay is expected to be higher.

References

1. Csendes A, Burdiles P, Burgos AM, Maluenda F, Diaz JC. Conservative management of anastomotic leaks after 557 open gastric bypasses. Obes Surg. 2005;15(9):1252–6.
2. Csendes A, Burgos AM, Braghetto I. Classification and management of leaks after gastric bypass for patients with morbid obesity: a prospective study of 60 patients. Obes Surg. 2012;22(6):855–62.
3. Ballesta C, Berindoague R, Cabrera M, Palau M, Gonzales M. Management of anastomotic leaks after laparoscopic Roux-en-Y gastric bypass. Obes Surg. 2008;18(6):623–30.
4. Fernandez AZ, DeMaria EJ, Tichansky DS, Kellum JM, Wolfe LG, Meador J, et al. Experience with over 3,000 open and laparoscopic bariatric procedures: multivariate analysis of factors related to leak and resultant mortality. Surg Endosc. 2004;18(2):193–7.
5. Podnos YD, Jimenez JC, Wilson SE, Stevens CM, Nguyen NT. Complications after laparoscopic gastric bypass: a review of 3464 cases. Arch Surg Chic Ill 1960. 2003;138(9):957–61.
6. Csendes A. Conservative management of anastomotic leaks. Obes Surg. 2006;16(3):375–6; author reply 376.
7. Csendes A, Díaz JC, Burdiles P, Braghetto I, Maluenda F, Nava O, et al. Classification and treatment of anastomotic leakage after extended total gastrectomy in gastric carcinoma. Hepatogastroenterology. 1990;37 Suppl 2:174–7.
8. Csendes A, Braghetto I, León P, Burgos AM. Management of leaks after laparoscopic sleeve gastrectomy in patients with obesity. J Gastrointest Surg Off J Soc Surg Aliment Tract. 2010;14(9):1343–8.
9. Jacobsen HJ, Nergard BJ, Leifsson BG, Frederiksen SG, Agajahni E, Ekelund M, et al. Management of suspected anastomotic leak after bariatric laparoscopic Roux-en-y gastric bypass. Br J Surg. 2014;101(4):417–23.
10. Gonzalez R, Nelson LG, Gallagher SF, Murr MM. Anastomotic leaks after laparoscopic gastric bypass. Obes Surg. 2004;14(10):1299–307.
11. Bertucci W, Yadegar J, Takahashi A, Alzahrani A, Frickel D, Tobin K, et al. Antecolic laparoscopic Roux-en-Y gastric bypass is not associated with higher complication rates. Am Surg. 2005;71(9):735–7.
12. Carrasquilla C, English WJ, Esposito P, Gianos J. Total stapled, total intra-abdominal (TSTI) laparoscopic Roux-en-Y gastric bypass: one leak in 1000 cases. Obes Surg. 2004;14(5):613–7.
13. Hamilton EC, Sims TL, Hamilton TT, Mullican MA, Jones DB, Provost DA. Clinical predictors of leak after laparoscopic Roux-en-Y gastric bypass for morbid obesity. Surg Endosc. 2003;17(5):679–84.

14. Edwards MA, Jones DB, Ellsmere J, Grinbaum R, Schneider BE. Anastomotic leak following antecolic versus retrocolic laparoscopic Roux-en-Y gastric bypass for morbid obesity. Obes Surg. 2007;17(3):292–7.
15. Ballesta-López C, Poves I, Cabrera M, Almeida JA, Macías G. Learning curve for laparoscopic Roux-en-Y gastric bypass with totally hand-sewn anastomosis: analysis of first 600 consecutive patients. Surg Endosc. 2005;19(4):519–24.
16. Schauer PR, Ikramuddin S, Gourash W, Ramanathan R, Luketich J. Outcomes after laparoscopic Roux-en-Y gastric bypass for morbid obesity. Ann Surg. 2000;232(4):515–29.
17. Oliak D, Ballantyne GH, Weber P, Wasielewski A, Davies RJ, Schmidt HJ. Laparoscopic Roux-en-Y gastric bypass: defining the learning curve. Surg Endosc. 2003;17(3):405–8.
18. Gonzalez R, Sarr MG, Smith CD, Baghai M, Kendrick M, Szomstein S, et al. Diagnosis and contemporary management of anastomotic leaks after gastric bypass for obesity. J Am Coll Surg. 2007;204(1):47–55.
19. Yurcisin BM, DeMaria EJ. Management of leak in the bariatric gastric bypass patient: reoperate, drain and feed distally. J Gastrointest Surg Off J Soc Surg Aliment Tract. 2009;13(9):1564–6.
20. Kolakowski S, Kirkland ML, Schuricht AL. Routine postoperative upper gastrointestinal series after Roux-en-Y gastric bypass: determination of whether it is necessary. Arch Surg Chic Ill 1960. 2007;142(10):930–4; discussion 934.
21. Mickevicius A, Sufi P, Heath D. Factors predicting the occurrence of a gastrojejunal anastomosis leak following gastric bypass. Wideochirur Inne Tech Małoinwazyjne Videosurgery Miniinvasive Tech Kwart Pod Patronatem Sekc Wideochirurgii TChP Oraz Sekc Chir Bariatrycznej TChP. 2014;9(3):436–40.
22. Lee S, Carmody B, Wolfe L, Demaria E, Kellum JM, Sugerman H, et al. Effect of location and speed of diagnosis on anastomotic leak outcomes in 3828 gastric bypass cases. J Gastrointest Surg Off J Soc Surg Aliment Tract. 2007;11(6):708–13.
23. Bellorin O, Abdemur A, Sucandy I, Szomstein S, Rosenthal RJ. Understanding the significance, reasons and patterns of abnormal vital signs after gastric bypass for morbid obesity. Obes Surg. 2011;21(6):707–13.
24. Schiesser M, Kressig P, Bueter M, Nocito A, Bauerfeind P, Gubler C. Successful endoscopic management of gastrointestinal leakages after laparoscopic Roux-en-Y gastric bypass surgery. Dig Surg. 2014;31(1):67–70.
25. Ece I, Yilmaz H, Alptekin H, Acar F, Yormaz S, Sahin M. Minimally invasive management of anastomotic leak after bariatric Roux-en-Y gastric bypass. J Minim Access Surg. 2015;11(2):160–2.

Prevention and Management of Bleeding After Sleeve Gastrectomy and Gastric Bypass

28

Vinoban Amirthalingam, Jaideepraj Rao, and Rachel Maria Gomes

28.1 Introduction

Bariatric Surgery has become one of the most successful and cost effective ways to manage the growing problem of obesity and its associated disorders. Today, close to 300 million adults worldwide are affected by obesity and the number is growing [1]. There are several options available in bariatric surgery and these are defined by certain principles. The procedures range from purely restrictive to purely malabsorptive, or a combination of both [2]. The most commonly performed bariatric procedures are the laparoscopic sleeve gastrectomy (LSG) and Laparoacopic roux en Y gastric bypass (LRYGB).

The aim of this chapter is to discuss the presentation, diagnosis, management and prevention of early bleeding following LSG and LRYGB.

28.2 Post-Operative Bleeding After Laparoscopic Sleeve Gastrectomy

Postsurgical complications after sleeve gastrectomy can be divided into acute and chronic. Hemorrhage, staple line leak and intra-abdominal abscess are considered acute complications [3]. Chronic complications include gastroesophageal reflux disease, nutritional deficiencies, bleeding etc [3]. Hemorrhage is one of the most common acute complications after sleeve gastrectomy as a result of the lengthy

V. Amirthalingam, MRCS (✉) • J. Rao, FRCS
Department of General Surgery, Tan Tock Seng Hospital, Singapore, Singapore
e-mail: vinoban@gmail.com; jaideeprajrao@gmail.com

R.M. Gomes, MS, FMAS
Bariatric Division, Upper Gastrointestinal Surgery and Minimal Access Surgery Unit, GEM Hospital and Research Centre, Coimbatore, India
e-mail: dr.gomes@rediffmail.com

P.R. Palanivelu et al. (eds.), *Bariatric Surgical Practice Guide*,
DOI 10.1007/978-981-10-2705-5_28

staple line and the change in intra-gastric pressure [4]. Another important risk factor for increased postoperative bleeding is preoperative low molecular weight heparins used for prevention of venous thromboembolism [5]. Chronic bleeding in LSG however is very uncommon and related to ulcers that may develop within the remnant stomach. Incidence of hemorrhage post LSG has been reported in 1.1–8.7 % of cases [3].

28.2.1 Presentation

Bleeding post LSG occurs, in the majority of cases, from the staple line, but may result from the resected greater omentum [6]. Some signs that aid in early recognition are hematemesis, blood loss through the nasogastric tube/drain (NG) and melena in stools[4] Clinical symptoms and signs of tachycardia (heart rate >100), pain, fever, hypotension (systolic blood pressure <100), mean hemoglobin count that has dropped at least 2 g/dl from what it was prior to the procedure should increase clinical suspicion of bleeding or staple line leak in the early post-operative period [4, 7].

Bleeding can be divided into intra-luminal and extra-luminal. Intraluminal bleeding presents as early hemorrhage, and it is the result of bleeding from the staple line, vessels nearby and gastric ulcers [8]. Early bleeding post-surgery is possibly due to technical failure in the operation [9]. Intraluminal bleeding from the staple line usually presents with an upper gastrointestinal bleed [9]. Extra-luminal hemorrhage presents in the abdominal cavity and early indication of extra-luminal bleeding will be through the abdominal drain [9]. Usual areas where extra-luminal bleeds occur are at the staple line, spleen, liver, or abdominal wall at trocar port sites [3]. As a result, there is an increased risk of developing hematoma and abscess formation. Early bleeding through drains or NG tube is called a sentinel bleed and it usually can occur within hours of surgery [9].

28.2.2 Diagnosis and Management

Acute management for hemorrhage involves fluid resuscitation, strict intake and output monitoring with Foley catheter [2]. Patient should receive adequate blood transfusion to stabilize hemoglobin level. Haemodynamically stable patients can be managed conservatively with serial hemoglobin monitoring and drain output. Majority of acute postoperative bleeds settle with conservative management. If there is clinical suspicion of an ongoing bleed, a Computed Tomography (CT) angiogram can demonstrate collections/hematomas and potentially identify the bleeding vessel. If active bleed is identified, angioembolization can be performed to control bleeding. If patient is unstable to proceed to radiology suite, then in the case of intraluminal bleeding the patient will need urgent endoscopic intervention – oesophagogastroduodenoscopy (OGD). Early endoscopic intervention has to be performed only by a trained bariatric endoscopist. Endoscopic evaluation allows for injection of adrenaline or insertion of clips to stop bleeding if detected. Endoscopic intervention should be attempted in the operating theatre in the event patient becomes unstable, and bleeding cannot be controlled endoscopically so that urgent surgery can be done.

In the case of intra-abdominal bleeding, hemodynamic instability warrants urgent re-operation. Diagnostic laparoscopy is an excellent option to allow direct visualization and to identify the bleeding source. It also allows evacuation of the hematoma and a thorough washout to prevent formation of an abscess. In some cases when no obvious source of bleeding is identified it may be advisable to oversew the entire staple line.

28.2.3 Intra-Operative Prevention of Bleeding

Several techniques have been established to control bleeding intraoperatively to identify the bleeder. One of the common methods used is intraoperative packing to help control bleeding and allow for hemostasis. Packing can be done with inserting a raytex gauze and helps to identify bleeding source. Another technique to help reduce bleeding is to increase abdominal pressure. Suction and irrigation can help to identify a source of bleeding, and allow for the application of a clip.

Various techniques have been developed when it comes to preventing bleeding from the staple line. Studies have shown 60 s of compression time instead of 20 s after closure of the stapler before firing has significantly reduced staple line bleeding [10]. It is extremely important to closely inspect the entire staple line after withdrawal of the bougie. Following these steps should significantly decrease the incidence of bleeding from the staple line. If any minor bleeding is detected in this area post-operatively, it can be easily controlled with small clips. However, post-operative bleeding may also be from the resected area of the omentum and the use of drains may aid in the detection of this type of intra-abdominal bleeding [4]. This will facilitate early treatment and the avoidance of the most serious consequences of bleeding [6].

Staple Line Reinforcement (SLR) is a routinely practiced technique today. Benefits of this has resulted in decreased bleeding and staple line leak postoperatively [3]. Concerns with SLR are that they can increase rate of stricture, increase operative time and costs for patients [3]. Different techniques are used for SLR:

1. Oversewing the staple line with running suture,
2. Buttressing it with specific material such as bovine pericardium strips, synthetic polyester, glycoside and trim ethylene carbonate copolymer, and applying glue/haemostatic agents.
3. Covering the staple line with omentum or jejunum [3]. Some surgeons report a reduction in bleeding by reinforcing the staple line by over sewing or by using buttressing material.

However, caution should be used with over sewing since some studies have shown an increased risk of tearing and bleeding at the point of suture penetration when using this technique [8]. Intraoperative placement of drain will help to identify intra-abdominal bleeding. Added benefits of drain placement include identification of leak, may allow converting a leak to a controlled fistula and allows removal of contaminated fluid for prevention of abscess formation [4].

28.2.4 Conclusion

Haemorrhage after sleeve gastrectomy can be intra-luminal or extra-luminal. While bleeding at the site of stapling is best treated by prevention during the surgical procedure, management of upper gastrointestinal bleeding requires a close monitoring and multidisciplinary care. If bleeding is suspected, it can be confirmed by endoscopy or contrast enhanced CT angiogram. Management of bleeding may include surgery or more conservative techniques such as fluid resuscitation and/ or blood transfusion. With proper surgical techniques and through prompt detection and treatment, bleeding following bariatric surgery can be minimized or even avoided.

28.3 Postoperative Bleeding After Roux-En-Y Gastric Bypass Patient

Bleeding is an uncommon but a potentially serious complication following Roux-en-Y gastric bypass. It presents as a very difficult clinical scenario because of the altered gastrointestinal anatomy. The commonly reported incidence is around 3.2–4.4% [11–14]. The frequency of postoperative hemorrhage is higher after laparoscopic than after open RYGB [15]. This increased bleeding with laparoscopic technique has been attributed to learning curve, stapler mechanics, less frequent oversewing of staple-lines and increasing use of venous thromboembolic prophylaxis [16]. Early bleeding after LRYGB is more common and has been attributed to staple line bleeding, iatrogenic visceral injury or mesenteric vessel bleeding [17]. Late postoperative bleeding after RYGB was usually secondary to marginal ulceration [17].

28.3.1 Presentation

The cause for hemorrhage after laparoscopic RYGB can be intraluminal or intrabdominal. Intraluminal bleeding is caused by staple line haemorrhage. There exist four potential sites of staple-line hemorrhage. These sites include the staple-lines at the gastric pouch, the gastrojejunostomy, the jejunojejunostomy, and the bypassed stomach [17]. Common sites of extraluminal bleeding include the divided jejunal mesentery, perigastric tissue and dissection planes, iatrogenic visceral injury and port sites. Staple line bleeding is commonest after RYGB and with manifestations of postoperative haemorrhage, it is often assumed that bleeding is from staple line unless proved otherwise.

The common signs of bleeding are tachycardia, hypotension, oliguria, bloody output from drains, haematemesis and hematochezia. Some clinical signs help differentiate intraluminal from intrabdominal bleeding. The presence of hematemesis points to the gastrojejunostomy or the gastric pouch as the source of bleeding whereas hematochezia points to bleeding from either the bypassed stomach or the jejunojejunostomy [16]. Bloody output from drains indicate intrabdominal bleeding [14].

Important diagnostic modalities are contrast enhanced computed tomography and upper gastrointestinal endoscopy. A CT scan can demonstrate intrabdominal collections/ haematomas and may identify the site of bleeding if active by presence of a blush/ contrast extravastion. Arteriography can be used to localize bleeding [18]. Endoscopy can be used to assess staple line bleeding but should be performed with caution to avoid staple line disruption.

28.3.2 Diagnosis and Management

The immediate management of post RYGB hemorrhage is evaluation of blood and coagulation profile, with fluid resuscitation, discontinuation of low molecular weight heparin and possible transfusion. Management is tailored according to clinical presentation. Patients who are hemodynamically stable can be managed by close observation and transfusions if necessary. In a literature review on 11 articles analyzing 2,895 patients Spaw et al. reported 89 patients (3.1 %) with postoperative bleeding. Twenty percent of patients had spontaneous resolution without the need for transfusion or therapy though the site of bleeding could not be confirmed in some [18]. Fifty-five percent of patients required transfusions [18]. Mehran et al. reported 85 % successfully treated with observation with transfusions when required [14].

In those with clinical severe bleeding with suspicion of intraluminal bleeding upper GI endoscopy is a less invasive option and may obviate the need for surgery. It is most successful for haemorrhage from the gastric pouch or gastrojujensotomy [16]. However even successful endoscopic control of haemorrhage at the jejunojejunostomy site has been reported [19]. Endoscopic therapeutic interventions include injection of epinephrine, thermal coagulation or endoclips [16]. Spaw et al reported upper GI endoscopy as diagnostic measure in 15.4 % with identification and control of bleeding in half of them [18]. Fernandez et al reported successful treatment of staple line bleeding by endoscopic injection of epinephrine alone or combined with polidocanol [20]. Tang et al reported successful treatment of staple line bleeding with application of endoclips [21]. Reported complications are aspiration and perforation at anastomotic site [22]. Importantly patient should undergo endoscopy in the operating room with endotracheal intubation and general anesthesia to avoid aspiration and to proceed with surgery if required [23]. A screening contrast study to be performed after any endoscopic intervention to rule perforation [16].

Early reoperation should be performed for patients with hemodynamic instability. Spaw et al reported operative intervention was required in 20.2 %. Operative interventions are source directed hemostasis in intrabdominal bleeding. In intraluminal bleeding where endoscopy was unsuccessful, luminal decompression is performed by gastrotomy or enterotomy with evacuation of clot with oversewing staple lines with/without decompressing gastrostomy tubes. This can be combined with with intraoperative endoscopy [23]. In many cases it may be difficult to identify the exact site of bleeding and oversewing the entire staple line may be necessary.

28.3.3 Prevention

As staple line bleeding is the most common cause of haemorrhage post RYGB several technical modifications have been described for prevention i.e. appropriate choice of staple size, holding pressure on the stapler before firing, oversewing staple lines, staple-line reinforcements, and use of hemostatic agents on staple lines.

A recent prospective, randomized trial showed that a shorter staple height (3.5 mm versus 4.8 mm) during construction of the gastrojejunostomy, showed a lower rate of GI bleeding [24]. In several randomized prospective trials, staple-line reinforcement has been shown to reduce staple-site bleeding after RYGB [25–27]. Fibrin sealants have been shown to achieve better hemostasis at the suture-line [28, 29].

Conclusion

Postoperative bleeding occurs in three to four percent of LRYGB cases and may be due in part to increased use of venous thromboembolism prophylaxis and use of staplers. Majority of patients can be successfully treated conservatively without the need for reoperation. Use of short staple heights and staple line buttressing may help in reducing the incidence of bleeding.

Recommendations

- Close monitoring and high index of suspicion is required to identify bleeding early.
- If bleeding is suspected, source can be confirmed by endoscopy or contrast enhanced CT angiogram.
- Management of bleeding in majority can be done successfully by observation with fluid resuscitation and/ or blood transfusion only
- If intervention is planned for ongoing/severe bleeding and if active bleed is identified, angioembolization can be performed to control bleeding.
- For intraluminal bleeding endoscopy is most successful for haemorrhage from the gastric pouch or gastrojujensotomy. Endoscopic therapeutic interventions include injection of epinephrine, thermal coagulation or endoclips. Contrast study should be performed post surgery to rule out perforation.
- Early reoperation should be performed for patients with hemodynamic instability with failure of other interventions

References

1. Deitel M. Overweight and obesity worldwide now estimated to involve 1.7 billion people. Obes Surg. 2003;13(3):329–30.
2. Sarkhosh K, Birch DW, Sharma A, Karmali S. Complications associated with laparoscopic sleeve gastrectomy for morbid obesity: a surgeon's guide. Can J Surg J Can Chir. 2013;56(5):347–52.
3. D'Ugo S, Gentileschi P, Benavoli D, Cerci M, Gaspari A, Berta RD, et al. Comparative use of different techniques for leak and bleeding prevention during laparoscopic sleeve gastrectomy: a multicenter study. Surg Obes Relat Dis Off J Am Soc Bariatr Surg. 2014;10(3):450–4.
4. Mittermair R, Sucher R, Perathoner A. Results and complications after laparoscopic sleeve gastrectomy. Surg Today. 2014;44(7):1307–12.
5. Zeni T, Rn ST, Roberts J. Bleeding rates are increased with preoperative lovenox administration in patients undergoing sleeve gastrectomy. Surg Obes Relat Dis. 2015;11(6):S17.
6. Aggarwal S, Sharma AP, Ramaswamy N. Outcome of laparoscopic sleeve gastrectomy with and without staple line oversewing in morbidly obese patients: a randomized study. J Laparoendosc Adv Surg Tech A. 2013;23(11):895–9.
7. Weiner RA, El-Sayes IA, Theodoridou S, Weiner SR, Scheffel O. Early post-operative complications: incidence, management, and impact on length of hospital stay. A retrospective comparison between laparoscopic gastric bypass and sleeve gastrectomy. Obes Surg. 2013;23(12):2004–12.
8. Baker RS, Foote J, Kemmeter P, Brady R, Vroegop T, Serveld M. The science of stapling and leaks. Obes Surg. 2004;14(10):1290–8.
9. Cuesta MA, Bonjer HJ, editors. Treatment of postoperative complications after digestive surgery [Internet]. London: Springer London; 2014 [Cited 18 Apr 2016]. Available from: http://link.springer.com/10.1007/978-1-4471-4354-3.
10. Kasalicky M, Michalsky D, Housova J, Haluzik M, Housa D, Haluzikova D, et al. Laparoscopic sleeve gastrectomy without an over-sewing of the staple line. Obes Surg. 2008;18(10):1257–62.
11. Nguyen NT, Rivers R, Wolfe BM. Early gastrointestinal hemorrhage after laparoscopic gastric bypass. Obes Surg. 2003;13(1):62–5.
12. Schauer PR, Ikramuddin S, Gourash W, Ramanathan R, Luketich J. Outcomes after laparoscopic Roux-en-Y gastric bypass for morbid obesity. Ann Surg. 2000;232(4):515–29.
13. Dillemans B, Sakran N, Van Cauwenberge S, Sablon T, Defoort B, Van Dessel E, et al. Standardization of the fully stapled laparoscopic Roux-en-Y gastric bypass for obesity reduces early immediate postoperative morbidity and mortality: a single center study on 2606 patients. Obes Surg. 2009;19(10):1355–64.
14. Mehran A, Szomstein S, Zundel N, Rosenthal R. Management of acute bleeding after laparoscopic Roux-en-Y gastric bypass. Obes Surg. 2003;13(6):842–7.
15. Podnos YD, Jimenez JC, Wilson SE, Stevens CM, Nguyen NT. Complications after laparoscopic gastric bypass: a review of 3464 cases. Arch Surg Chic Ill 1960. 2003;138(9):957–61.
16. Nguyen NT, Longoria M, Chalifoux S, Wilson SE. Gastrointestinal hemorrhage after laparoscopic gastric bypass. Obes Surg. 2004;14(10):1308–12.
17. Heneghan HM, Meron-Eldar S, Yenumula P, Rogula T, Brethauer SA, Schauer PR. Incidence and management of bleeding complications after gastric bypass surgery in the morbidly obese. Surg Obes Relat Dis Off J Am Soc Bariatr Surg. 2012;8(6):729–35.
18. Spaw AT, Husted JD. Bleeding after laparoscopic gastric bypass: case report and literature review. Surg Obes Relat Dis Off J Am Soc Bariatr Surg. 2005;1(2):99–103.
19. Moretto M, Mottin CC, Padoin AV, Berleze D, Repetto G. Endoscopic management of bleeding after gastric bypass – a therapeutic alternative. Obes Surg. 2004;14(5):706.
20. Fernandez AZ, DeMaria EJ, Tichansky DS, Kellum JM, Wolfe LG, Meador J, et al. Experience with over 3,000 open and laparoscopic bariatric procedures: multivariate analysis of factors related to leak and resultant mortality. Surg Endosc. 2004;18(2):193–7.

21. Tang S-J, Rivas H, Tang L, Lara LF, Sreenarasimhaiah J, Rockey DC. Endoscopic hemostasis using endoclip in early gastrointestinal hemorrhage after gastric bypass surgery. Obes Surg. 2007;17(9):1261–7.
22. Jamil LH, Krause KR, Chengelis DL, Jury RP, Jackson CM, Cannon ME, et al. Endoscopic management of early upper gastrointestinal hemorrhage following laparoscopic Roux-en-Y gastric bypass. Am J Gastroenterol. 2008;103(1):86–91.
23. Rabl C, Peeva S, Prado K, James AW, Rogers SJ, Posselt A, et al. Early and late abdominal bleeding after Roux-en-Y gastric bypass: sources and tailored therapeutic strategies. Obes Surg. 2011;21(4):413–20.
24. Nguyen NT, Dakin G, Needleman B, Pomp A, Mikami D, Provost DA, et al. Effect of staple height on gastrojejunostomy during laparoscopic gastric bypass: a multicenter prospective randomized trial. Surg Obes Relat Dis Off J Am Soc Bariatr Surg. 2010;6(5):477–82.
25. Nguyen NT, Longoria M, Welbourne S, Sabio A, Wilson SE. Glycolide copolymer staple-line reinforcement reduces staple site bleeding during laparoscopic gastric bypass: a prospective randomized trial. Arch Surg Chic Ill 1960. 2005;140(8):773–8.
26. Miller KA, Pump A. Use of bioabsorbable staple reinforcement material in gastric bypass: a prospective randomized clinical trial. Surg Obes Relat Dis Off J Am Soc Bariatr Surg. 2007;3(4):417–21; discussion 422.
27. Angrisani L, Lorenzo M, Borrelli V, Ciannella M, Bassi UA, Scarano P. The use of bovine pericardial strips on linear stapler to reduce extraluminal bleeding during laparoscopic gastric bypass: prospective randomized clinical trial. Obes Surg. 2004;14(9):1198–202.
28. Sapala JA, Wood MH, Schuhknecht MP. Anastomotic leak prophylaxis using a vapor-heated fibrin sealant: report on 738 gastric bypass patients. Obes Surg. 2004;14(1):35–42.
29. Silecchia G, Boru CE, Mouiel J, Rossi M, Anselmino M, Morino M, et al. The use of fibrin sealant to prevent major complications following laparoscopic gastric bypass: results of a multicenter, randomized trial. Surg Endosc. 2008;22(11):2492–7.

Part VII

Revisional Bariatric Surgery

29 Revisional Surgical Options After Laparoscopic Adjustable Gastric Banding

Siddharth Bhatacharya and Praveen Raj Palanivelu

29.1 Introduction

Laparoscopic adjustable gastric banding (LAGB) is the most commonly performed bariatric surgical procedure. It has gained a lot of popularity because of the relative simplicity of the procedure, reversibility and ability to achieve durable weight loss. Although the morbidity of LAGB is low in comparison to other more complex bariatric procedures, it has a very high failure rate of 40–50 % with revision rates of 20–30 % [1–3].

Indications for revision surgery after LAGB include:

Band related problems
- Band slippage
- Tubing problems – leakage, breakage, disconnection
- Port site problems – inversion, hernia, infection
- Band erosion

Motility problems
- Pouch dilatation
- Esophageal dysmotility, dilatation

Miscellaneous
- Inadequate weight loss (BMI >35 or %EWL <50 %)
- Wound infection
- Psychological band intolerance

S. Bhatacharya, MS, FMAS (✉) • P.R. Palanivelu, MS, DNB, DNB (SGE), FALS, FMAS
Bariatric Division, Upper Gastrointestinal Surgery and Minimal Access Surgery Unit,
GEM Hospital and Research Centre, Coimbatore, India
e-mail: drsiddharthabhattacharya@gmail.com; drraj@geminstitute.in

P.R. Palanivelu et al. (eds.), *Bariatric Surgical Practice Guide*,
DOI 10.1007/978-981-10-2705-5_29

Types of revision include:

Conversion
Corrective
Reversal

The aim of this chapter is to focus only on the revision options for inadequate weightloss/weight regain based on existing literature. Selection of the appropriate revisional procedure will depend on several factors including patient characteristics, intraoperative findings, response to primary LAGB and patient tolerability to LAGB. Accordingly the various options include,

Rebanding
Laparoscopic Roux-en-Y gastric bypass (LRYGB)
Laparoscopic sleeve gastrectomy (LSG)
Biliopancreatic diversion-Duodenal switch (BPD/DS)
Others (Eg: Minigastric bypass etc.)

29.2 Laparoscopic Roux-en-Y Gastric Bypass

LRYGB is the most common revision surgery performed following failure of LAGB [4]. Elnahas et al. in their review comparing revisional LSG, RYGB, BPD have shown that LRYGB can achieve successful weight loss following LAGB with relatively low complication rate [4]. In a systematic review on re-operative bariatric surgery by American society for metabolic and bariatric surgery revision task force the reported incidence of conversion from LAGB to RYGB was between 2 and 28.8 % with the medium-term (upto 4 year) weight loss outcomes comparable to primary RYGB with complication rates being slightly higher than primary RYGB [5]. A systematic review of 15 studies (588 patients) reported an overall complication rate (major and minor) of 8.5 % with anastomotic leak and bleeding rates of 0.9 % and 1.8 %, respectively [6]. Robert et al. in their experience of 85 patients who underwent revisional LRYGB have concluded that conversion to LRYGB currently remains the choice of procedure in case of LAGB failure with satisfactory results and acceptable morbidity [7]. Topart et al. compared the results of revisional RYGB to primary RYGB and concluded that when RYGB is performed after an LAGB failure to restore weight loss or because of a complication, the weight loss curve was similar to that after primary RYGB [8]. Mongols et al. in their experience of 70 revisional RYGB concluded that laparoscopic conversion of LAGB to RYGBP is a technically challenging procedure that can be safely performed with good short-term results [9].

LRYGB also adheres to the principle of adding a malabsorptive component to a failed restrictive procedure. LRYGB also offers the extra advantage of treating reflux in patients with associated GERD [10]. In addition LRYGB may also offer resolution or improvement of glycemic control in patients who had T2DM and did not respond to LAGB [11].

Another consideration during revisional RYGB is whether to perform in one stage or as a two stage procedure. Stroh et al. in their data analysis of the German bariatric surgery registry found that the incidence of anastomotic leak after a one stage RYGB following LAGB was actually lower (1.9 %) than after the two stage procedure (2.6 %) making single stage procedure a more prudent choice [12].

29.3 Laparoscopic Sleeve Gastrectomy

Traditionally LRYGB has been considered the optimal revisional surgery for failed LAGB. LSG by principle is a restrictive procedure and hence considered to be inappropriate for another failed restrictive procedure like LAGB. Elnahas et al. have shown in their systematic review that %EWL after LSG at 2 years follow up is inferior to LRYGB/BPD [4]. But reports from many other authors have challenged this by reporting good outcomes following LSG as well. Also the metabolic effects of LSG have now been well established and it is not considered anymore as a purely restrictive bariatric procedure [13]. In a systematic review on reoperative bariatric surgery by American society for metabolic and bariatric surgery revision task force, conversion of LAGB to LSG was the most commonly performed revision surgery for inadequate weight loss [5].

Yazbek et al. in their review of 90 patients who underwent LSG following failed LAGB have shown that successful weight loss can be achieved with mean postoperative %EWL of 61.3 % (n=60), 53.0 % (n=30), 55.3 % (n=20), and 54.1 % (n=10) at 1, 2, 3, and 4 years, respectively [14]. Jacobs et al. in their experience of 32 patients of revisional LSG also showed it is a feasible and acceptable alternative for failed LAGB [15]. Khoursheed et al. in a retrospective review of 95 patients who underwent revisional surgery after failed LAGB, 42 patients underwent LSG and 53 underwent LRYGB. They concluded that both the procedures had similar weight loss but LSG may be superior to LRYGB in terms of long term nutritional consequences [16]. Acholonu et al. concluded that LSG could provide good short-term weight loss after previously failed LAGB, but prone to more complications compared to a primary LSG [17]. Alqahtani et al. in their retrospective review comparing revisional LSG after failed LAGB with primary LSG concluded that single stage conversion of LAGB to LSG is a safe and efficient procedure and achieves similar outcomes as primary LSG surgery alone [18].

But the complication rate following revisional LSG was higher than primary LSG in the form of leaks and staple line bleed [5]. A recent systematic review of 8 studies (286 patients) evaluating conversion of LAGB to SG reported an overall complication rate (major and minor) of 12.2 % with staple line leak rate of 5.6 % [6]. This is postulated to be a result of the scar tissue at the angle of His that occurs after banding. Conversion to LSG can be performed as a single-stage procedure or in two stages with band removal and interval conversion to LSG [19].

29.4 Biliopancreatic Diversion with Duodenal Switch

BPD-DS has also been performed as a revisional surgery after failed LAGB. But the numbers are small to arrive at a reasonable conclusion. Elnahas et al. in their review of 71 patients from 3 case series have found the %EWL for the BPD-DS group was 18 % (12), 47.1 % (14), and 78.4 % (25) at 6–12, 12–24, and 24–48 months, respectively with the mean BMI being 33 kg/m^2 and 28 kg/m^2 at 12–24 and 24–48 months, respectively [4]. In the review on reoperative bariatric surgery by American society for metabolic and bariatric surgery revision task force, conversion to BPD or BPD/DS resulted in weight loss similar to a primary malabsorptive procedure, but with the complication rates being higher than a primary BPD/DS [5].

A modification of BPD-DS which has been explored by some authors in the revisional setting following failed LAGB is to convert it into a BPD-DS with the gastric band in situ without sleeve gastrectomy. This offers the extra advantage of not having to operate in the area of band where the dense adhesions are present and creating the anastomosis in a virgin site, hence reducing the possible chances of leak. Slater et al. have reported successful weight loss in 11 patients with this procedure [20]. But with such small numbers it is difficult to come to a conclusion for the results of this modified technique.

29.5 Rebanding

Vijgen et al. analyzed 94 patients who underwent revision LAGB following failed LAGB. Revision was mainly necessary due to anterior slippage (46 %) and symmetrical pouch dilatation (36 %), which could be resolved by replacing (70 %) or re-fixing the band (27 %). Weight loss significantly increased after revision. After revision, 23 patients (24 %) needed a second re-operation. Patients converted to other procedures (16 %) during the second operation showed better weight loss than the revised group [21]. Muller et al. also showed that patients who underwent revision LRYGB had a significantly better weight loss than patients with a rebanding operation [22].

29.6 Mini Gastric Bypass

Data on LMGB after LAGB is limited but it may be considered as an alternate option. Piazza et al. in their experience of 48 patients who underwent LMGB after failure of LAGB have concluded that LMGB is a safe, feasible, effective and easy-to-perform revisional procedure for failed LAGB [23].

Conclusion

The ideal revisional procedure after failure of LAGB is still debatable. Most commonly performed procedure is LRYGB followed by LSG. As discussed above, both LRYGB and LSG have provided good results in the revisional setting but with an overall increase in complication rate when compared to primary surgery. The decision regarding which surgery should be offered to which patient needs to be tailored. If a patient has had good weight loss following LAGB but with the procedure failing due to band related complications then rebanding or LSG may be more appropriate. On the other hand, if a patient has not had adequate weight loss and/or has GERD and/or has poor response to diabetes following LAGB, LRYGB may be a more appropriate choice. Whether to perform a single stage procedure or a two stage procedure depends on intraoperative findings and surgeons preference except in cases of band erosion where a two stage procedure with band removal and repair as the first stage followed by a definitive procedure as a second stage. The complication rate following revisional procedure will be higher than primary surgery and hence appropriate precautions to be undertaken. Revisional surgery should be done only by experienced surgeons with adequate expertise.

Recommendations

- Single stage LSG, LRYGB can both achieve successful weight loss following LAGB but with complication rates slightly higher than a primary procedure.
- LRYGB offers the advantage of treating associated GERD and both LSG and LRYGB result in better resolution or improvement of glycemic control in T2DM.
- Lap BPD –DS/MGB are less commonly used but also can achieve successful weight loss following LAGB but with complication rates slightly higher than a primary procedure
- Rebanding is an option with band slippage and pouch dilatation (36 %) but with weight loss outcomes expected to be inferior compared to other procedures.

References

1. Gagner M, Gentileschi P, de Csepel J, Kini S, Patterson E, Inabnet WB, et al. Laparoscopic reoperative bariatric surgery: experience from 27 consecutive patients. Obes Surg. 2002;12(2):254–60.
2. Mittermair RP, Obermüller S, Perathoner A, Sieb M, Aigner F, Margreiter R. Results and complications after Swedish adjustable gastric banding-10 years experience. Obes Surg. 2009;19(12):1636–41.
3. Suter M, Calmes JM, Paroz A, Giusti V. A 10-year experience with laparoscopic gastric banding for morbid obesity: high long-term complication and failure rates. Obes Surg. 2006;16(7):829–35.
4. Elnahas A, Graybiel K, Farrokhyar F, Gmora S, Anvari M, Hong D. Revisional surgery after failed laparoscopic adjustable gastric banding: a systematic review. Surg Endosc. 2013;27(3):740–5.
5. Brethauer SA, Kothari S, Sudan R, Williams B, English WJ, Brengman M, et al. Systematic review on reoperative bariatric surgery: American Society for Metabolic and Bariatric Surgery Revision Task Force. Surg Obes Relat Dis Off J Am Soc Bariatr Surg. 2014;10(5):952–72.

6. Coblijn UK, Verveld CJ, van Wagensveld BA, Lagarde SM. Laparoscopic Roux-en-Y gastric bypass or laparoscopic sleeve gastrectomy as revisional procedure after adjustable gastric band – a systematic review. Obes Surg. 2013;23(11):1899–914.
7. Robert M, Poncet G, Boulez J, Mion F, Espalieu P. Laparoscopic gastric bypass for failure of adjustable gastric banding: a review of 85 cases. Obes Surg. 2011;21(10):1513–9.
8. Topart P, Becouarn G, Ritz P. One-year weight loss after primary or revisional Roux-en-Y gastric bypass for failed adjustable gastric banding. Surg Obes Relat Dis Off J Am Soc Bariatr Surg. 2009;5(4):459–62.
9. Mognol P, Chosidow D, Marmuse J-P. Laparoscopic conversion of laparoscopic gastric banding to Roux-en-Y gastric bypass: a review of 70 patients. Obes Surg. 2004;14(10):1349–53.
10. Zundel N, Hernandez JD. Revisional surgery after restrictive procedures for morbid obesity. Surg Laparosc Endosc Percutan Tech. 2010;20(5):338–43.
11. Ngiam KY, Khoo VYH, Kong L, Cheng AKS. Laparoscopic adjustable gastric banding revisions in Singapore: a 10-year experience. Obes Surg. 2015;26(5):1069–74.
12. Stroh C, Weiner R, Wolff S, Lerche C, Knoll C, Keller T, et al. One versus two-step Roux-en-Y gastric bypass after gastric banding – data analysis of the German Bariatric Surgery Registry. Obes Surg. 2015;25(5):755–62.
13. Shabbir A, Dargan D. The success of sleeve gastrectomy in the management of metabolic syndrome and obesity. J Biomed Res. 2015;29(2):93–7.
14. Yazbek T, Safa N, Denis R, Atlas H, Garneau PY. Laparoscopic sleeve gastrectomy (LSG)-a good bariatric option for failed laparoscopic adjustable gastric banding (LAGB): a review of 90 patients. Obes Surg. 2013;23(3):300–5.
15. Jacobs M, Gomez E, Romero R, Jorge I, Fogel R, Celaya C. Failed restrictive surgery: is sleeve gastrectomy a good revisional procedure? Obes Surg. 2011;21(2):157–60.
16. Khoursheed M, Al-Bader I, Mouzannar A, Al-Haddad A, Sayed A, Mohammad A, et al. Sleeve gastrectomy or gastric bypass as revisional bariatric procedures: retrospective evaluation of outcomes. Surg Endosc. 2013;27(11):4277–83.
17. Acholonu E, McBean E, Court I, Bellorin O, Szomstein S, Rosenthal RJ. Safety and short-term outcomes of laparoscopic sleeve gastrectomy as a revisional approach for failed laparoscopic adjustable gastric banding in the treatment of morbid obesity. Obes Surg. 2009;19(12):1612–6.
18. Alqahtani AR, Elahmedi M, Alamri H, Mohammed R, Darwish F, Ahmed AM. Laparoscopic removal of poor outcome gastric banding with concomitant sleeve gastrectomy. Obes Surg. 2013;23(6):782–7.
19. Stroh C, Benedix D, Weiner R, Benedix F, Wolff S, Knoll C, et al. Is a one-step sleeve gastrectomy indicated as a revision procedure after gastric banding? Data analysis from a quality assurance study of the surgical treatment of obesity in Germany. Obes Surg. 2014;24(1):9–14.
20. Slater GH, Fielding GA. Combining laparoscopic adjustable gastric banding and biliopancreatic diversion after failed bariatric surgery. Obes Surg. 2004;14(5):677–82.
21. Vijgen GHEJ, Schouten R, Pelzers L, Greve JW, van Helden SH, Bouvy ND. Revision of laparoscopic adjustable gastric banding: success or failure? Obes Surg. 2012;22(2):287–92.
22. Müller MK, Attigah N, Wildi S, Hahnloser D, Hauser R, Clavien P-A, et al. High secondary failure rate of rebanding after failed gastric banding. Surg Endosc. 2008;22(2):448–53.
23. Piazza L, Di Stefano C, Ferrara F, Bellia A, Vacante M, Biondi A. Revision of failed primary adjustable gastric banding to mini-gastric bypass: results in 48 consecutive patients. Updates Surg. 2015;67(4):433–7.

Revisional Surgical Options After Laparoscopic Sleeve Gastrectomy

30

Praveen Raj Palanivelu

30.1 Introduction

With increasing rates of obesity and its related co morbidities, the number of bariatric procedures has also steadily increased [1–3]. Over the years many new procedures have been introduced and many have become obsolete. Laparoscopic sleeve gastrectomy (LSG), which was initially performed as the first stage of a laparoscopic biliopancreatic diversion with duodenal switch (LBPD-DS) has now gained tremendous popularity as a independent bariatric procedure due to its comparable results with roux-en-Y gastric bypass (RYGB), both in terms of weight loss and resolution of co- morbidities [4–8]. A recent review of long term weight loss results showed that the overall mean percentage of excess weight loss was 55 % at the end of 8 years [9]. This has been encouraging reflecting on the increasing numbers of LSG being performed today. The popularity could also be attributed to the relative safety and reproducibility associated with the procedure [3].

Similar to any bariatric procedure, LSG has also been reported with insufficient weight loss, weight regain and other complications like gastro-esophageal reflux disease (GERD), strictures etc. requiring revisional procedures. Although the strategies for management of the latter mentioned complications are better defined, the strategies for weight regain and inadequate weight loss after LSG has not been appropriately defined [10–12].

In this chapter, we have analyzed the existing literature on revisional options after sleeve gastrectomy to guide the choice of the appropriate surgical procedure for patients with weight regain or failure after LSG when surgical management is considered appropriate.

P.R. Palanivelu, MS, DNB, DNB (SGE), FALS, FMAS
Bariatric Division, Upper Gastrointestinal Surgery and Minimal Access Surgery Unit, GEM Hospital and Research Centre, Coimbatore, India
e-mail: drraj@geminstitute.in

P.R. Palanivelu et al. (eds.), *Bariatric Surgical Practice Guide*,
DOI 10.1007/978-981-10-2705-5_30

30.2 Definitions of Success or Failure of Bariatric Procedures

The success or failure of LSG can be expressed in many ways. Based upon the percentage of excess weight loss, >65 % is considered an excellent outcome, 50–65 % is considered a good outcome and <50 % is considered as a failure [13]. Based upon the bariatric analysis and reporting outcome system (BAROS) score, a score of >3 is considered a success [14]. According to the Reinhold criteria a postoperative BMI <35 is considered successful and according to the Biron criteria which is similar to Reinhold criteria a BMI <40 in extremely obese and <35 in obese following surgery is considered successful [15, 16].

30.3 Evaluation of Patients with Failure After Sleeve Gastrectomy

The reasons for failure could be either patient related factors, technique related factors or a combination of both. Hence, the principles of management of any patient with inadequate weight loss or weight regain is to understand the patient related factors and provide appropriate lifestyle management and also to identify anatomical factors which could possibly be corrected surgically [17, 18].

Evaluation of any patient with inadequate weight loss or weight regain would include identification of patient factors related to eating habits, psychological factors and identification of anatomical factors which could require potential surgical correction [19]. This would include dilatation of the stomach and assessment of residual gastric volume (RGV) [17, 18].

Dilatation can be primary or secondary [17]. Primary dilatation refers to a dilated posterior gastric pouch which was incompletely dissected and removed during the initial procedure. This stresses the importance of a thorough posterior dissection and adequate excision of the fundus [20]. Primary dilatation can be identified in the immediate or early post-operative period by upper GI series showing a large proximal remnant which progressively dilates over time. Secondary dilatation refers to a homogeneously dilated stomach tube, which was normal in the initial post-operative period and identified during the course of follow up. This could be a natural phenomenon at the level of the LSG, secondary to patients eating habits or could be precipitated by a narrowing at the level of the incisura with upstream dilatation [17].

Deguines JB et al. have shown that a residual gastric volume of over 250 cc has correlated significantly with inferior results following LSG and have also shown that laproscopic re-sleeve gastrectomy (LRSG) to provide good results in patients with higher RGV [10, 18]. Similar results have also been shown by Noel et al. who had a mean CT volumetry of 387.76 cc (275–555 cc) in 21 patients prior to LRSG [17]. The RGV can be studied using a combination of sodium bicarbonate and tartaric acid [18].

Evaluation of a patient with inadequate weight loss or weight regain should also include a good understanding of the patients eating pattern. This could be volume eating (hyperphagia) and frequent eating (polyphagia) [21]. Hyperphagia would correlate with gastric dilatation and would necessitate additional restriction. Polypahgia necessitates a behavioral therapy followed by addition of a malabsorptive procedure if necessary [21, 22]. This was the basis of selection of the procedure by Dapri et al. who had performed LRSG in patients with hyperphagia and LBPD-DS in patients with polyphagia.

30.4 Strategies for Management of Weight Regain or Failure After Sleeve Gastrectromy

In patients with inadequate weight loss or weight regain, no specific guidelines exist on the appropriate management strategy. Many different procedures have been attempted in this set of patients including LRSG, LRYGB, Lap Omega loop gastric bypass (LOGB), placement of adjustable band over the sleeve, butterfly gastroplasty and LBPD-DS. With many different procedures being reported with varying success rates, no specific criteria exist to appropriately choose the type of procedure.

30.4.1 Laparoscopic Revisional Sleeve Gastrectomy (LRSG)

LRSG is one of the commonly reported procedures following LSG especially in patients with dilated/large gastric pouch [6, 10, 17, 21, 23, 24]. It is based on the principle of adding more restriction hence reducing the RGV. LRSG was first described by Gagner and Rogula in a patient operated for LBPD/DS with a dilated gastric pouch, with excellent results [24]. Baltasar later reported two cases of LRSG with large fundus in one patient and antral dilatation in another [23]. Ianelli et al. showed an increase in %EWL from 46.5 to 71.4 % following LRSG in 13 patients with large gastric fundus and/or body/antrum as noted in upper GI series [6]. Rebibo et al. had shown mean %EWL of 65.95 % at 12 months following LRSG in patients with RGV above 250 cc, with the mean BMI dropping from 43 to 33 [10]. In the series from Dapri et al., seven patients underwent a LRSG achieving a %EWL of 43.7 % with a mean follow up of 23.2 months [21]. Noel et al. reported a %EWL of 58.5 % following LRSG with a mean follow up of 19.9 months [17]. This was specifically performed on patients with higher RGV.

Although the results have been encouraging, the incidence of complications after LRSG have been high. Rebibo et al. had reported two patients (13.3 %) with gastric leak, one patient with post operative bleeding and one post operative death [10]. Dapri et al. had reported one patient (14.2 %) with sleeve leak and Noel et al. had one patient with perigastric hematoma [17, 21]. Trelles et al. had reported a complicated gastrocolic fistula following LRSG in a prior LBPD-DS patient [25]. This incidence was much higher compared to the primary sleeve gastrectomy group [26].

30.4.2 Laparoscopic Roux-en-Y Gastric Bypass

LRYGB is another procedure which has shown promising results in patients with failure of LSG. Revisional LSG to LRYGB was first performed by Regan et al. as a planned first stage procedure for super obese patients [27]. Recent series on LSG conversion to LRYGB for LSG failure has shown excellent results. Idan Carmelli et al. retrospectively reported ten patients who underwent a revisional LSG to LRYGB with % EWL of 66.6 % with a mean follow-up of 16 months [28]. One case of stomal ulcer with bleeding was reported which was managed conservatively. Gautier et al. reported nine patients with revisional LRYGB who had a % EWL of 59 % with a mean followup of 15.5 months [29]. One patient in this series reported small bowel injury with subsequent peritonitis.

Van Rutte et al. reported 37 patients with a revisional LRYGB, of which 14 had the initial sleeve as a staged procedure, 5 after a secondary sleeve and 18 after a primary sleeve with failure [11]. The patients had a % EWL of 45.9, 52.5 and 80.3 % in each of the groups respectively. Their series had one patient with enterocutaneous fistula in the second group, two patients with post operative bleeding, two with anastamotic leakage and one internal hernia in the third group.

The recent systematic review by Cheung et al. on revisional surgery following LSG showed no signifiant difference between patients undergoing LRSG and LRYGB with an %EWL of 48 vs 44 % [30]. However the series of LRSG were specifically performed in patients with a large dilated fundus and those of the LRYGB series had no specific mention. This could be that the patients in the LRYGB group might not have had significant dilatation making LRSG not a feasible option.

From the above data we now understand that both LRSG and LRYGB does provide convincing weight loss in these subset of patients and LRSG is a possible alternative in patients with hyperphagia, dilated gastric fundus or with a RGV of over 250 cc [6, 10, 17, 21, 23]. But caution has to be exerted as a much higher incidence of complications have been reported in both the LRSG and LRYGB group [10, 11, 17, 21, 25, 29].

30.4.3 Laparoscopic Bilio-Pancreatic Diversion with Duodenal Switch

Conversion of LSG to LBPD-DS has also shown promising results but most of the series have been for planned conversion where LSG was performed as a first stage procedure [4, 5]. But this is a potential option where the primary restriction has failed as understood by a non dilated sleeve. But as mentioned above, polyphagia, if present needs to be corrected by a behavior therapy before contemplating a surgical approach. Again the incidence of complications are higher than primary LBPD-DS as shown by Dapri et al. who had 1 patient with post-operative bleeding, one with duodenoileostomy leak and one with duodenoileostomy stricture among 19 patients who had a revision [21]. They also had reported better weight loss in patients who underwent a BPD-DS compared to the ones who had a LRSG, but with higher late complications like hypo-proteinemia in two patients and ventral hernia in one patient, who eventually required surgical intervention. Idan Carmeli et al. had shown an %EWL of 80.3 % in patients who had a BPD-DS which was better compared to RYGB who had 66.6 % [28].

Although the results looks encouraging from the aspect of weight loss, caution has to be exerted in selecting patients for a BPD-DS owing to its higher rates of complications [21, 28, 31, 32].

30.4.4 Other Procedures

The other procedures that have been reported are laparoscopic one-anastomosis gastric bypass, placement of adjustable band over the sleeve, laparoscopic butterfly gastroplasty and laparoscopic ileal interposition with varying success [27, 33]. With endoluminal approaches gaining popularity in bariatric practice, may find potential use in the revisional setting too in the future [34]. Endosocopic sleeve plication has also been recently reported [35]. With limited data on these procedures, no firm conclusion can be arrived until larger and long term data become available.

Conclusion

With increasing numbers of bariatric surgeries being performed, the numbers of revisional procedure are also expected to rise. Lifestyle and behavior modification would hold key as the first line of management. If these measures fail, then surgical intervention can be considered. The two most commonly performed procedure are LRSG and LRYGB. LRSG can be effective in patients with primary/secondary dilatation with a RGV of over 250 cc, who present with hyperphagia. Lap BPD-DS can be selectively performed with strict follow-up to monitor for nutritional complications. Other procedures are still in its infancy and cannot be advocated as standard of care based on current data.

Recommendations

- Patients need to be evaluated for patient factors, technical factors or both.
- Correction of patient factors is crucial before planning for surgery.
- Evaluation for dilatation of the stomach and the residual gastric volume is needed.
- Patients with a dilated sleeve defined as a RGV of >250 cc, or with hyperphagia (volume eating) or endoscopy suggestive of a dilated fundus may benefit from a re-sleeve gastrectomy/LRYGB but with higher complication rates than a primary procedure.
- In patients without any dilatation, LRYGB or DS are the options to be considered. Malabsorptive procedure like BPD-DS has shown better outcomes compared to LRYGB, but with the expense of higher nutritional and surgical complications.

References

1. Ogden CL, Carroll MD, Kit BK, Flegal KM. Prevalence of childhood and adult obesity in the United States, 2011–2012. JAMA. 2014;311(8):806–14.
2. Buchwald H, Williams SE. Bariatric surgery worldwide 2003. Obes Surg. 2004;14(9):1157–64.
3. Buchwald H, Oien DM. Metabolic/bariatric surgery worldwide 2011. Obes Surg. 2013;23(4):427–36.
4. Milone L, Strong V, Gagner M. Laparoscopic sleeve gastrectomy is superior to endoscopic intragastric balloon as a first stage procedure for super-obese patients (BMI > or =50). Obes Surg. 2005;15(5):612–7.
5. Basso N, Casella G, Rizzello M, Abbatini F, Soricelli E, Alessandri G, et al. Laparoscopic sleeve gastrectomy as first stage or definitive intent in 300 consecutive cases. Surg Endosc. 2011;25(2):444–9.
6. Iannelli A, Facchiano E, Gugenheim J. Internal hernia after laparoscopic Roux-en-Y gastric bypass for morbid obesity. Obes Surg. 2006;16(10):1265–71.
7. Keidar A, Hershkop KJ, Marko L, Schweiger C, Hecht L, Bartov N, et al. Roux-en-Y gastric bypass vs sleeve gastrectomy for obese patients with type 2 diabetes: a randomised trial. Diabetologia. 2013;56(9):1914–8.
8. Yaghoubian A, Tolan A, Stabile BE, Kaji AH, Belzberg G, Mun E, et al. Laparoscopic Roux-en-Y gastric bypass and sleeve gastrectomy achieve comparable weight loss at 1 year. Am Surg. 2012;78(12):1325–8.
9. Diamantis T, Apostolou KG, Alexandrou A, Griniatsos J, Felekouras E, Tsigris C. Review of long-term weight loss results after laparoscopic sleeve gastrectomy. Surg Obes Relat Dis Off J Am Soc Bariatr Surg. 2014;10(1):177–83.
10. Rebibo L, Fuks D, Verhaeghe P, Deguines J-B, Dhahri A, Regimbeau J-M. Repeat sleeve gastrectomy compared with primary sleeve gastrectomy: a single-center, matched case study. Obes Surg. 2012;22(12):1909–15.
11. van Rutte PWJ, Smulders JF, de Zoete JP, Nienhuijs SW. Indications and short-term outcomes of revisional surgery after failed or complicated sleeve gastrectomy. Obes Surg. 2012;22(12):1903–8.
12. Burgos AM, Csendes A, Braghetto I. Gastric stenosis after laparoscopic sleeve gastrectomy in morbidly obese patients. Obes Surg. 2013;23(9):1481–6.
13. Deitel M, Greenstein RJ. Recommendations for reporting weight loss. Obes Surg. 2003;13(2):159–60.
14. Oria HE, Moorehead MK. Bariatric analysis and reporting outcome system (BAROS). Obes Surg. 1998;8(5):487–99.
15. Reinhold RB. Critical analysis of long term weight loss following gastric bypass. Surg Gynecol Obstet. 1982;155(3):385–94.
16. Biron S, Hould F-S, Lebel S, Marceau S, Lescelleur O, Simard S, et al. Twenty years of biliopancreatic diversion: what is the goal of the surgery? Obes Surg. 2004;14(2):160–4.
17. Noel P, Nedelcu M, Nocca D, Schneck A-S, Gugenheim J, Iannelli A, et al. Revised sleeve gastrectomy: another option for weight loss failure after sleeve gastrectomy. Surg Endosc. 2014;28(4):1096–102.
18. Deguines J-B, Verhaeghe P, Yzet T, Robert B, Cosse C, Regimbeau J-M. Is the residual gastric volume after laparoscopic sleeve gastrectomy an objective criterion for adapting the treatment strategy after failure? Surg Obes Relat Dis Off J Am Soc Bariatr Surg. 2013;9(5):660–6.
19. Rutledge T, Groesz LM, Savu M. Psychiatric factors and weight loss patterns following gastric bypass surgery in a veteran population. Obes Surg. 2011;21(1):29–35.
20. Kueper MA, Kramer KM, Kirschniak A, Königsrainer A, Pointner R, Granderath FA. Laparoscopic sleeve gastrectomy: standardized technique of a potential stand-alone bariatric procedure in morbidly obese patients. World J Surg. 2008;32(7):1462–5.
21. Dapri G, Cadière GB, Himpens J. Laparoscopic repeat sleeve gastrectomy versus duodenal switch after isolated sleeve gastrectomy for obesity. Surg Obes Relat Dis Off J Am Soc Bariatr Surg. 2011;7(1):38–43.

22. Weineland S, Arvidsson D, Kakoulidis TP, Dahl J. Acceptance and commitment therapy for bariatric surgery patients, a pilot RCT. Obes Res Clin Pract. 2012;6(1):e1–90.
23. Baltasar A, Serra C, Pérez N, Bou R, Bengochea M. Re-sleeve gastrectomy. Obes Surg. 2006;16(11):1535–8.
24. Gagner M, Rogula T. Laparoscopic reoperative sleeve gastrectomy for poor weight loss after biliopancreatic diversion with duodenal switch. Obes Surg. 2003;13(4):649–54.
25. Trelles N, Gagner M, Palermo M, Pomp A, Dakin G, Parikh M. Gastrocolic fistula after re-sleeve gastrectomy: outcomes after esophageal stent implantation. Surg Obes Relat Dis Off J Am Soc Bariatr Surg. 2010;6(3):308–12.
26. Zellmer JD, Mathiason MA, Kallies KJ, Kothari SN. Is laparoscopic sleeve gastrectomy a lower risk bariatric procedure compared with laparoscopic Roux-en-Y gastric bypass? A meta-analysis. Am J Surg. 2014;208(6):903–10; discussion 909–10.
27. Regan JP, Inabnet WB, Gagner M, Pomp A. Early experience with two-stage laparoscopic Roux-en-Y gastric bypass as an alternative in the super-super obese patient. Obes Surg. 2003;13(6):861–4.
28. Carmeli I, Golomb I, Sadot E, Kashtan H, Keidar A. Laparoscopic conversion of sleeve gastrectomy to a biliopancreatic diversion with duodenal switch or a Roux-en-Y gastric bypass due to weight loss failure: our algorithm. Surg Obes Relat Dis Off J Am Soc Bariatr Surg. 2015;11(1):79–85.
29. Gautier T, Sarcher T, Contival N, Le Roux Y, Alves A. Indications and mid-term results of conversion from sleeve gastrectomy to Roux-en-Y gastric bypass. Obes Surg. 2013;23(2):212–5.
30. Cheung D, Switzer NJ, Gill RS, Shi X, Karmali S. Revisional bariatric surgery following failed primary laparoscopic sleeve gastrectomy: a systematic review. Obes Surg. 2014;24(10):1757–63.
31. Buchwald H, Estok R, Fahrbach K, Banel D, Sledge I. Trends in mortality in bariatric surgery: a systematic review and meta-analysis. Surgery. 2007;142(4):621–32; discussion 632–5.
32. Kim W-W, Gagner M, Kini S, Inabnet WB, Quinn T, Herron D, et al. Laparoscopic vs. open biliopancreatic diversion with duodenal switch: a comparative study. J Gastrointest Surg Off J Soc Surg Aliment Tract. 2003;7(4):552–7.
33. Moszkowicz D, Rau C, Guenzi M, Zinzindohoué F, Berger A, Chevallier J-M. Laparoscopic omega-loop gastric bypass for the conversion of failed sleeve gastrectomy: early experience. J Visc Surg. 2013;150(6):373–8.
34. Çelik A, Ugale S, Ofluoğlu H. Laparoscopic diverted resleeve with ileal transposition for failed laparoscopic sleeve gastrectomy: a case report. Surg Obes Relat Dis Off J Am Soc Bariatr Surg. 2015;11(1):e5–7.
35. Majumder S, Birk J. A review of the current status of endoluminal therapy as a primary approach to obesity management. Surg Endosc. 2013;27(7):2305–11.

Revisional Surgical Options After Laparoscopic Roux-en-Y Gastric Bypass

31

Praveen Raj Palanivelu and Saravana Kumar

31.1 Introduction

Laparoscopic Roux-en-Y gastric bypass (LRYGB) is one of the most commonly performed bariatric procedures worldwide [1]. LRYGB has also been proven to be an effective bariatric procedure in terms of weight loss and resolution of comorbidities. But a significant percentage of patients may require surgical revision or reversal for inadequate weight loss, weight recidivism or complications related to nutrition (deficiencies, protein energy malnutrition) or surgery (dumping, persistent nausea/vomiting) etc. [2–4]. In fact, the most common reason for re- operative bariatric surgery after LRYGB is inadequate weight loss. Long- term studies have shown that at 10-year follow up, RYGB failure rates were between 15–35 % [5]. The definitions for failure have been described in the earlier chapter on revision after Laparoscopic sleeve gastrectomy (LSG).

The assessment of the bariatric patient at this point must begin with a thorough history and physical examination. The reasons for failure are multifactorial and these patients need to be evaluated for anatomic, behavioral, psychological, hormonal and metabolic reasons for their weight regain by a multidisciplinary team. Appropriate further investigations should include either an esophagogastroduodenoscopy or upper gastrointestinal study to rule out a gastro-gastric fistula, hiatal hernia, or gastric pouch/anastomotic dilatation.

The aim of this chapter is to review the current literature on surgical options for failure or weight regain after LRYGB due to anatomical complications.

The several surgical strategies attempted include laparoscopic adjustable gastric banding (LAGB), pouch or anastomotic revision with or without endoluminal

P.R. Palanivelu, MS, DNB, DNB (SGE), FALS, FMAS (✉) • S. Kumar, DNB(Gen. Surg), FMAS
Bariatric Division, Upper Gastrointestinal Surgery and Minimal Access Surgery Unit,
GEM Hospital and Research Centre, Coimbatore, India
e-mail: drraj@geminstitute.in; drsakubariatric@gmail.com

P.R. Palanivelu et al. (eds.), *Bariatric Surgical Practice Guide*,
DOI 10.1007/978-981-10-2705-5_31

techniques and conversion to a LDRYGB or a laparoscopic bilio-pancreatic diversion with duodenal switch (BPD-DS).

31.1.1 Laparoscopic Adjustable Gastric Banding

Pouch dilation is a frequent finding after LRYGB even in patients who maintain good weight loss [6]. This procedure involves placing a LAGB on the gastric pouch of the RYGB in an attempt to promote greater gastric restriction for the patient especially recommended for hyperphagic patients. The safety and efficacy of LAGB for failed LRYGB has been well demonstrated wherein LAGB provides external reinforcement to help regulate the pouch size over time [6–9]. As a result, it may reduce hunger and increase satiety in patients who fail to lose weight [10]. Bessler et al. found that LAGB after LRYGB produced an EWL of 38 % and 44 % at 12 and 24 months, respectively [6]. A larger study by Irani et al. reported a mean EWL of 38.3 % on 42 patients with a mean follow-up of 26 months (range 6–66) after LAGB placement [11]. However complications of LAGB (erosion/slippage) were to an extent of 10 %. The study also noted a higher complication rate compared with primary LAGB patients, which was expected given that band placements were part of a revisional procedure. It is also to be noted that salvage banding is technically challenging due to dense adhesions carrying significant morbidity. This approach may still be an option in carefully selected patients who have a dilated pouch and/or stoma following RYGB [12].

31.1.2 Pouch or Anastomotic Revision with Surgery or Endoluminal Techniques

Some small series have shown that pouch resizing and anastomotic revision can be performed safely with reasonably good outcomes [13–15]. Surgical or endoluminal re-creation versus banding allows addressing all the dilated components i.e. the pouch, stoma and the alimentary limb, all of which function as one unit. These revisions have been performed in many different ways. Muller et al. reported a technique of dividing the pouch proximal to the anastomosis and resection the anastomosis with a portion of the alimentary limb and creating a new gastrojejunostomy [16]. This technique has been shown to help in further weight loss and also improvement of symptoms related to poor pouch emptying. Parikh et al. evaluated another type of revisional procedure, termed "gastro-jejunal sleeve reduction." wherein an orogastric bougie (e.g., 40F) is guided into the jejunum and a linear stapler is serially fired trimming the alimentary limb, gastrojejunostomy (GJ) and the gastric pouch toward the left crus. However this technique did not appear to offer any significant therapeutic benefit with only 12 % EWL at 1 year [17]. León et al. had demonstrated a technique of gastro-jejunal reduction by performing a hand-sewn double-layer gastro-jejunal plication (GJP) [14].

A few endoscopic techniques have also been described to revise pouches. Spaulding et al. had performed circumferential sclerotherapy injections (1 mL of 5 % morrhuate sodium) into the muscular wall at the gastrojejunostomy to decrease the diameter [18]. Although this was 100 % successful in reducing the size of the stoma, more than one session was often required and the clinical effect in terms of weight loss was only marginal. The risk of chemical esophagitis, stricture, or fatal hemorrhage if injected into the aorta has to be considered.

Endoscopic suturing devices have also been developed to endoluminally reduce the pouch or stoma size after LRYGB [19]. This was shown to be effective in the short term [20]. However the long-term benefits are still unknown as the sutures could be lost within a year and the stoma likely re-distends [21]. A large prospective trial by Horgan et al. using expandable tissue anchors made of biocompatible, non-absorbable suture and nitinol to create stomal and pouch tissue folds had shown that 88 % of patients had stopped regaining weight at 6 months of follow-up, with an average EWL of 18 % [19]. Early results of Stomaphy X, another new surgical endoscopic device has demonstrated 19.5 % EWL at 1 year. This device suctions the surrounding tissue and fires polypropylene H-fasteners to form a circular pleat of tissue slightly proximal to the anastomosis resulting in a reduced stomal diameter [22]. Although recent studies have demonstrated that the above-mentioned endoscopic techniques are safe and effective, further evaluation is necessary given that their long-term benefits are unknown.

31.1.3 Laparoscopic Distal Roux-en-Y Gastric Bypass (LDRYGB)

Revision of LRYGB to a Laparoscopic distal Roux-en-Y gastric bypass (LDRYGB) has been the most common revision performed for inadequate weight loss after LRYGB which works by increasing the malabsorptive element and is preferred in polyphagic patients [23]. In a conventional LRYGB, the Roux limb is between 75 and 150 cm, preserving most of the small bowel for absorption of nutrients. In a LDRYGB the alimentary is made longer and the length of the common channel is significantly reduced thereby increasing the malabsorption. However, this is associated with a higher risk of developing protein malnutrition and significant diarrhea [24]. Therefore, patients who undergo revisional LDRYGB require more frequent monitoring and nutritional supplementation. It has also been recommended to supplement fat-soluble vitamins and calcium to prevent night blindness and osteoporosis. Patients can also develop symptoms of bacterial overgrowth (i.e., diarrhea, fever, and malaise) in their bypassed intestine [25]. Sugerman et al. converted LRYGB patients with less than 40 % EWL to a distal gastric bypass achieving an EWL of 61 % at 1 year and 69 % at 5 years after revision [25]. The common channel was 50 cm from the ileocecal valve in five patients and 150 cm from the ileocaecal valve in 22 patients. Malnutrition occurred in all five patients with a 50 cm "common tract" requiring further parenteral nutrition and revision back to long-limb LRYGB. Two of these patients died of hepatic failure. Three of 22 patients with a 150 cm common channel required revision for malnutrition. Therefore, the study concluded that a 50 cm common channel LDRYGB should not be used because of an unacceptable morbidity and mortality henceby recommending a 150 cm common tract. Even with 150 cm common channel, it is important to recognize that revision to a LDRYGB is also potentially dangerous and mandates a close follow up in the long-term. A recent study by Caruana et al. had concluded that revision of RYGB to distal bypass when it is <70 % of a patient's total small bowel length results in an acceptable balance of weight loss with safety.

31.1.4 Laparoscopic Biliopancreatic Diversion with Duodenal Switch

Conversion of a failed LRYGB for inadequate weight loss or weight regain to a more malabsorptive option is possible by converting to a LBPD-DS which again acts by increasing the malabsorptive element. But this is a more technically complex operation with only small numbers reporting long-term results [23]. Parikh et al. had reported this technique to be highly effective with 63 % EWL at 11 months [4]. Keshishian et al. also reported an EWL of 69 % at 30 months and suggested LBPD-DS appears to be the most effective bariatric operation producing the most sustained weight loss without the unwanted side effects seen in other bariatric operations [26]. However this series reported a leak rate of 15 %. The authors also concluded that patients with surgical complications such as dumping syndrome, intolerance to solids, or persistent nausea and vomiting would benefit from this conversion. However it was cautioned that for patients who present with weight gain or inappropriate weight loss with a preoperative BMI lower than the guidelines set by the National Institute of Health, should not be converted to a LBPD-DS due to unjustifiable risk of serious complications.

Recommendations

- Patients need to be evaluated for patient factors, technical factors or both.
- Correction of patient factors is crucial before planning for surgery.
- LAGB on the gastric pouch, surgical revision of the pouch with/without stoma revision can be performed with a dilated pouch and/or stoma and/or hyperphagia following RYGB.
- In patients without any dilatation, Laparoscopic distal Roux-en-Y gastric bypass or biliopancreatic diversion are the options to be considered. Both the procedures have high chances of nutritional complications necessitating close follow up.

References

1. Angrisani L, Santonicola A, Iovino P, Formisano G, Buchwald H, Scopinaro N. Bariatric surgery worldwide 2013. Obes Surg. 2015;25(10):1822–32.
2. Vilallonga R, van de Vrande S, Himpens J. Laparoscopic reversal of Roux-en-Y gastric bypass into normal anatomy with or without sleeve gastrectomy. Surg Endosc. 2013;27(12):4640–8.
3. Campos GM, Ziemelis M, Paparodis R, Ahmed M, Davis DB. Laparoscopic reversal of Roux-en-Y gastric bypass: technique and utility for treatment of endocrine complications. Surg Obes Relat Dis Off J Am Soc Bariatr Surg. 2014;10(1):36–43.
4. Parikh M, Pomp A, Gagner M. Laparoscopic conversion of failed gastric bypass to duodenal switch: technical considerations and preliminary outcomes. Surg Obes Relat Dis Off J Am Soc Bariatr Surg. 2007;3(6):611–8.
5. Christou NV, Look D, Maclean LD. Weight gain after short- and long-limb gastric bypass in patients followed for longer than 10 years. Ann Surg. 2006;244(5):734–40.
6. Bessler M, Daud A, DiGiorgi MF, Olivero-Rivera L, Davis D. Adjustable gastric banding as a revisional bariatric procedure after failed gastric bypass. Obes Surg. 2005;15(10):1443–8.
7. Gobble RM, Parikh MS, Greives MR, Ren CJ, Fielding GA. Gastric banding as a salvage procedure for patients with weight loss failure after Roux-en-Y gastric bypass. Surg Endosc. 2008;22(4):1019–22.
8. Chin PL, Ali M, Francis K, LePort PC. Adjustable gastric band placed around gastric bypass pouch as revision operation for failed gastric bypass. Surg Obes Relat Dis Off J Am Soc Bariatr Surg. 2009;5(1):38–42.
9. Bessler M, Daud A, DiGiorgi MF, Inabnet WB, Schrope B, Olivero-Rivera L, et al. Adjustable gastric banding as revisional bariatric procedure after failed gastric bypass – intermediate results. Surg Obes Relat Dis Off J Am Soc Bariatr Surg. 2010;6(1):31–5.
10. Dixon AFR, Dixon JB, O'Brien PE. Laparoscopic adjustable gastric banding induces prolonged satiety: a randomized blind crossover study. J Clin Endocrinol Metab. 2005;90(2):813–9.
11. Irani K, Youn HA, Ren-Fielding CJ, Fielding GA, Kurian M. Midterm results for gastric banding as salvage procedure for patients with weight loss failure after Roux-en-Y gastric bypass. Surg Obes Relat Dis Off J Am Soc Bariatr Surg. 2011;7(2):219–24.
12. Aminian A, Corcelles R, Daigle CR, Chand B, Brethauer SA, Schauer PR. Critical appraisal of salvage banding for weight loss failure after gastric bypass. Surg Obes Relat Dis Off J Am Soc Bariatr Surg. 2015;11(3):607–11.
13. Al-Bader I, Khoursheed M, Al Sharaf K, Mouzannar DA, Ashraf A, Fingerhut A. Revisional laparoscopic gastric pouch resizing for inadequate weight loss after Roux-en-Y gastric bypass. Obes Surg. 2015;25(7):1103–8.
14. León F, Maiz C, Daroch D, Quezada N, Gabrielli M, Muñoz C, et al. Laparoscopic hand-sewn revisional gastrojejunal plication for weight loss failure after Roux-en-Y gastric bypass. Obes Surg. 2015;25(4):744–9.
15. Nguyen D, Dip F, Huaco JA, Moon R, Ahmad H, LoMenzo E, et al. Outcomes of revisional treatment modalities in non-complicated Roux-en-Y gastric bypass patients with weight regain. Obes Surg. 2015;25(5):928–34.
16. Müller MK, Wildi S, Scholz T, Clavien P-A, Weber M. Laparoscopic pouch resizing and redo of gastro-jejunal anastomosis for pouch dilatation following gastric bypass. Obes Surg. 2005;15(8):1089–95.
17. Parikh M, Heacock L, Gagner M. Laparoscopic "gastrojejunal sleeve reduction" as a revision procedure for weight loss failure after roux-en-y gastric bypass. Obes Surg. 2011;21(5):650–4.
18. Spaulding L. Treatment of dilated gastrojejunostomy with sclerotherapy. Obes Surg. 2003;13(2):254–7.
19. Horgan S, Jacobsen G, Weiss GD, Oldham JS, Denk PM, Borao F, et al. Incisionless revision of post-Roux-en-Y bypass stomal and pouch dilation: multicenter registry results. Surg Obes Relat Dis Off J Am Soc Bariatr Surg. 2010;6(3):290–5.

20. Gitelis M, Ujiki M, Farwell L, Linn J, Wang C, Miller K, et al. Six month outcomes in patients experiencing weight gain after gastric bypass who underwent gastrojejunal revision using an endoluminal suturing device. Surg Endosc. 2015;29(8):2133–40.
21. Thompson CC, Slattery J, Bundga ME, Lautz DB. Peroral endoscopic reduction of dilated gastrojejunal anastomosis after Roux-en-Y gastric bypass: a possible new option for patients with weight regain. Surg Endosc. 2006;20(11):1744–8.
22. Mikami D, Needleman B, Narula V, Durant J, Melvin WS. Natural orifice surgery: initial US experience utilizing the StomaphyX device to reduce gastric pouches after Roux-en-Y gastric bypass. Surg Endosc. 2010;24(1):223–8.
23. Gumbs AA, Pomp A, Gagner M. Revisional bariatric surgery for inadequate weight loss. Obes Surg. 2007;17(9):1137–45.
24. Fobi MA, Lee H, Igwe D, Felahy B, James E, Stanczyk M, et al. Revision of failed gastric bypass to distal Roux-en-Y gastric bypass: a review of 65 cases. Obes Surg. 2001;11(2):190–5.
25. Sugerman HJ, Kellum JM, DeMaria EJ. Conversion of proximal to distal gastric bypass for failed gastric bypass for superobesity. J Gastrointest Surg Off J Soc Surg Aliment Tract. 1997;1(6):517–24; discussion 524–6.
26. Keshishian A, Zahriya K, Hartoonian T, Ayagian C. Duodenal switch is a safe operation for patients who have failed other bariatric operations. Obes Surg. 2004;14(9):1187–92.

Part VIII

Nutritional Management in Bariatric Surgery

Perioperative Diet Management in Bariatric Surgery

32

Parimala Devi and Praveen Raj Palanivelu

Bariatric surgery is an effective weight loss procedure in morbidly obese people. A short term pre-operative energy restrictive diet or 'liver shrinkage diet' is widely accepted practice to reduce the fatty liver mass and to improve the liver flexibility [1]. This occurs by reduction of glycogen and lipid stores and reduction of visceral adipose tissue depots. This enables easy access to the upper stomach and oesophagus during liver retraction [1–4]. Preoperative weight loss has been shown to improve control of co-morbidities, decrease operative times and improve percentage of excess weight loss in the short term [5]. In addition some studies have also demonstrated a decrease in postoperative complications [6, 7].

A recent observational study from UK reported that 59 % practitioners used a low energy, food based low carbohydrate and liquid diet, 18 % used a milk/yogurt diet, 18 % used a meal replacement liquid diet and 2 % used a clear liquid diet. The preoperative diet period varied from 7 to 42 days [8]. Although the pre-surgical caloric restriction has been widely followed in many centers around the world, however the type of diet and duration of the diet markedly varies and there exists no standard guidelines.

The aim of this chapter is to understand the importance of the pre-operative bariatric dietary program and the type of diet/duration needed based on existing literature.

P. Devi, MSc (✉) • P.R. Palanivelu, MS, DNB, DNB (SGE), FALS, FMAS
Bariatric Division, Upper Gastrointestinal Surgery and Minimal Access Surgery Unit, GEM Hospital and Research Centre, Coimbatore, India
e-mail: parimalaswamy30@gmail.com; drraj@geminstitute.in

P.R. Palanivelu et al. (eds.), *Bariatric Surgical Practice Guide*,
DOI 10.1007/978-981-10-2705-5_32

32.1 Choice of Pre-operative Diet

The pre-operative diet can be either a partial or complete formula based diet or meal replacement and a food based diet [1–4]. A randomized trial of a very low calorie diet showed formula based diets and standard diets are both capable of achieving comparable results on preoperative weight loss before bariatric surgery However patient compliance, tolerance and acceptance were all significantly better after a standard diet [9]. Another study showed that a partial use of a formula diet is more effective in reducing body weight than food-based diets alone perhaps due to a balanced composition of the formula and improved compliance [10]. Whatever be type of diet is used the selection of the amount of carbohydrate intake is most important as it may directly affect the level of the liver fat and liver volume [11]. It has also been shown that a low carbohydrate diet results in reduction of insulin resistance too [12]. Fluid recommendations should be given with all diets from an additional 1 l of fluids to 3.5 l dependent on the type of diet. Micronutrient supplementation is essential in this preoperative phase. Emerging evidence also suggests that immunonutrition formulas may be even better than high protein formulas or regular diet of similar caloric intake [13].

The duration of a preoperative diet varies from 2 to 12 weeks [1–4]. However it has been shown that 80% of expected liver volume reduction will occur in the first 2 weeks of a very low energy restrictive diet [1]. It has also been demonstrated that compliance to diet restriction will reduce over time relative to the severity of energy restriction [14].

Thus a short term energy restrictive diet or liver shrinkage diet (food based or formula based) of around 2 weeks can be used in the pre surgery period.

32.2 Post Bariatric Surgery Diet

The principles of post bariatric surgery nutritional management are diet modifications based on the food texture, consistency and volume. The goal is to provide adequate energy and nutrition while reducing symptoms like dumping syndrome and early satiety [15–17]. Post nutritional requirement was not documented and was not stressed until protein malnutrition and other nutritional deficiencies had appeared [18–22]. In general, post-operative bariatric diet is comprised of four stages each providing a more advanced form of food texture than the previous starting from liquid to solid diet [23].

Stage 1: This is the stage of clear liquid diet composed of a low calorie, low sugar beverages which is started few hours after surgery. These beverages are free of caffeine, carbonation and alcohol. This will last for 1–2 days.

Stage 2: This stage comprises of full liquids containing high protein, low caloric beverages with low sugar content to prevent dumping syndrome especially in gastric bypass patients. This stage usually lasts for 2 weeks slowly advancing to mashed or pureed food.

Stage 3: Also called the pureed stage, the texture is soft, moist, minced, diced, grounded or pureed. If the patient does not tolerate this stage then they may remain on liquid diet for some time. This stage lasts for around 2 weeks.

Stage 4: This stage is the eventual transition to a solid-food diet, for which the dietitian will focus on monitoring eating speeds and volume, encouraging healthy eating for life. In addition, patients must separate solid foods from liquids with an interval of 30 min for better tolerability.

32.3 Macronutritient Requirements

The recommended dietary allowance for carbohydrate is 130 g/day for adults providing between 45 and 65 % of total energy intake (TEI). The role of carbohydrate in weight loss has been related to glycemic load but the outcomes have been varied. Moize et al. proposed a food pyramid model for bariatric surgery, in which a CHO intake of between 40 and 45 % of daily TEI was recommended [24].

Protein intake should be individualized, assessed, and guided by an experienced dietitian, with reference to gender, age, and weight. A minimal protein intake of 60 g/d and up to 1.5 g/kg ideal body weight per day should be adequate; higher amounts of protein intake – up to 2 g/kg ideal body weight per day – may be required in special situations. The importance of protein intake has been discussed later in chapter 33.

When the stomach size is reduced during bariatric surgery, there is an increase in pH secondary to the reduction of pepsin thereby limiting the early steps in fat digestion. Also malabsorptive procedures like bilio-pancreatic diversion (BPD) have been shown to decrease fat absorption by upto 72 %. This increases the risk for essential fatty acid and fat soluble vitamin deficiencies. Essential fatty acid deficiency symptoms includes dry scaly skin, hair loss, decreased immunity, increased susceptibility to infections, anemia, mood changes, and unexplained cardiac, hepatic, gastrointestinal and neurological dysfunction.

Researchers have shown that high fat diet (50 % of calories) resulted in fat storage and impaired suppression of carbohydrate oxidation. No relationship with oxidation was noted with low (20 % of energy derived from fats) or moderate (30 % of energy derived from fat) fat diets [25]. Thus fats should provide 20–30 % of the total energy. Saturated fat should be decreased and replace it with poly and monounsaturated fats.

32.4 Common Post-surgery Nutritional Problems

Dumping syndrome is commonly reported which mainly occurs after consumption of foods with a high sugar and carbohydrate content, resulting in symptoms of early dumping syndrome such as nausea, dizziness, weakness, rapid pulse, cold sweats, fatigue, cramps, and diarrhea 10–30 min after eating [26]. Some RYGB patients experience late dumping, which occurs 1–3 h after a meal as a result of an exaggerated insulin release and reactive hypoglycemia [26]. To prevent dumping syndrome sugar consumption should be less than 25 g per serving. Hence concentrated sugar containing drinks like soda, juices and frosts should be avoided and natural sugars like dairy and whole fruits can be included.

Nausea, vomiting, dehydration are the commonly seen early post operative complications due to eating and drinking methods. They tend to occur if patients eat fast or eat more or advance to solid foods quicker than the actual time and dietitians should guide them regarding their eating quantity, time and the frequency. If the symptoms continue, a diagnosis of stricture, pregnancy and ketosis should be looked for. In extremely nauseated patients, anti-emetics will prevent dehydration. A good daily goal of fluid is 64 ounces which equates to approximately 2 L [17]. When symptoms like dark coloured urine, tiredness, nausea, dizziness and extreme weight loss is seen, patients must be encouraged to drink clear liquids (e.g. water, tender coconut water) frequently by sipping slowly even though they do not have any interest in drinking.

Bariatric surgery patients often have diarrhea as a symptom of lactose intolerance, which can occur sometimes after gastric pass surgery and lactose should be avoided. If the symptoms persist after lactose elimination then other organic causes of diarrhea should be looked for.

32.5 Foods to Be Avoided After Surgery

Caffeine is an acid-secretion stimulator, and can cause gastric irritation and, when consumed in increased quantities it can precipitate dehydration [27]. Caffeine can also stimulate epinephrine release, which can negatively influence insulin sensitivity [28]. There is no clear evidence to avoid caffeine post surgery but caution should be taken against frequent consumption. Also, carbonated beverages can cause abdominal discomfort and reflux problems [20]. Although there's no clear evidence, it is suggested that carbonated drinks may stretch the gastric pouch and these are best avoided. In addition to these, alcohol consumption should be avoided due to decreased tolerance and the risk of ulcer formation after surgery [29].

Conclusion

Post-operative diet is based on food texture and nutrients and involves four stages of progression: sugar free clear liquid diet for 1–2 days, full liquid diet for 1–2 weeks, semisolid or pureed diet for the next 2 weeks followed by soft diet. Common problems in the postoperative period are nausea and vomiting, dumping syndrome and diarrhea which can be managed by eating time, pattern, frequency and type/texture of food. If persistent then organic causes are to be looked for. Caffeine, carbonated beverages and alcohol are best avoided in the postoperative period.

Recommendations

- A minimum period of 2 weeks of pre-operative low calorie diet reduces the fatty liver mass, improves co-morbidities, decreases operative times and improves percentage of excess weight loss in the short term.
- A postoperative liquid diet for 2 weeks is recommended before progressing onto pureed food, soft food and then more normal textured food along with a high protein intake and adequate multivitamin and mineral supplementation.

References

1. Colles SL, Dixon JB, Marks P, Strauss BJ, O'Brien PE. Preoperative weight loss with a very-low-energy diet: quantitation of changes in liver and abdominal fat by serial imaging. Am J Clin Nutr. 2006;84(2):304–11.
2. Collins J, McCloskey C, Titchner R, Goodpaster B, Hoffman M, Hauser D, et al. Preoperative weight loss in high-risk superobese bariatric patients: a computed tomography-based analysis. Surg Obes Relat Dis Off J Am Soc Bariatr Surg. 2011;7(4):480–5.
3. Edholm D, Kullberg J, Haenni A, Karlsson FA, Ahlström A, Hedberg J, et al. Preoperative 4-week low-calorie diet reduces liver volume and intrahepatic fat, and facilitates laparoscopic gastric bypass in morbidly obese. Obes Surg. 2011;21(3):345–50.
4. Fris RJ. Preoperative low energy diet diminishes liver size. Obes Surg. 2004;14(9):1165–70.
5. Alami RS, Morton JM, Schuster R, Lie J, Sanchez BR, Peters A, et al. Is there a benefit to preoperative weight loss in gastric bypass patients? A prospective randomized trial. Surg Obes Relat Dis Off J Am Soc Bariatr Surg. 2007;3(2):141–5; discussion 145–6.
6. Benotti PN, Still CD, Wood GC, Akmal Y, King H, El Arousy H, et al. Preoperative weight loss before bariatric surgery. Arch Surg. 2009;144(12):1150–5.
7. Van Nieuwenhove Y, Dambrauskas Z, Campillo-Soto A, et al. Preoperative very low-calorie diet and operative outcome after laparoscopic gastric bypass: a randomized multicenter study. Arch Surg. 2011;146(11):1300–5.
8. Baldry EL, Leeder PC, Idris IR. Pre-operative dietary restriction for patients undergoing bariatric surgery in the UK: observational study of current practice and dietary effects. Obes Surg. 2014;24(3):416–21.
9. Schouten R, van der Kaaden I, van't Hof G, Feskens PGBM. Comparison of preoperative diets before bariatric surgery: a randomized, single-blinded, non-inferiority trial. Obes Surg. 2015;26(8):1743–9.
10. Shirai K, Saiki A, Oikawa S, Teramoto T, Yamada N, Ishibashi S, et al. The effects of partial use of formula diet on weight reduction and metabolic variables in obese type 2 diabetic patients – multicenter trial. Obes Res Clin Pract. 2013;7(1):e43–54.
11. Browning JD, Baker JA, Rogers T, Davis J, Satapati S, Burgess SC. Short-term weight loss and hepatic triglyceride reduction: evidence of a metabolic advantage with dietary carbohydrate restriction. Am J Clin Nutr. 2011;93(5):1048–52.
12. Kirk E, Reeds DN, Finck BN, Mayurranjan SM, Mayurranjan MS, Patterson BW, et al. Dietary fat and carbohydrates differentially alter insulin sensitivity during caloric restriction. Gastroenterology. 2009;136(5):1552–60.
13. Ruiz-Tovar J, Zubiaga L, Diez M, Murcia A, Boix E, Muñoz JL, et al. Preoperative regular diet of 900 kcal/day vs balanced energy high-protein formula vs immunonutrition formula: effect on preoperative weight loss and postoperative pain, complications and analytical acute phase reactants after laparoscopic sleeve gastrectomy. Obes Surg. 2015;26(6):1221–7.

14. Del Corral P, Chandler-Laney PC, Casazza K, Gower BA, Hunter GR. Effect of dietary adherence with or without exercise on weight loss: a mechanistic approach to a global problem. J Clin Endocrinol Metab. 2009;94(5):1602–7.
15. Allied Health Sciences Section Ad Hoc Nutrition Committee, Aills L, Blankenship J, Buffington C, Furtado M, Parrott J. ASMBS allied health nutritional guidelines for the surgical weight loss patient. Surg Obes Relat Dis Off J Am Soc Bariatr Surg. 2008;4(5 Suppl):S73–108.
16. Elliot K. Nutritional considerations after bariatric surgery. Crit Care Nurs Q. 2003;26(2):133–8.
17. Mechanick JI, Youdim A, Jones DB, Garvey WT, Hurley DL, McMahon MM, et al. Clinical practice guidelines for the perioperative nutritional, metabolic, and nonsurgical support of the bariatric surgery patient – 2013 update: cosponsored by American Association of Clinical Endocrinologists, The Obesity Society, and American Society for Metabolic & Bariatric Surgery. Obes Silver Spring Md. 2013;21 Suppl 1:S1–27.
18. Avinoah E, Ovnat A, Charuzi I. Nutritional status seven years after Roux-en-Y gastric bypass surgery. Surgery. 1992;111(2):137–42.
19. Kushner R. Managing the obese patient after bariatric surgery: a case report of severe malnutrition and review of the literature. JPEN J Parenter Enteral Nutr. 2000;24(2):126–32.
20. Moize V, Geliebter A, Gluck ME, Yahav E, Lorence M, Colarusso T, et al. Obese patients have inadequate protein intake related to protein intolerance up to 1 year following Roux-en-Y gastric bypass. Obes Surg. 2003;13(1):23–8.
21. Brolin RE, Gorman JH, Gorman RC, Petschenik AJ, Bradley LB, Kenler HA, et al. Prophylactic iron supplementation after Roux-en-Y gastric bypass: a prospective, double-blind, randomized study. Arch Surg. 1998;133(7):740–4.
22. Wardé-Kamar J, Rogers M, Flancbaum L, Laferrère B. Calorie intake and meal patterns up to 4 years after Roux-en-Y gastric bypass surgery. Obes Surg. 2004;14(8):1070–9.
23. Isom KA. Standardizing the evolution of the postoperative bariatric diet. Diabetes Spectr. 2012;25(4):222–8.
24. Moizé VL, Pi-Sunyer X, Mochari H, Vidal J. Nutritional pyramid for post-gastric bypass patients. Obes Surg. 2010;20(8):1133–41.
25. Astrup A, Buemann B, Christensen NJ, Toubro S. Failure to increase lipid oxidation in response to increasing dietary fat content in formerly obese women. Am J Physiol. 1994;266(4 Pt 1):E592–9.
26. Ukleja A. Dumping syndrome: pathophysiology and treatment. Nutr Clin Pract Off Publ Am Soc Parenter Enter Nutr. 2005;20(5):517–25.
27. Weiss C, Rubach M, Lang R, Seebach E, Blumberg S, Frank O, et al. Measurement of the intracellular ph in human stomach cells: a novel approach to evaluate the gastric acid secretory potential of coffee beverages. J Agric Food Chem. 2010;58(3):1976–85.
28. Keijzers GB, De Galan BE, Tack CJ, Smits P. Caffeine can decrease insulin sensitivity in humans. Diabetes Care. 2002;25(2):364–9.
29. Holstege A. Effects of nicotine, alcohol and caffeine on the incidence, healing and recurrence rate of peptic ulcer. Z Für Gastroenterol. 1987;25 Suppl 3:33–40.

Importance of Protein After Bariatric Surgery

33

Parimala Devi and Praveen Raj Palanivelu

Protein is an essential macronutrient vital for transporting molecules, speeding up biochemical processes and supporting the immune system [1, 2]. In bariatric surgery patients proteins are an important dietary component for weight loss and fat-free mass (FFM) maintenance [2, 3]. It has also been noted that a high-protein diet may be effective in preventing weight regain that can occur a few years after bariatric surgery [4].

Proteins also play a beneficial role in energy regulation, glucose homeostasis and blood pressure regulation. A recent meta-analysis showed that partial replacement of dietary carbohydrate with protein may be important for the prevention and treatment of hypertension [5]. A randomized study, demonstrated that a low-carbohydrate, protein-rich diet increased high-density lipoprotein levels and decreased glycated hemoglobin levels in overweight and obese individuals over a 2 year follow up [7]. Several other studies have also shown reductions in triglycerides, blood pressure, cholesterol levels, waist circumference and fasting blood glucose with the long-term consumption of higher-protein diets [2, 6]. Thus in a morbidly obese patients, proteins may play a vital role in optimization of co-morbidities.

In this chapter we aim to understand the importance of protein intake in the post bariatric surgery patients with recommendations for adequate supplementation.

P. Devi, MSc (✉) • P.R. Palanivelu, MS, DNB, DNB (SGE), FALS, FMAS
Bariatric Division, Upper Gastrointestinal Surgery and Minimal Access Surgery Unit, GEM Hospital and Research Centre, Coimbatore, India
e-mail: parimalaswamy30@gmail.com; drraj@geminstitute.in

P.R. Palanivelu et al. (eds.), *Bariatric Surgical Practice Guide*,
DOI 10.1007/978-981-10-2705-5_33

33.1 Protein Energy Malnutrition (PEM) After Bariatric Surgery

Protein is absorbed across the entire intestinal tract, but is primarily absorbed in the mid-ileum, which is bypassed in many bariatric procedures. After bowel bypass only 57 % of ingested protein is estimated to be absorbed [8]. Research has shown that protein malabsorption occurs in 7–21 % after biliopancreatic diversion (BPD)/roux en Y gastric bypass (RYGB) and this is accompanied by a large loss of fat free mass [8–10]. Interestingly protein malabsorption can also occur after laparoscopic adjustable gastric banding (LAGB), vertical banded gastroplasty (VBG) and laparoscopic sleeve gastrectomy (LSG) [11–13]. Thus not just malabsorption but many other factors may also be involved in protein calorie malnutrition in bariatric patients including lack of adequate intake, food intolerance, food aversions, socio-economic status, vomiting, and diarrhea [14]. Therefore, most bariatric patients irrespective of the type of bariatric procedure will be at a risk of protein malnutrition.

It has been shown that post bariatric patients with inadequate protein intake find it difficult to lose weight and maintain weight [2]. Loss of lean body mass is more than expected with a consequent reduction in basal metabolic rate and physiological damage. Conversely, a protein-rich diet can lead to increased satiety, enhance weight loss and improved body composition. Hence increased consumption of dietary protein improves body weight management and prevention of weight regain in post bariatric surgery patients [2].

33.2 Dietary Protein Recommendation of After Bariatric Surgery

Motivating protein consumption post surgery is really difficult as protein-rich foods are difficult to chew and swallow, inducing aversion more easily than foods rich in carbohydrates, and even tend to reduce appetite [15, 16]. Dry or tough pork, poultry and red meat are protein sources that tend to be more difficult to tolerate but the tolerance of protein-rich foods tends to improve at 1 year after bariatric surgery [17].

It has been shown that the addition of 0.5 g protein/kg ideal weight increased the serum albumin levels by 0.11 g/dl indicating that the visceral protein status of bariatric surgery patients can be easily improved by consuming an adequate protein diet [19]. In a study on complicated post–bariatric surgery patients requiring artificial nutritional support, high protein low calorie feedings resulted in positive nitrogen balance, better wound healing along with weight loss [20].

A prospective study on daily protein intake of >1 g/kg/day resulted in increased weight loss, decreased percentage of body fat and improved percentage of lean mass 1 year after laparoscopic RYGB [18]. For bariatric surgery patients, the recommended daily protein consumption is 1.5 g/kg ideal weight which is about 60–120 g of protein daily to maintain adequate FFM during weight loss [21]. However a higher protein intake of 1.5–2.0 g of protein/kg ideal body weight per day is encouraged after malabsorptive procedures like BPD/DS patients. For Indian patients, a protein intake of 1–1.5 g/kg ideal body weight for restricted procedures and 1.5–2 g/kg ideal body weight for malabsorptive procedure such as the duodenal switch, BPD and long limb RYGB is recommended [22].

An important point to note is that a protein-rich diet usually includes at least 25–30 % of proteins expressed as percentage of energy from protein for a normal calorie diet. However for a low calorie diet this percentage of energy from protein may not meet the requirements in absolute terms (i.e., grams of protein) and the proportion of proteins need to be increased [23]. For example, a 2866 kcal/day diet can achieve a protein intake of 67–100 g (10–15 % protein), whereas for a 478-kcal/day very-low-calorie diet 47 % of calories should come from protein to obtain 52 g protein.

It is also to be noted that a balanced intake of protein is important. It was shown that 30 g of protein every meal helps maintain healthy bones and muscles. It is also suggested that patients should consume a high protein intake for breakfast to relieve the catabolic state of overnight fasting and that protein rich foods should be consumed before carbohydrate and fat foods [24]. Several other authors also have supported the intake of a generous and balanced protein at each meal (>30 g) for optimal protein synthesis in the muscle [25, 26]. Also consumption of high protein meals throughout the day prolongs satiety compared with consuming standard-protein meals. A randomized cross over study showed a protein rich breakfast might be a useful strategy to improve satiety in overweight or obese teenage girls [27]. Consumption of a moderate amount of protein at each meal stimulated 24 h muscle protein synthesis more effectively than taking protein in an evening meal [28].

The quality of protein each meal also needs to be considered. Protein quality is measured by its essential amino acid (EAA) content, unique amino acid profile, and the digestibility of each essential amino acid in the protein [29]. Animal origin foods such as meat, fish, eggs, poultry and dairy products are rich sources of protein but are also high in fat. Lean meat, egg white, skimmed milk and nonfat cheese are rich sources of protein but are low in fat. Plant foods like legumes, nuts, soy and grains are also rich in protein. Protein supplements have high protein with low carbohydrate and fat content. However it has been demonstrated that plant based proteins such as soy and wheat resulted in lower muscle protein synthesis than animal based proteins [30]. This could be due to lower anabolic properties of plant proteins and lack of specific essential amino acids such as leucine, arginine and citruline [31].

Several studies have underscored the importance of leucine-rich diet [32]. Many studies have suggested that high protein diets are beneficial partly due to branched chain amino acids especially leucine, which favors the maintenance of muscle mass. It has been shown that during catabolic periods particularly in a post bariatric situation, muscle protein synthesis is stimulated by leucine supplementation. Also, leucine plays a role in the insulin signaling pathway which maintains protein synthesis [32]. The richest source of leucine is whey protein (14 %) followed by casein (10.1 %), egg protein (8.5 %), isolated soy proteins (8 %) and wheat protein (7 %). A protein rich and leucine rich diet promotes long term weightloss and improved body composition It has been estimated that stimulation of muscle protein synthesis would be optimized with 18 g Indispensible Amino Acids (IAA) or Essential Amino Acids (EAA), including 2.5 g leucine, at each of the three meals per day [33].

Hence, it's to be concluded that protein management is an important and integral part of post bariatric dietary management and adequate monitoring and supplementation should be guided by the bariatric dietitian for better post-operative outcomes.

Conclusion

Proteins are important macronutrients involved in the regulation of various bodily processes. High protein diet has a beneficial role in prevention of various cardiovascular risk factors. Also, high protein diet plays a major role in maintenance of fat free mass and weight management. Protein energy malnutrition is possible after all kinds of bariatric procedures due to insufficient and inefficient intake, although more common with malabsorptive procedures with increasing losses. Protein rich diet may help in better weight loss and also in preventing weight regain after bariatric surgery. The recommended protein requirement after bariatric surgery is 1–1.5 g/kg/day for restrictive procedures and 1.5–2 g/kg/day for malabsorptive procedures. Also balanced protein intake with approximately 30 g/meal helps maintain healthy bones and muscles. Animal proteins have a better muscle protein synthetic response compared to plant based protein. Leucine supplementation also helps in muscle protein synthesis helping in better weightloss and body composition in the post bariatric setting.

Recommendations

- High protein diet is needed for maintenance of fat free mass and weight management.
- Recommended protein requirement after bariatric surgery is 1–1.5 g/kg/day for restrictive procedures and 1.5–2 g/kg/day for malabsorptive procedures.
- Balanced protein intake with approximately 30 g/meal is recommended
- Animal proteins are better than plant based protein.
- Leucine supplementation helps in muscle protein synthesis

References

1. Wolfe RR, Miller SL, Miller KB. Optimal protein intake in the elderly. Clin Nutr Edinb Scotl. 2008;27(5):675–84.
2. Westerterp-Plantenga MS, Nieuwenhuizen A, Tomé D, Soenen S, Westerterp KR. Dietary protein, weight loss, and weight maintenance. Annu Rev Nutr. 2009;29:21–41.
3. Farnsworth E, Luscombe ND, Noakes M, Wittert G, Argyiou E, Clifton PM. Effect of a high-protein, energy-restricted diet on body composition, glycemic control, and lipid concentrations in overweight and obese hyperinsulinemic men and women. Am J Clin Nutr. 2003;78(1):31–9.

4. Faria SL, de Oliveira Kelly E, Lins RD, Faria OP. Nutritional management of weight regain after bariatric surgery. Obes Surg. 2010;20(2):135–9.
5. Rebholz CM, Friedman EE, Powers LJ, Arroyave WD, He J, Kelly TN. Dietary protein intake and blood pressure: a meta-analysis of randomized controlled trials. Am J Epidemiol. 2012;176 Suppl 7:S27–43.
6. Layman DK, Shiue H, Sather C, Erickson DJ, Baum J. Increased dietary protein modifies glucose and insulin homeostasis in adult women during weight loss. J Nutr. 2003;133(2): 405–10.
7. Wycherley TP, Moran LJ, Clifton PM, Noakes M, Brinkworth GD. Effects of energy-restricted high-protein, low-fat compared with standard-protein, low-fat diets: a meta-analysis of randomized controlled trials. Am J Clin Nutr. 2012;96(6):1281–98.
8. Fujioka K, DiBaise JK, Martindale RG. Nutrition and metabolic complications after bariatric surgery and their treatment. JPEN J Parenter Enteral Nutr. 2011;35(5 Suppl):52S–9.
9. Parkes E. Nutritional management of patients after bariatric surgery. Am J Med Sci. 2006;331(4):207–13.
10. Mango VL, Frishman WH. Physiologic, psychologic, and metabolic consequences of bariatric surgery. Cardiol Rev. 2006;14(5):232–7.
11. Moizé V, Andreu A, Flores L, Torres F, Ibarzabal A, Delgado S, et al. Long-term dietary intake and nutritional deficiencies following sleeve gastrectomy or Roux-En-Y gastric bypass in a mediterranean population. J Acad Nutr Diet. 2013;113(3):400–10.
12. Friedrich AE, Damms-Machado A, Meile T, Scheuing N, Stingel K, Basrai M, et al. Laparoscopic sleeve gastrectomy compared to a multidisciplinary weight loss program for obesity – effects on body composition and protein status. Obes Surg. 2013;23(12): 1957–65.
13. Damms-Machado A, Friedrich A, Kramer KM, Stingel K, Meile T, Küper MA, et al. Pre- and postoperative nutritional deficiencies in obese patients undergoing laparoscopic sleeve gastrectomy. Obes Surg. 2012;22(6):881–9.
14. Ziegler O, Sirveaux MA, Brunaud L, Reibel N, Quilliot D. Medical follow up after bariatric surgery: nutritional and drug issues. General recommendations for the prevention and treatment of nutritional deficiencies. Diabetes Metab. 2009;35(6 Pt 2):544–57.
15. Midkiff EE, Bernstein IL. Targets of learned food aversions in humans. Physiol Behav. 1985;34(5):839–41.
16. Weigle DS, Breen PA, Matthys CC, Callahan HS, Meeuws KE, Burden VR, et al. A high-protein diet induces sustained reductions in appetite, ad libitum caloric intake, and body weight despite compensatory changes in diurnal plasma leptin and ghrelin concentrations. Am J Clin Nutr. 2005;82(1):41–8.
17. Moize V, Geliebter A, Gluck ME, Yahav E, Lorence M, Colarusso T, et al. Obese patients have inadequate protein intake related to protein intolerance up to 1 year following Roux-en-Y gastric bypass. Obes Surg. 2003;13(1):23–8.
18. Rinaldi Schinkel E, Pettine SM, Adams E, Harris M. Impact of varying levels of protein intake on protein status indicators after gastric bypass in patients with multiple complications requiring nutritional support. Obes Surg. 2006;16(1):24–30.
19. Ortega J, Ortega-Evangelio G, Cassinello N, Sebastia V. What are obese patients able to eat after Roux-en-Y gastric bypass? Obes Facts. 2012;5(3):339–48.
20. Beebe ML, Crowley N. Can hypocaloric, high-protein nutrition support be used in complicated bariatric patients to promote weight loss? Nutr Clin Pract Off Publ Am Soc Parenter Enter Nutr. 2015;30(4):522–9.
21. Marcason W. What are the dietary guidelines following bariatric surgery? J Am Diet Assoc. 2004;104(3):487–8.
22. Remedios C, Bhasker AG, Dhulla N, Dhar S, Lakdawala M. Bariatric nutrition guidelines for the Indian population. Obes Surg. 2015;26(5):1057–68.
23. Heber D, Greenway FL, Kaplan LM, Livingston E, Salvador J, Still C, et al. Endocrine and nutritional management of the post-bariatric surgery patient: an Endocrine Society Clinical Practice Guideline. J Clin Endocrinol Metab. 2010;95(11):4823–43.

24. Layman DK, Anthony TG, Rasmussen BB, Adams SH, Lynch CJ, Brinkworth GD, et al. Defining meal requirements for protein to optimize metabolic roles of amino acids. Am J Clin Nutr. 2015; pii: ajcn084053.
25. Symons TB, Sheffield-Moore M, Wolfe RR, Paddon-Jones D. A moderate serving of high-quality protein maximally stimulates skeletal muscle protein synthesis in young and elderly subjects. J Am Diet Assoc. 2009;109(9):1582–6.
26. Pennings B, Groen B, de Lange A, Gijsen AP, Zorenc AH, Senden JMG, et al. Amino acid absorption and subsequent muscle protein accretion following graded intakes of whey protein in elderly men. Am J Physiol Endocrinol Metab. 2012;302(8):E992–9.
27. Hoertel HA, Will MJ, Leidy HJ. A randomized crossover, pilot study examining the effects of a normal protein vs. high protein breakfast on food cravings and reward signals in overweight/obese "breakfast skipping", late-adolescent girls. Nutr J. 2014;13:80.
28. Mamerow MM, Mettler JA, English KL, Casperson SL, Arentson-Lantz E, Sheffield-Moore M, et al. Dietary protein distribution positively influences 24-h muscle protein synthesis in healthy adults. J Nutr. 2014;144(6):876–80.
29. Young VR, Taylor YS, Rand WM, Scrimshaw NS. Protein requirements of man: efficiency of egg protein utilization at maintenance and submaintenance levels in young men. J Nutr. 1973;103(8):1164–74.
30. Van Vliet S, Burd NA, van Loon LJC. The skeletal muscle anabolic response to plant- versus animal-based protein consumption. J Nutr. 2015;145(9):1981–91.
31. Jonker R, Engelen MPKJ, Deutz NEP. Role of specific dietary amino acids in clinical conditions. Br J Nutr. 2012;108 Suppl 2:S139–48.
32. Layman DK. The role of leucine in weight loss diets and glucose homeostasis. J Nutr. 2003;133(1):261S–7.
33. Layman DK. Protein quantity and quality at levels above the RDA improves adult weight loss. J Am Coll Nutr. 2004;23(6 Suppl):631S–6.

Anemia and Related Deficiencies in Bariatric Surgery

34

Parimala Devi and Praveen Raj Palanivelu

34.1 Introduction

Anemia is considered a global disease, with the incidence being especially very high in developing countries. After bariatric surgery, almost two-thirds of the population may be affected by anaemia with preoperative existing deficiency being an important contributing factor besides the consequences of bariatric surgery like pouch hypoacidity, bypassed small bowel, red meat intolerance etc.

Anemia can be microcytic (which is usually due to iron deficiency) or macrocytic anaemia (which is usually due to vitamin B12 and/or folate deficiency). While iron, vitamin B12 and folate are the most commonly associated deficiencies, a significant number of anemias may be secondary to chronic inflammation and micronutrient deficiencies such as copper, zinc, vitamins A and E etc.

The aim of this chapter is to understand the reasons for the development of anemia and the most commonly related deficiencies of iron, vitamin B12 and folic acid and its prevention/management in post bariatric surgical patients.

34.2 Importance of Iron, Folic Acid and B12

Iron is an essential mineral vital to make hemoglobin and myoglobin and plays a role in metabolic processes like oxygen transport, DNA synthesis and electron transport [1]. It is obtained as nonheme iron from vegetables and haeme iron from meat. Vitamin B12 is a key B vitamin important for proper brain development and deficiency causes central nervous system development disorders and dementia [2]. Folate is a water soluble B vitamin (also known as vitamin B9) essential for amino

P. Devi, MSc (✉) • P.R. Palanivelu, MS, DNB, DNB (SGE), FALS, FMAS
Bariatric Division, Upper Gastrointestinal Surgery and Minimal Access Surgery Unit, GEM Hospital and Research Centre, Coimbatore, India
e-mail: parimalaswamy30@gmail.com; drraj@geminstitute.in

P.R. Palanivelu et al. (eds.), *Bariatric Surgical Practice Guide*,
DOI 10.1007/978-981-10-2705-5_34

acid metabolism, DNA synthesis, repair and methylation [3]. Folate includes endogenous food folate and its synthetic form folic acid [4]. Bioavailability of folic acid is 70 % higher than the natural folate present in the foods [5].

34.3 Etiology of Post-bariatric Surgery Anemia

Several factors have been implicated in the occurrence of anaemia after bariatric surgery. These include (1) preoperative existing deficiency (2) malabsorption due to the surgical procedure (3) inadequate dietary intake in the post-operative period (4) altered drug bioavailability (5) reduced hematopoiesis (6) inflammation related to obesity (increased hepcidin) (7) altered absorption and metabolism of other nutrients.

Premenopausal women have higher risk of post-operative development of anemia [6, 7]. The most common non-malabsorptive types of anemia were inflammation and dysfunctional uterine bleeding [8]. The incidences have also been less common with better follow up profile [9].

Of all of the above factors preoperative existing deficiency of iron, folic acid and vitamin B12 is the major factor predicting post-operative deficiency and secondary anemia [7]. Preoperatively, the incidence of anemia is 5–21.5 %, iron deficiency of 20–47 %, of folate deficiency of 21–32 % and vitamin B12 deficiency of 13 % [10–13]. Hence, identification and appropriate correction of preoperative deficiency is of paramount importance.

Post bariatric surgery, the absorption of iron may be disrupted due to the reduction of $Fe3^{+}$ by gastric acid to $Fe2^{+}$ would be altered, which is the more easily absorbed form. Malabsorptive procedures further reduce iron absorption by diverting the food away from the duodenum and proximal intestine where iron absorption majorly occurs. Altered dietary intake in the post-operative period and reduced bioavailability of oral supplements further increase the chances of development of anemia [6, 7]. Dietary intake of iron following surgery is also noted to be lower than the recommended amount because patients generally avoid red meat which is a good dietary source of heme iron [6]. It is also suggested the possibility of reduced haematopoiesis (due to frequent association with leucopenia and thrombocytopenia) as predisposing factor for anemia [14]. Inflammation secondary to obesity has also been suggested as a contributing factor [15]. Iron absorption and metabolism can be affected by zinc, vitamin C and copper as excessive dietary intake of zinc can compete with iron for absorption and copper is needed for ceruloplasmin which catalyses $Fe2^{+}$ to $Fe3^{+}$ and vitamin C which increases nonheme iron absorption.

Bariatric procedures with significant malabsorption like biliopancreatic diversion with and without duodenal switch (BPD/BPD-DS) have been shown to have higher incidences for developing post operating anemia [16]. Laparoscopic roux en Y gastric bypass (LRYGB) has been the most commonly reported procedure associated with nutritional deficiencies and anemia [9, 17]. Some authors have demonstrated no iron deficiency after laparoscopic sleeve gastrectomy (LSG) but many others have shown deficiencies in iron [18–20]. A recent meta-analysis demonstrated higher chance of vitamin B12 deficiency with RYGB compared to LSG but with similar risk of anemia and iron deficiency, necessitating prophylactic supplementation even after LSG [21].

34.4 Identification and Management of Iron, Vitamin B12 and Folate Deficiency

Identifying iron deficiency in bariatric patients include symptoms like extreme lethargy, increased shortness of breath or new onset shortness of breath with unknown etiology, cravings for red meat and/or other significant sources of dietary iron. Pica mainly pagophagia (eating of ice) and/or Pica for dirt, paper or other nonfood items is also commonly seen in post bariatric surgery patients. RYGB is commonly seen to trigger pica in these patients [22, 23]. Findings of pallor and spoon shaped nails (koilonychia) may be detected on examination.

Vitamin B12 deficiency can cause various gastrointestinal, hematologic and neurological disorders and the latter when left untreated can cause permanent damage [24]. Symptoms of vitamin B12 deficiency are tingling and numbness of the extremities, gait abnormalities, severe joint pain, visual disturbances, megaloblastic anemia, progressive short breath, depression, paranoia, delusions, memory loss, dementia, incontinence and loss of taste and smell. Folic acid deficiency is mostly asymptomatic and similar to vitamin B12 deficiency with symptoms like muscle weakness, irritability and memory loss.

Since these deficiencies have been reported in spite of regular supplementation based on the existing guidelines, more intense follow up and management of any deficiencies is necessary. The identification and treatment of post operative anemia is important not just to prevent anemia related complications but it helps identify patients with complications like GJ stomal ulcer etc. which needs to be looked for in the workup. Total iron binding capacity or serum transferring receptor are better measures of iron deficiency when compared with serum iron or ferritin as ferritin may be elevated even in inflammatory conditions, such as obesity [25]. Elevated methylmalonic acid (MMA) and total homocysteine concentrations are considered as sensitive metabolic markers for vitamin B12 deficiency as Vitamin B12 by itself is a poor predictor of functional B12 status, as deficiencies might occur within the reference limits and MMA will identify the deficiency at intracellular levels [22, 24].

34.5 Treatment and Supplementation for Anemia

Iron Dietary iron is present in heme and nonheme sources. The primary sources of heme iron are liver, eggs (especially yolk), lean red meat (especially beef), poultry, and fish like salmon, tuna, oysters and sources of nonheme are whole grains, pulses, dried beans, fruits, dried fruits, and vegetables. Haeme iron is absorbed two to three times better than non-haem iron. Vitamin C improves the dietary iron availability whereas phytates and calcium in milk inhibits iron absorption.

Vitamin B12 Liver and kidney are the best sources and beef, mutton, chicken, pork, ham, fish, and whole egg are good sources of vitamin B12. Milk, yogurt, cheese are the vegetarian sources and plant foods like rice and soy beverages, ready to eat breakfast cereals and nutritional yeast can be fortified with vitamin B12.

Folate Folic acid is present in broccoli, sprouts, peas, asparagus, chick peas and brown rice.

The American Society of Metabolic and Bariatric Surgery (ASMBS) guidelines advise 18–36 mg iron per day for patients after RYGB as part of one to two multivitamin/mineral tablets with additional 18–27 mg per day for menstruating women. However several studies have shown that this supplementation is inadequate to avoid deficiency. A recent triple blinded randomized controlled study showed that post RYGB, iron supplementation of five times the RDA (70 mg) resulted in fewer deficiencies [26].

For iron deficiency anemia oral ferrous iron (ferrous fumerate, sulfate or gluconate) with 150–200 mg of elemental iron is preferred for post-surgery patients with added ascorbic acid to enhance the iron absorption. It has also been shown that only 1 out of 23 patients showed sufficient absorption on an oral iron challenge [27]. Hence it is suggested that IV iron supplements be used to restore the lost iron status more rapidly and reliably. Several studies have demonstrated successful intravenous iron supplementation but cautioned against iron overload [28].

Studies have shown that oral treatment of post-operative vitamin B12 deficiencies was successful in more than 80 % of the patients in contrast to oral treatment of iron deficiency which was only successful in 62.5 % of the patients [12]. Intramuscular vitamin B12 is the gold standard therapy for vitamin B12 deficiency especially in symptomatic patients [12]. In select patients with asymptomatic vitamin B12 deficiency after RYGB, high-dose oral cyanocobalamin can be considered [29]. Oral supplementation of vitamin B12 at a dosage of 1000 μg daily may be used to maintain normal vitamin B12 levels. Intranasally administered vitamin B12, 500 μg weekly, may also be considered. Parenteral (intramuscular or subcutaneous) B12 supplementation, 1000–3000 μg every 6–12 months to 1000 μg every month, is indicated if B12 sufficiency cannot be maintained using oral or intranasal routes [30]. Folic acid supplementation (400 μg/d) as part of a multivitamin preparation and a separate supplement to childbearing women to prevent fetal neural tube defects is recommended post surgically [30].

The recommended dietary allowance for iron, vitamin B12 and folate

Nutrients	Country	Males	Females
Iron (mg/day)	RDA* (India) (53)	17	21
	RDA* (US) (54)	8	18
	RNI** (UK) (55)	8.7	14.8
	NRV*** (Australia/New Zealand) (56)	8	18
Folate (mcg/day)	RDA* (India) (53)	200	200
	RDA* (US) (54)	400	400
	RNI** (UK) (55)	200	200
	NRV*** (Australia/New Zealand) (56)	400	400
Vitamin B12 (mcg/day)	RDA* (India) (53)	1.0	1.0
	RDA* (US) (54)	2.4	2.4
	RNI** (UK) (55)	1.5	1.5
	NRV*** (Australia/New Zealand) (56)	2.4	2.4

*RDA** recommended dietary allowances, *RNI*** reference nutrient intake, *NRV**** nutrient reference value

Recommendations

- Preoperative existing deficiency of iron, folic acid and vitamin B12 is the major factor predicting post-operative deficiency and secondary anemia.
- Iron supplementation should be five times the RDA.
- Vitamin B12 and folic acid supplementation can be given as part of a multivitamin preparation.
- Similar replacements have to be considered after sleeve gastrectomy.
- Even with regular supplementation intense follow up and management of deficiencies is necessary.
- Total iron binding capacity or serum transferring receptor are better measures of iron deficiency than serum iron or ferritin
- Elevated methylmalonic acid and total homocysteine concentrations are better measures of vitamin B12 deficiency than vitamin B12 levels.
- With iron deficiency IV iron supplements restore the lost iron status more rapidly and reliably than oral iron supplements.
- Asymptomatic vitamin B12 deficiency can be treated with oral or intranasal vitamin B12 reserving parenteral supplementation for symptomatic or severe deficiencies.

References

1. Aisen P, Enns C, Wessling-Resnick M. Chemistry and biology of eukaryotic iron metabolism. Int J Biochem Cell Biol. 2001;33(10):940–59.
2. Reynolds E. Vitamin B12, folic acid, and the nervous system. Lancet Neurol. 2006;5(11): 949–60.
3. Tamura T, Picciano MF. Folate and human reproduction. Am J Clin Nutr. 2006;83(5):993–1016.
4. Crider KS, Bailey LB, Berry RJ. Folic acid food fortification-its history, effect, concerns, and future directions. Nutrients. 2011;3(3):370–84.
5. McNulty H, Pentieva K. Folate bioavailability. Proc Nutr Soc. 2004;63(4):529–36.
6. Salgado W, Modotti C, Nonino CB, Ceneviva R. Anemia and iron deficiency before and after bariatric surgery. Surg Obes Relat Dis Off J Am Soc Bariatr Surg. 2014;10(1):49–54.
7. Kotkiewicz A, Donaldson K, Dye C, Rogers AM, Mauger D, Kong L, et al. Anemia and the Need for Intravenous Iron Infusion after Roux-en-Y Gastric Bypass. Clin Med Insights Blood Disord. 2015;8:9–17.
8. Del Villar Madrigal E, Neme-Yunes Y, Clavellina-Gaytan D, Sanchez HA, Mosti M, Herrera MF. Anemia after Roux-en-Y gastric bypass. How feasible to eliminate the risk by proper supplementation? Obes Surg. 2015;25(1):80–4.
9. Karefylakis C, Näslund I, Edholm D, Sundbom M, Karlsson FA, Rask E. Prevalence of anemia and related deficiencies 10 years after gastric bypass – a retrospective study. Obes Surg. 2015;25(6):1019–23.
10. Ben-Porat T, Elazary R, Yuval JB, Wieder A, Khalaileh A, Weiss R. Nutritional deficiencies after sleeve gastrectomy: can they be predicted preoperatively? Surg Obes Relat Dis Off J Am Soc Bariatr Surg. 2015;11(5):1029–36.
11. Van Rutte PWJ, Aarts EO, Smulders JF, Nienhuijs SW. Nutrient deficiencies before and after sleeve gastrectomy. Obes Surg. 2014;24(10):1639–46.
12. Van der Beek ESJ, Monpellier VM, Eland I, Tromp E, van Ramshorst B. Nutritional deficiencies in gastric bypass patients; incidence, time of occurrence and implications for postoperative surveillance. Obes Surg. 2015;25(5):818–23.

13. Vargas-Ruiz AG, Hernández-Rivera G, Herrera MF. Prevalence of iron, folate, and vitamin B12 deficiency anemia after laparoscopic Roux-en-Y gastric bypass. Obes Surg. 2008;18(3):288–93.
14. Dallal RM, Leighton J, Trang A. Analysis of leukopenia and anemia after gastric bypass surgery. Surg Obes Relat Dis Off J Am Soc Bariatr Surg. 2012;8(2):164–8.
15. Wisse BE. The inflammatory syndrome: the role of adipose tissue cytokines in metabolic disorders linked to obesity. J Am Soc Nephrol. 2004;15(11):2792–800.
16. Homan J, Betzel B, Aarts EO, Dogan K, van Laarhoven KJHM, Janssen IMC, et al. Vitamin and mineral deficiencies after biliopancreatic diversion and biliopancreatic diversion with duodenal switch – the rule rather than the exception. Obes Surg. 2015;25(9):1626–32.
17. Obinwanne KM, Fredrickson KA, Mathiason MA, Kallies KJ, Farnen JP, Kothari SN. Incidence, treatment, and outcomes of iron deficiency after laparoscopic Roux-en-Y gastric bypass: a 10-year analysis. J Am Coll Surg. 2014;218(2):246–52.
18. Saif T, Strain GW, Dakin G, Gagner M, Costa R, Pomp A. Evaluation of nutrient status after laparoscopic sleeve gastrectomy 1, 3, and 5 years after surgery. Surg Obes Relat Dis Off J Am Soc Bariatr Surg. 2012;8(5):542–7.
19. Damms-Machado A, Friedrich A, Kramer KM, Stingel K, Meile T, Küper MA, et al. Pre- and postoperative nutritional deficiencies in obese patients undergoing laparoscopic sleeve gastrectomy. Obes Surg. 2012;22(6):881–9.
20. Aarts EO, Janssen IMC, Berends FJ. The gastric sleeve: losing weight as fast as micronutrients? Obes Surg. 2011;21(2):207–11.
21. Kwon Y, Kim HJ, Lo Menzo E, Park S, Szomstein S, Rosenthal RJ. Anemia, iron and vitamin B12 deficiencies after sleeve gastrectomy compared to Roux-en-Y gastric bypass: a meta-analysis. Surg Obes Relat Dis Off J Am Soc Bariatr Surg. 2014;10(4):589–97.
22. Kushner RF, Shanta Retelny V. Emergence of pica (ingestion of non-food substances) accompanying iron deficiency anemia after gastric bypass surgery. Obes Surg. 2005;15(10):1491–5.
23. Kushner RF, Gleason B, Shanta-Retelny V. Reemergence of pica following gastric bypass surgery for obesity: a new presentation of an old problem. J Am Diet Assoc. 2004;104(9):1393–7.
24. Stabler SP, Allen RH, Dolce ET, Johnson MA. Elevated serum S-adenosylhomocysteine in cobalamin-deficient elderly and response to treatment. Am J Clin Nutr. 2006;84(6):1422–9.
25. Zimmermann MB, Hurrell RF. Nutritional iron deficiency. Lancet Lond Engl. 2007;370(9586):511–20.
26. Dogan K, Aarts EO, Koehestanie P, Betzel B, Ploeger N, de Boer H, et al. Optimization of vitamin suppletion after Roux-en-Y gastric bypass surgery can lower postoperative deficiencies: a randomized controlled trial. Medicine Baltimore. 2014;93(25):e169.
27. Gesquiere I, Lannoo M, Augustijns P, Matthys C, Van der Schueren B, Foulon V. Iron deficiency after Roux-en-Y gastric bypass: insufficient iron absorption from oral iron supplements. Obes Surg. 2014;24(1):56–61.
28. Malone M, Barish C, He A, Bregman D. Comparative review of the safety and efficacy of ferric carboxymaltose versus standard medical care for the treatment of iron deficiency anemia in bariatric and gastric surgery patients. Obes Surg. 2013;23(9):1413–20.
29. Majumder S, Soriano J, Louie Cruz A, Dasanu CA. Vitamin B12 deficiency in patients undergoing bariatric surgery: preventive strategies and key recommendations. Surg Obes Relat Dis Off J Am Soc Bariatr Surg. 2013;9(6):1013–9.
30. Mechanick JI, Youdim A, Jones DB, Garvey WT, Hurley DL, McMahon MM, et al. Clinical practice guidelines for the perioperative nutritional, metabolic, and nonsurgical support of the bariatric surgery patient – 2013 update: cosponsored by American Association of Clinical Endocrinologists, The Obesity Society, and American Society for Metabolic & Bariatric Surgery. Obes Silver Spring Md. 2013;21 Suppl 1:S1–27.

Calcium and Vitamin D Deficiencies in Bariatric Surgery

35

Parimala Devi and Praveen Raj Palanivelu

35.1 Introduction

Nutritional deficiencies are common after all kinds of bariatric procedures and can be due to both macronutrient and micronutrient deficiencies [1–4]. This can be attributed to vomiting, decreased food intake, food intolerance, reduction of gastric secretions, bypass of absorption surface areas and altered drug bioavailability that occur after bariatric procedures [5, 6]. Bypass of absorption surface areas is perhaps the most important factor in the cause of nutritional deficiencies and the risk of developing these deficiencies seems to be proportional to the length of bypassed proximal intestine [7].

One micronutrient of importance in the morbidly obese when considering bariatric surgery is calcium [8]. Understanding calcium metabolism in these patients is important because some bariatric procedures can lead to vitamin D malabsorption, hypocalcaemia and hyperparathyroidism.

This chapter aims to understand the alterations in calcium and vitamin D metabolism after different types of bariatric procedures and the appropriate supplementation required to maintain a proper calcium homeostasis.

35.2 Calcium Homestasis

Calcium is the most abundant mineral and constitutes 2% of the body mass. It is involved in muscle contraction/relaxation, blood clotting, nerve function, regulation of blood pressure, cell signaling and in bone and teeth mineralization.

P. Devi, MSc (✉) • P.R. Palanivelu, MS, DNB, DNB (SGE), FALS, FMAS
Bariatric Division, Upper Gastrointestinal Surgery and Minimal Access Surgery Unit, GEM Hospital and Research Centre, Coimbatore, India
e-mail: parimalaswamy30@gmail.com; drraj@geminstitute.in

P.R. Palanivelu et al. (eds.), *Bariatric Surgical Practice Guide*,
DOI 10.1007/978-981-10-2705-5_35

The main site of absorption of calcium is the duodenum. Calcium from diets is absorbed by the intestine through two pathways: transcellular absorption and paracellular transport of calcium. In the duodenum, transcellular absorption is responsible for 80 % calcium uptake in low-calcium diets and less than 10 % calcium uptake in high-calcium diets and the rest will be by paracellular transport [9].

Vitamin D is important for calcium homeostasis as it regulates the calcium absorption in the small intestine [10, 11]. Vitamin D regulates calcium metabolism, insulin action, immune function and cell proliferation [12]. Magnesium is also needed for calcium absorption and to retain calcium by suppressing parathyroid hormone and by stimulating calcitonin. But excess calcium can prevent magnesium from being absorbed. Hence calcium intake should be supplemented with adequate magnesium to prevent both calcium malabsorption and magnesium deficiency, as magnesium is not stored well.

Parathyroid hormone (PTH) secretion (secreted by parathyroid glands) is controlled by calcium concentration and it has biological effects on the bones, kidneys and intestinal mucosa [13, 14]. A decrease in ionized calcium stimulates the release of PTH, which maintains calcium homeostasis by (1) increasing bone mineral dissolution, thus releasing calcium and phosphorus, (2) increasing renal reabsorption of calcium and excretion of phosphorus, and (3) enhancing the gastrointestinal absorption of both calcium and phosphorus indirectly through its effects on the synthesis of 1,25$(OH)_2$D (calcitriol) in the body [13].

35.3 Bariatric Surgery and Calcium and Vitamin D Metabolism

Bariatric surgery has been reported to be closely associated with altered calcium metabolism and changes in the bone mineral density [15, 16]. Bypass of the duodenum and/or nutritional inadequacy in the immediate post-operative period are the main factors that lead to calcium malabsorption which could potentiate secondary hyperparathyroidism.

After bariatric surgery low levels of circulating calcium leads to increased parathyroid hormones and a reduction in bone mass, particularly a depletion of calcium and phosphorous in order to increase the blood calcium levels. At the same time, the kidney increases the phosphorus and calcitrol excretion and reduces calcium excretion. This whole mechanism causes secondary hyperparathyroidism [16]. Vitamin D deficiency secondary to less sunlight exposure and inadequate vitamin D rich food intake may worsen secondary hyperparathyroidism.

Studies have shown a significant fall in bone mineral density (BMD), bone mineral content (BMC) and increased bone remodeling within the first year post-bariatric surgery [17]. This fall in BMD has been demonstrated after all kinds of bariatric procedures [18–20]. It has been noted that these changes in BMD are closely associated with the change in body composition following weight loss. For non-surgical weight loss therapies every 10 % weight loss leads to a bone mass reduction by 1–2 % [21]. But with more significant weight loss following bariatric surgery this fall has been found to be significantly higher [22]. It has also been demonstrated that this fall in BMD persisted beyond the first year, with bone loss continuing throughout the second year at all skeletal sites with the serum calcium levels, vitamin D3 and PTH levels maintained within normal limits during this period [21].

Thus, several mechanisms have been suggested for changes in BMD besides nutritional inadequacy. One mechanism suggested is that a reduced mechanical load on the skeleton leads to secondary reduction in bone mass [21]. The other possible explanations are alterations in gut derived hormones like GLP-1, Peptide YY and Ghrelin which can lead to bone loss in association with fall in levels of leptin and elevated adiponectin [23–26].

The distribution of BMD reduction has been researched in several studies. A recent meta-analysis comparing all kinds of bariatric procedures showed that this BMD was significantly low only at the femoral neck and not at the lumbar spine [27]. Another study in post sleeve gastrectomy patients also showed significant fall in BMD in the hip and femoral neck and not in the spine [19]. The clinical implications of this distribution are uncertain. A recent population based study showed that following bariatric surgery the risk of fracture was increased two fold [28]. A population based retrospective study from UK showed that bariatric surgery increased fracture risk at 3–5 years after surgery, but this was not statistically significant [29]. In another study on bariatric surgery and bone loss it was demonstrated that there was no increased risk of fractures [30].

This stresses the importance of adequate replacements of calcium and vitamin D3 that needs to be initiated in the first months of surgery itself, which is the period, associated with severe muscle loss and increased bone turnover [31]. The BABS study (Bone metabolism after bariatric surgery) demonstrated that pre-operative loading of vitamin D along with ongoing vitamin D and calcium supplementation with adequate protein supplementation with physical exercise decelerates the loss of both BMD and LBM (lean body mass) after bariatric surgery [32].

35.4 Choice of Procedure in Patients with Pre-existing Deficiency

With regard to the choice of procedure in patients with pre-existing deficiency, procedures like biliopancreatic diversion with duodenal switch (BPD-DS) may be avoided as it is associated with significant malabsorption, wherein hypovitaminosis D and secondary hyperparathyroidism is difficult to manage in spite of adequate supplementation [33].

Amongst the rest of the commonly performed bariatric procedures, there is conflicting data on whether roux en Y gastric bypass (RYGB) causes more significant effects compared to sleeve gastrectomy (LSG). With no clear recommendations available and with the understanding that the changes are closely associated with the body composition, either procedure should be considered based on other clinical parameters and RYGB would not be a contra-indication.

35.5 Calcium Recommendation in Bariatric Surgery

Major food sources of calcium include dairy products, low-oxalate vegetables like cabbage, cauliflower, cucumber, mushrooms, peas, radish (to avoid high oxalate vegetables like beetroot, carrot, eggplant, ladies finger (okra), potato, sweet potato, legumes and sesame seeds) and fortified foods. For vitamin D primary sources are fortified dairy products, egg yolk and fatty fish [14]. Magnesium is found in nuts (especially almonds, cashews), seeds, whole grains, seafood, legumes tofu, yogurt, green leafy vegetables such as spinach, fruits like avocado, figs and banana.

Adequate dietary intake of calcium, magnesium and vitamin D rich food substances needs to be ensured. More importantly food interactions need to be noted. High fat in foods hinder calcium absorption and reduce the bioavailability of calcium. Oxalic acid in vegetables, phytic acid in cereal bran, and caffeine in coffee also decreases calcium absorption. Phosphorus in cola and processed foods, high protein and sodium impairs calcium absorption by increasing calcium excretion through the kidneys. Magnesium levels can be lowered by high intake of coffee, soda, alcohol, salt, during heavy menstrual periods, excessive sweating and prolonged stress. As high protein decreases the bone mass due to its acid nature more concern should be given to increase the intake of alkalining fruits and vegetables rather reducing protein sources [34]. Also high protein diets particularly with animal protein actually result in greater bone mass.

In addition to dietary sources, medical supplementation becomes important in order to replace ongoing losses especially in malabsorptive procedures. It has been demonstrated that calcium and vitamin D supplementation may attenuate the risk of bone loss following bariatric surgery [35, 36]. Expert recommendations for daily supplementation are 1200–1500 mg calcium and at least 3000 international units of vitamin D. Calcium citrate is safer than calcium carbonate that in large quantities can evoke a 'milk-alkali' syndrome [37]. Calcium citrate also reduces the risk of kidney stone formation [38]. This is of importance in RYGB procedures that appear to increase the risk of urinary stone disease [39]. Magnesium oxide and citrate are commonly used magnesium supplementations, but in case of intolerance, this can be replaced for IM or IV injections (magnesium sulphate, 100 mg/mL; 5 and 10 mL ampoules). Hence encouraging adequate intake with replacements with appropriate treatment of deficiencies is of prime importance.

The recommended dietary allowance for calcium, phosphorus, vitamin D, magnesium

Nutrients	Country	Males	Females
Calcium (mg/day)	RDA* (India) (39) RDA* (US) (40) RNI** (UK) (41) NRV*** (Australia/New Zealand) (42)	600 1000 700 1000	600 1000 700 1000
Vitamin D (mcg/day)	RDA* (India) (39) RDA* (US) (40) RNI** (UK) (41) NRV*** (Australia/New Zealand) (42)	10 15 5 5–10	10 15 5 5–10
Phosphorus (mg/day)	RDA* (India) (39) RDA* (US) (40) RNI** (UK/EU) (41) NRV*** (Australia/New Zealand) (42)	600 700 550 1000	600 700 550 1000
Magnesium (mg/day)	RDA* (India) (39) RDA* (US) (40) RNI** (UK) (41) NRV*** (Australia/New Zealand) (42)	340 420 300 400–420	310 320 270 310–320

*RDA** recommended dietary allowances, *RNI*** reference nutrient intake, NRV*** nutrient reference value

Recommendations

- There is a significant fall in bone mineral density, bone mineral content and increased bone remodeling within the first year post all kinds of bariatric procedures.
- Daily supplementation of 1200–1500 mg calcium and at least 3000 international units of vitamin D is recommended. Calcium citrate is safer than calcium carbonate
- Similar replacements have to be considered after sleeve gastrectomy.
- Even with regular supplementation intense follow up and management of deficiencies is necessary.
- BPD-DS should be avoided with pre-existing deficiency as hypovitaminosis D and secondary hyperparathyroidism is difficult to manage in spite of adequate supplementation.

References

1. Bloomberg RD, Fleishman A, Nalle JE, Herron DM, Kini S. Nutritional deficiencies following bariatric surgery: what have we learned? Obes Surg. 2005;15(2):145–54.
2. Brolin RE, Leung M. Survey of vitamin and mineral supplementation after gastric bypass and biliopancreatic diversion for morbid obesity. Obes Surg. 1999;9(2):150–4.
3. Alvarez-Leite JI. Nutrient deficiencies secondary to bariatric surgery. Curr Opin Clin Nutr Metab Care. 2004;7(5):569–75.
4. Clements RH, Katasani VG, Palepu R, Leeth RR, Leath TD, Roy BP, et al. Incidence of vitamin deficiency after laparoscopic Roux-en-Y gastric bypass in a university hospital setting. Am Surg. 2006;72(12):1196–202; discussion 1203–4.
5. Schweiger C, Keidar A. Nutritional deficiencies in bariatric surgery patients: prevention, diagnosis and treatment. Harefuah. 2010;149(11):715–20, 748.
6. Stein J, Stier C, Raab H, Weiner R. Review article: the nutritional and pharmacological consequences of obesity surgery. Aliment Pharmacol Ther. 2014;40(6):582–609.
7. Gracia J-A, Martinez M, Aguilella V, Elia M, Royo P. Postoperative morbidity of biliopancreatic diversion depending on common limb length. Obes Surg. 2007;17(10):1306–11.
8. Gletsu-Miller N, Wright BN. Mineral malnutrition following bariatric surgery. Adv Nutr. 2013;4(5):506–17.
9. Christakos S, Dhawan P, Porta A, Mady LJ, Seth T. Vitamin D and intestinal calcium absorption. Mol Cell Endocrinol. 2011;347(1–2):25–9.
10. Weaver CM, Fleet JC. Vitamin D requirements: current and future. Am J Clin Nutr. 2004;80(6 Suppl):1735S–9.
11. Fleet JC, Schoch RD. Molecular mechanisms for regulation of intestinal calcium absorption by vitamin D and other factors. Crit Rev Clin Lab Sci. 2010;47(4):181–95.
12. Holick MF. Vitamin D, deficiency. N Engl J Med. 2007;357(3):266–81.
13. DiGiorgi M, Daud A, Inabnet WB, Schrope B, Urban-Skuro M, Restuccia N, et al. Markers of bone and calcium metabolism following gastric bypass and laparoscopic adjustable gastric banding. Obes Surg. 2008;18(9):1144–8.
14. Ross AC, Manson JE, Abrams SA, Aloia JF, Brannon PM, Clinton SK, et al. The 2011 report on dietary reference intakes for calcium and vitamin D from the Institute of Medicine: what clinicians need to know. J Clin Endocrinol Metab. 2011;96(1):53–8.
15. Von Mach M-A, Stoeckli R, Bilz S, Kraenzlin M, Langer I, Keller U. Changes in bone mineral content after surgical treatment of morbid obesity. Metabolism. 2004;53(7):918–21.
16. Vilarrasa N, San José P, García I, Gómez-Vaquero C, Miras PM, de Gordejuela AGR, et al. Evaluation of bone mineral density loss in morbidly obese women after gastric bypass: 3-year follow-up. Obes Surg. 2011;21(4):465–72.
17. Vilarrasa N, Gómez JM, Elio I, Gómez-Vaquero C, Masdevall C, Pujol J, et al. Evaluation of bone disease in morbidly obese women after gastric bypass and risk factors implicated in bone loss. Obes Surg. 2009;19(7):860–6.
18. Maghrabi AH, Wolski K, Abood B, Licata A, Pothier C, Bhatt DL, et al. Two-year outcomes on bone density and fracture incidence in patients with T2DM randomized to bariatric surgery versus intensive medical therapy. Obes Silver Spring Md. 2015;23(12):2344–8.
19. Adamczyk P, Bužga M, Holéczy P, Švagera Z, Zonča P, Sievänen H, et al. Body size, bone mineral density, and body composition in obese women after laparoscopic sleeve gastrectomy: a 1-year longitudinal study. Horm Metab Res Horm Stoffwechselforschung Horm Métabolisme. 2015;47(12):873–9.
20. Hsin M-C, Huang C-K, Tai C-M, Yeh L-R, Kuo H-C, Garg A. A case-matched study of the differences in bone mineral density 1 year after 3 different bariatric procedures. Surg Obes Relat Dis Off J Am Soc Bariatr Surg. 2015;11(1):181–5.
21. Liu C, Wu D, Zhang J-F, Xu D, Xu W-F, Chen Y, et al. Changes in bone metabolism in morbidly obese patients after bariatric surgery: a meta-analysis. Obes Surg. 2016;26(1):91–7.

22. Yu EW, Bouxsein ML, Putman MS, Monis EL, Roy AE, Pratt JSA, et al. Two-year changes in bone density after Roux-en-Y gastric bypass surgery. J Clin Endocrinol Metab. 2015;100(4):1452–9.
23. Al-Rasheid N, Gray R, Sufi P, Marina-Gonzalez N, Al-Sayrafi M, Atherton E, et al. Chronic elevation of systemic glucagon-like peptide-1 following surgical weight loss: association with nausea and vomiting and effects on adipokines. Obes Surg. 2015;25(2):386–91.
24. Oliván B, Teixeira J, Bose M, Bawa B, Chang T, Summe H, et al. Effect of weight loss by diet or gastric bypass surgery on peptide YY3-36 levels. Ann Surg. 2009;249(6):948–53.
25. Chen J, Pamuklar Z, Spagnoli A, Torquati A. Serum leptin levels are inversely correlated with omental gene expression of adiponectin and markedly decreased after gastric bypass surgery. Surg Endosc. 2012;26(5):1476–80.
26. Bose M, Teixeira J, Olivan B, Bawa B, Arias S, Machineni S, et al. Weight loss and incretin responsiveness improve glucose control independently after gastric bypass surgery. J Diabetes. 2010;2(1):47–55.
27. Ko B-J, Myung SK, Cho K-H, Park YG, Kim SG, Kim DH, et al. Relationship between bariatric surgery and bone mineral density: a meta-analysis. Obes Surg. 2015;26(7):1414–21.
28. Nakamura KM, Haglind EGC, Clowes JA, Achenbach SJ, Atkinson EJ, Melton LJ, et al. Fracture risk following bariatric surgery: a population-based study. Osteoporos Int J Establ Result Coop Eur Found Osteoporos Natl Osteoporos Found USA. 2014;25(1):151–8.
29. Lalmohamed A, de Vries F, Bazelier MT, Cooper A, van Staa T-P, Cooper C, et al. Risk of fracture after bariatric surgery in the United Kingdom: population based, retrospective cohort study. BMJ. 2012;345:e5085.
30. Scibora LM, Ikramuddin S, Buchwald H, Petit MA. Examining the link between bariatric surgery, bone loss, and osteoporosis: a review of bone density studies. Obes Surg. 2012;22(4):654–67.
31. Costa TL, Paganotto M, Radominski RB, Kulak CM, Borba VC. Calcium metabolism, vitamin D and bone mineral density after bariatric surgery. Osteoporos Int J Establ Result Coop Eur Found Osteoporos Natl Osteoporos Found USA. 2015;26(2):757–64.
32. Muschitz C, Kocijan R, Haschka J, Zendeli A, Pirker T, Geiger C, et al. The impact of vitamin D, calcium, protein supplementation, and physical exercise on bone metabolism after bariatric surgery: the BABS study. J Bone Miner Res Off J Am Soc Bone Miner Res. 2015;31(3):672–82.
33. Topart P, Becouarn G, Sallé A, Ritz P. Biliopancreatic diversion requires multiple vitamin and micronutrient adjustments within 2 years of surgery. Surg Obes Relat Dis Off J Am Soc Bariatr Surg. 2014;10(5):936–41.
34. Heaney RP, Layman DK. Amount and type of protein influences bone health. Am J Clin Nutr. 2008;87(5):1567S–70.
35. Mechanick JI, Youdim A, Jones DB, Garvey WT, Hurley DL, McMahon MM, et al. Clinical practice guidelines for the perioperative nutritional, metabolic, and nonsurgical support of the bariatric surgery patient – 2013 update: cosponsored by American Association of Clinical Endocrinologists, The Obesity Society, and American Society for Metabolic & Bariatric Surgery. Obes Silver Spring Md. 2013;21 Suppl 1:S1–27.
36. Mahdy T, Atia S, Farid M, Adulatif A. Effect of Roux-en Y gastric bypass on bone metabolism in patients with morbid obesity: mansoura experiences. Obes Surg. 2008;18(12):1526–31.
37. Sakhaee K, Bhuket T, Adams-Huet B, Rao DS. Meta-analysis of calcium bioavailability: a comparison of calcium citrate with calcium carbonate. Am J Ther. 1999;6(6):313–21.
38. Sakhaee K, Poindexter J, Aguirre C. The effects of bariatric surgery on bone and nephrolithiasis. Bone. 2016;84:1–8.
39. Jayram G, Matlaga APBR. Bariatric surgery and stone disease: help or hindrance? In: Pearle MS, Nakada SY, editors. Practical controversies in medical management of stone disease. New York: Springer; 2014. p. 63–70. [Internet] [cited 2016]. Available from: http://link.springer.com/chapter/10.1007/978-1-4614-9575-8_5.

Other Micronutrient Deficiencies in Bariatric Surgery

36

Parimala Devi and Praveen Raj Palanivelu

As the obesity epidemic continues and the number of patients undergoing bariatric surgery rises, it is important to optimize long-term nutrition after bariatric surgery in addition to monitoring weight and co-morbidities outcomes. It is important for clinicians to be aware of both pre-existing and new onset nutritional deficiencies in obese patients, to screen for and recognize symptoms of deficiency, prescribe appropriate supplementation and treat deficiencies that may emerge both in the short term and long-term post-operatively.

The aim of this chapter is to serve as guideline for the identification, assessment and treatment of potential vitamin and mineral deficiencies post bariatric surgery. Thiamine, Copper, Selenium, Vitamin A, E and K have been covered in this chapter. Iron Vitamin B12, Folic acid, Calcium and Vitamin D have been discussed in the earlier chapters.

36.1 Thiamine

Thiamine (Vitamin B1) was one of the first B vitamins identified and constitutes one of the eight essential water soluble B vitamins. It serves as a coenzyme that helps the body to convert macronutrients (carbohydrates, fat and protein) into energy and is vital for proper functioning of the central and peripheral nervous system [1].

Primary absorption of thiamine occurs in the duodenum by an active process which requires magnesium as a cofactor; hence hypomagnesaemia can precipitate thiamine deficiency. Conventional cooking methods may destroy thiamine content by 50 % in food sources. Tea and coffee contain thiaminase, an enzyme that breaks

P. Devi, MSc (✉) • P.R. Palanivelu, MS, DNB, DNB(SGE), FALS, FMAS
Bariatric Division, Upper Gastrointestinal Surgery and Minimal Access Surgery Unit, GEM Hospital and Research Centre, Coimbatore, India
e-mail: parimalaswamy30@gmail.com; drraj@geminstitute.in

P.R. Palanivelu et al. (eds.), *Bariatric Surgical Practice Guide*,
DOI 10.1007/978-981-10-2705-5_36

down ingested thiamin. Excessive alcohol ingestion can significantly alter thiamine absorption. Surgical stress, trauma and pregnancy increase thiamine requirements.

Thiamine deficiency results in dry beriberi-a peripheral neuropathy, wet beriberi-a cardiomyopathy with edema and lactic acidosis, and Wernicke—Korsakoff syndrome, whose manifestations consist of nystagmus, ophthalmoplegia, ataxia, confusion, retrograde amnesia, cognitive impairment, and confabulation. The most common cause of thiamine deficiency in affluent countries is alcoholism [2]. In nonalcoholic patients the commonest cause is malnutrition/prolonged vomiting [3–5]. Patients on a thiamine-deficient diet display a state of severe depletion within 9–18 days which corresponds to its short half-life. Prolonged vomiting also results in rapid depletion of thiamine.

Whole blood thiamine levels are not reliable for the diagnosis of thiamine deficiency, though these levels are commonly estimated. In individuals with suspicion of thiamine deficiency (a high index of suspicion must be maintained because of the varied clinical presentations), more sensitive markers such as thiamine diphosphate or erythrocyte transketolase activity may be required to confirm the diagnosis [6].

36.1.1 Thiamine Deficiency in Bariatric Surgery

Thiamine deficiency after bariatric surgery is commonly associated with nausea, vomiting and constipation (thiamine deficiency is a known cause of colonic dilation). All types of bariatric procedures can be associated with thiamine deficiency [7, 8]. Only 16–38 % of patients present with classical symptoms of Wernicke's encephalopathy. The rest present only with atypical symptoms requiring a high index of clinical suspicion in patients with prior history of bariatric surgery, unbalanced diet and progressing neurological symptoms [9, 10].

A condition called 'bariatric beriberi' has been described in post Roux-en-Y gastric bypass (RYGB) patients in which thiamine deficiency exists but is not corrected by supplementation [8]. Bacterial overgrowth in the small intestine is responsible for this form of beriberi, and the diagnosis is supported by an increase of serum folate or an increase of breath hydrogen after oral glucose administration. 'Bariatric beriberi' needs to be corrected by intramuscular vitamin supplementation concomitantly with antibiotic therapy to counteract the bacterial overgrowth [8].

The recommended Dietary Allowance for Thiamine

Thiamine	Males	Females
RDA* (India) [16]	1.2–1.7 mg/day	1.0–1.4 mg/day
RDA*(US) [17]	1.2 mg/day	1.1 mg/day
RNI**(UK) [18]	1.3 mg/day	1.1 mg/day
NRV***(Australia/New Zealand) [19]	1.2 mg/day	1.1 mg/day

*RDA** recommended dietary allowances, *RNI*** reference nutrient intake, *NRV**** nutrient reference value

36.1.2 Thiamine Recommendation Post-bariatric Surgery

Dietary sources of thiamine are whole grain cereals (brown rice and bran), meat (pork, poultry), eggs, nuts, legumes (dried beans, peas), soybeans and vegetables (green leafy vegetables, beetroot, and potatoes).

Thiamine should be part of a routine multivitamin with mineral preparation prescribed post bariatric surgery. Also routine thiamine screening is not recommended following bariatric surgery [11]. Empiric thiamine supplementation and/or screening for thiamine deficiency should be considered in post bariatric surgery patients with rapid weight loss, protracted vomiting, parenteral nutrition, excessive alcohol use, neuropathy, encephalopathy, or heart failure [11].

Patients with severe thiamine deficiency (suspected or established) should be treated with intravenous thiamine, 500 mg/day, for 3–5 days, followed by 250 mg/day for 3–5 days or until resolution of symptoms, and then to consider treatment with 100 mg/day, orally, usually indefinitely or until risk factors have resolved. Mild deficiency can be treated with intravenous thiamine, 100 mg/day, for 7–14 days. It is important to note that thiamine supplementation requires in addition 300–400 mg/day of elemental magnesium supplementation [11].

For Wernicke's encephalopathy most authors agree on a dosage scheme of 500 mg of intravenous thiamine three times daily for 2–3 days, followed by 250 mg intravenously daily until improvement [4, 10]. Dramatic improvement with thiamine administration practically confirms the diagnosis. Timely recognition of affected patients can be difficult but is of utmost importance, since intense supplementation of thiamine may completely reverse symptoms. Thiamine administration should not be delayed until diagnosis is confirmed as delay in treatment inadvertently leads to permanent neurological deficits or even death [9]. However, even with replacement therapy, almost half the patients will still exhibit permanent cognitive impairment [9].

36.2 Copper

Copper is an essential micronutrient which acts as a cofactor in several oxidative enzymes vital to the function of hematopoietic, skeletal, vascular tissues as well as the structure and function of the nervous system [12].

Copper is mainly absorbed in the stomach and duodenum. In the small intestine, copper is bound to metallothionein with greater affinity than zinc or other metal ions. Excessive intake of zinc may result in decreased copper levels and sideroblastic anaemia [13].

Due to the malabsorptive nature of procedures like RYGB, biliopancreatic diversion with/without duodenal switch (BPD-DS) copper deficiency is more common in these procedures. Gastric acid is involved in freeing copper from food, and the risk of copper deficiency increases as the stomach and duodenum are bypassed. Diarrhea caused by BPD-DS can cause excess loss of copper in addition to malabsorption [14]. One study reported that in post BPD-DS patients 50.6% of 89 BPD patients had at least once, a low copper level, and half of them repeatedly had low levels during a 5-year period. Several cases of copper deficiency after RYGB have also been reported [14, 15]. The prevalence and incidence of copper deficiency following RYGB surgery was determined to be 9.6 % and 18.8 %, respectively, with many patients experiencing mild-to-moderate symptoms.

The symptoms of copper deficiency include hematologic abnormalities like anaemia, neutropenia, leucopenia and myeloneuropathy. Myeloneuropathy is rare and often unrecognized complication of copper deficiency.

Also copper and vitamin B12 deficiency may coexist as acquired copper deficiency in humans has been described, causing a syndrome similar to the subacute combined degeneration of vitamin B_{12} deficiency. Ataxia and myelopathy secondary to acquired copper deficiency are rare complications. Early recognition and therapy with oral or parenteral copper may lead to a decrease in both neurologic and hematologic consequences.

36.2.1 Copper Recommendation After Bariatric Surgery

The highest diet rich sources of copper include organ meats, shellfish, nuts and seeds like sesame seeds, cashew, sunflower seeds, walnuts, pumpkin seeds, peanuts, almonds, flax seeds, chocolate soy beans, shiitake mushroom, crimini mushroom, spinach, kale, summer squash, tempeh, tofu, kidney beans, sweet potatoes, grapes, pineapple, tomatoes and egg plant.

The recommended Dietary Allowance for Copper

Copper	Males	Females
RDA* (India) [16]	1.35 mg/day	1.35 mg/day
RDA*(US) [17]	0.9 mg/day	0.9 mg/day
RNI**(UK) [18]	1.2 mg/day	1.2 mg/day
NRV***(Australia,New Zealand) [19]	1.7 mg/day	1.2 mg/day

*RDA** recommended dietary allowances, *RNI*** reference nutrient intake, *NRV**** nutrient reference value

Despite the lack of consensus concerning supplementation dosing, routine copper supplementation is recommended. At least 2 mg of copper per day is advised in the form of copper gluconate or sulfate as part of a vitamin and mineral supplement for BPD-DS and RYGB patients. Patients being treated for zinc deficiency or using supplemental zinc for hair loss should receive 1 mg of copper for each 8–15 mg of zinc as zinc replacement can cause copper deficiency. Copper levels are not routinely monitored but need to be evaluated in patients with neuropathy and normal vitamin B12 levels [16, 17]. The literature reports the use of oral copper gluconate in mild to moderate deficiency and IV copper infusion in severe deficiency [18–22]. For mild to moderate deficiency, the recommended oral administration is of 3–8 mg/d of copper gluconate until copper indices return to normal. Severe deficiency should be treated with 2–4 mg/d IV copper for 6 days or until neurological symptoms resolve and serum levels return to normal. Continuous monitoring of copper status is necessary every 3 months after deficiency is treated [23].

36.3 Selenium

Selenium is an essential trace element and a vital constituent of antioxidant enzymes that participate in various physiological activities and protects the cell against the deleterious effects of free radicals by modulating the cell response. The role of selenium has been explored in normal thyroid functioning, enhancing immune function, carcinogenesis, cardiovascular diseases, in the prevention of pre-eclampsia, diabetes mellitus and male reproduction etc.

It has been reported that obese people have lower serum selenium levels [23]. The actual incidence of selenium deficiency after bariatric surgery is not well documented, hence it's difficult to get a clear picture of its deficiency state but post bariatric patients can be at a risk of selenium deficiency secondary to reduction in nutrient intake and altered absorption as selenium is mainly absorbed in the duodenum.

Selenium is assimilated more effectively from plant food than animal products but some dietary constituents (vitamin C and vitamin E) generally affect its absorption. Also, other factors like, copper, magnesium, zinc, vitamin B, lipoic acid and some amino acids such as cysteine, glutamine, and methionine may play a role that affect the level of selenium.

A recent study following bariatric surgery showed that even with multivitamin and mineral supplements, a reduction in selenium concentration was noted in the early post-operative period which normalised during the first year after surgery [24].

Selenium deficiency is uncommon, but severe deficiency can cause symptoms and diseases including myopathy, cardiomyopathy, arrhythmia, muscle wasting, impaired immunity, low thyroid function, loss of skin and hair pigmentation, whitened nail beds, and progressive encephalopathy. There is an indication that selenium deficiency may contribute to the progression of viral infections.

Plasma erythrocyte and whole blood selenium, plasma selenoproteins P, and plasma platelet and whole blood glutathione activity are good biomarkers of selenium status in the body. In humans the selenoenzyme methionine sulfoxide reductase B1 (MsrB1) is the most sensitive protein marker of selenium status [25].

The recommended Dietary Allowance for Selenium

Selenium	Males	Females
RDA* (India) [16]	40 mcg	40 mcg
RDA*(US) [17]	55 mcg	55 mcg
RNI**(UK) [18]	75 mcg	60 mcg
NRV***(Australia,Newzealand) [19]	70 mcg	60 mcg

*RDA** recommended dietary allowances, *RNI*** reference nutrient intake, *NRV**** nutrient reference value

36.3.1 Selenium Recommendation After Bariatric Surgery

Plant foods are the major sources of selenium and it varies tremendously according to its concentrations in soil which varies regionally. Animals that eat grains or plants that were grown in selenium rich soil have higher levels of selenium in their muscle and is widely distributed in all tissues. Selenium is present in foods like brazil nuts, walnuts, almonds, peanuts, cashew nuts, pistachios, pine nuts, hazelnuts, sunflower seeds, grains (wheat germ, barley, brown rice, oats), fresh water and salt water fish (tuna, halibut, sardines, flounder, salmon), shellfish (oysters, mussels, shrimp, clams, scallops), meat (beef, lamb, pork, liver), poultry (chicken, turkey), eggs and mushroom (button, crimini, shiitake) [45].

A prospective pilot study ($n=39$) showed that RYGB and laparoscopic adjustable gastric banding (LAGB) procedures increase the risk for disturbances of selenium and GTP homeostasis and suggested that consideration of selenium supplementation at higher levels of current RDA (i.e. 55 mcg) during the first 3 months and perhaps longer may be needed [26].

However, there is insufficient evidence for routine selenium screening or supplementation but patients with malabsorptive bariatric surgeries who have unexplained anemia or fatigue, persistent diarrhea, cardiomyopathy or bone metabolic diseases, selenium levels should be checked.

36.4 Zinc

Zinc is an abundant essential trace element and important for cell function as well as metabolism, protein synthesis, detoxification, thyroid function, blood clotting, cognitive functions, fetal growth, immune response, growth and maintenance, sperm production, signaling transduction and gene regulation and essential for over 300 enzymatic reactions. Zinc is also an essential antioxidant and anti-inflammatory agent [27].

Zinc deficiency can either be genetic or can be acquired and can happen due to low intake, intestinal malabsorption (e.g. RYGB, inflammatory bowel disease (IBD), celiac disease, chronic diarrhea) or increased depletion (infection, pregnancy, burns, alcoholism, stress) [28, 29]. Serum zinc levels can also be lowered by medicines like penicillamine, diuretics, antimetabolites and valproate [28].

A moderate zinc deficiency can be seen as growth retardation, male hypoganadism in adolescents, rough skin, poor appetite, mental lethargy, delayed wound healing, cell mediated immune dysfunctions and abnormal neurosensory changes. Manifestations of severe deficiency include bullous pustular dermatitis, alopecia, diarrhea, pica, significant dysgeusia, emotional disorders, weight loss, intercurrent infections. If the deficiency is not treated then it may lead to a fatal situation [27].

36.4.1 Zinc Deficiency and Bariatric Surgery

Zinc deficiency is common after bariatric surgery as the main absorption sites such as duodenum and proximal jejunum are being bypassed and also the deficiency rates may vary depending on the type of surgery. After surgery, reduced stomach acid which is essential for zinc bioavailability, reduced protein intake, food intolerance and impaired zinc absorption may worsen the situation and may lead to zinc deficiency [30, 31]. In addition, regular iron and calcium supplementation can also contribute to insufficient zinc absorption [32, 33]. Zinc deficiency can also be associated with pregnancy and can lead to reduced birth weight, preterm delivery and congenital abnormalities and can induce hypertension in the mother [34–36].

A recent retrospective study showed that patients ($n=272$) who underwent RYGB, LSG and BPD-DS, 99 % had zinc deficiency preoperatively [31]. Studies at 2 years follow up after RYGB reported 20–35 % and Sleeve with 18–34 % and higher deficiency rates were found with BPD (74–91 %) with serum or plasma zinc levels [15, 37, 38]. It was found that, zinc deficiency persisted in patients even after 5 years follow up with 12.5 % after sleeve, 21–33 % after RYGB and 45 % after BPD. Rojas et al. stated that at 6 months, post bariatric surgery patients have an increased hair loss with lower intakes of zinc and iron requiring monitoring and supplementation [39].

36.4.2 Zinc Recommendation After Bariatric Surgery

Liver (beef, chicken, lamb, pork), red meat (beef, lamb, pork), sea foods like crab, lobsters, oysters and scallops, wheat germ, spinach, pumpkin, sesame and squash seeds, cashew nuts, mushrooms, chick peas, lentils, black beans, tofu, and whole grains are good dietary sources of zinc.

Copper and zinc compete for the same transport mechanism, so the excess of one might determine the deficiency of the other. Hence post bariatric patients should be advised oral zinc gluconate or acetate to provide 8–15 mg of zinc and 1 mg of copper for each 8–15 mg of zinc given.

The recommended Dietary Allowance for Zinc

Zinc	Males	Females
RDA* (India) [18]	12 mg	10 mg
RDA*(US) [19]	11 mg	8 mg
RNI**(UK) [20]	11.3 mg	14.8 mg
NRV***(Australia/New Zealand) [21]	14 mg	8 mg

*RDA** recommended dietary allowances, *RNI*** reference nutrient intake, *NRV**** nutrient reference value

36.5 Vitamin A

Vitamin A (includes retinol, B-carotene and caroteniods), is an essential fat soluble vitamin absorbed through the small intestine either as retinal (animal derived) or carotene (plant and vegetable derived) and is stored in the liver. Vitamin A is essential to eyes and immune system and it plays an important role in the cellular proliferation process and also in the protection against free radicals hence protecting against development of certain chronic diseases. Vitamin A can also affect iron metabolism contributing to iron deficiency. Zinc deficiency can affect vitamin A metabolism as it is essential for the synthesis of retinol binding protein (RBP) in both the liver and the plasma and the oxidation of retinol to retinal [40]. Iron deficiency also compromises the function of the intestinal mucosa, affecting the absorption of vitamin A and iron deficiency should be corrected in order to normalize vitamin A levels [41].

Vitamin A deficiency causes night blindness which evolves into destruction of the cornea (keratomalacia) and total blindness. The other problems include impaired immunity, hypokeratosis, squamous metaplasia of the bladder and respiratory tract epithelium and enamel hypoplasia. Vitamin A deficiency is associated with a low serum concentration of prealbumin and deficiency should be suspected in those with evidence of protein-calorie malnutrition.

After bariatric surgery vitamin A deficiency occurs because of various factors such as (1) surgical bypass of duodenum and first portion of jejunum leading to an iatrogenically induced malabsorption (2) significant decrease in the dietary intake particularly in the early post-op period (3) low fat dietary recommendation after bariatric surgery particularly in malabsorptive procedures like gastric bypass, BPD/BPD-DS limits the fat soluble vitamin absorption. The risk may increase due to confounding factors such as nonalcoholic fatty liver disease NAFLD or cirrhosis which both can interfere with the maintenance of vitamin A storage and production. Higher levels of oxidative stress can also interfere with vitamin A absorption [41].

Around 60–70 % of BPD with or without DS patients and 10 % of distal RYGB patients had low of vitamin A level despite a compliance with multivitamin supplementation on long term follow up [42–44]. Few clinical cases of vitamin A deficiency after bariatric surgery have been reported with night blindness and ocular xerosis [45]. Low levels was reported preoperatively in 12.5 % of adults undergoing bariatric surgery which increased post operatively [46].

Routine screening for vitamin A deficiency, which may present as ocular complications, is recommended after malabsorptive bariatric procedures, such as BPD or BPD/DS, and supplementation alone or in combination with other fat-soluble vitamins (D, E, and K) may be indicated in this setting [23]. Vitamin A is found naturally in milk, eggs, liver, fish oils, green and bright colored green (leafy) vegetables such as spinach, bell peppers, fruits like mango, papaya, apricots, tomatoes, cantaloupe, melon and carrots, sweet potatoes and butter.

The recommended Dietary Allowance for Vitamin A

Vitamin A	Males	Females
RDA* (India) [16]	600 mcg	600 mcg
RDA*(US) [17]	900 mcg	700 mcg
RNI**(UK) [18]	700 mcg	600 mcg
NRV***(Australia/New Zealand) [19]	900 mcg	700 mcg

*RDA** recommended dietary allowances, *RNI*** reference nutrient intake, *NRV**** nutrient reference value

The suggested post operative supplementation after LABD and LSG is 100 % RDA (600–900 mcg) and 200 % (1200–1800 mcg) for BPD/DS patients.

36.6 Vitamin E

Vitamin E (tocopherols and tocotrienols) functions as a cell oxidant and protects cell membranes from oxidation by reacting with lipid radicals produced in the lipid peroxidation chain reaction providing a high level of skin protection against ultraviolet radiation and enhance immune response [47]. Vitamin E can be found in high concentrations in avocado, eggs, milk, nuts, green leafy vegetables, vegetable oils and whole grain foods. Vitamin E deficiency includes visual symptoms like retinopathy and neurologic symptoms like muscle weakness and hematological conditions like anemia and hemolytic anemia. Reports of symptomatic deficiencies after bariatric surgery are lacking. Vitamin E deficiency appears to be more common after BPD due to significant fat malabsorption and was reported in 7.1 % of patients [42].

The recommended Dietary Allowance for Vitamin E

Vitamin E	Males	Females
RDA* (India) [16]	7.5–10 mg	7.5–10 mg
RDA*(US) [17]	15 mg	15 mg
RNI**(UK) [18]	12 mg	12 mg
NRV***(Australia/New Zealand) [19]	10 mg	7 mg

*RDA** recommended dietary allowances, *RNI*** reference nutrient intake, *NRV**** nutrient reference value

36.7 Vitamin K in Bariatric Surgery

Vitamin K plays an essential role in the blood coagulation regulation through the formation of prothrombin (factor II, VII, IX. X protein C and protein S). Other functions are bone metabolism regulation (in particular osteocalcin) and regulation of vascular biology.

Vitamin K is absorbed in the jejunum and ileum in the presence of bile and pancreatic juice. Fifty percent of the daily requirement of this vitamin is derived from the intestinal flora biosynthesis and it is present in food sources such as green leafy vegetables, avocado, kiwi fruit, liver, soy and vegetable oils [48].

Vitamin K deficiency may be secondary to low intake (anorexia, alcoholics, elderly patients), fat malabsorption (e.g. cystic fibrosis, biliary atresia, gastrointestinal surgeries such as bariatric surgery), use of antibiotics that alter the intestinal bacterial flora (e.g. cephalsporins, isoniazid, rifampicin) and intake of vitamin K inhibiting drugs (e.g. phenytoin, cholestryramine) [48].

Low levels of vitamin K have been noted in 69 % of BPD/DS patients despite routine supplementation, with the deficiency being commonly asymptomatic [49].

Vitamin K deficiency results in bleeding coagulation disorders presenting as purpura, petechiae, ecchymoses, and bruising. Post bariatric pregnant females having excessive vomiting or fat malabsorption have a higher risk of vitamin K deficiency related bleeding disorders in the neonates [37]. Fetal cerebral hemorrhage was reported due to maternal vitamin K deficiency following vomiting after gastric band slippage [50]. Maternal vitamin K deficiency and related complications were documented by Eerdekens et al. in five patients with severe intracranial bleeding and skeletal malformations similar to warfarin fetopathy (Rhizomelic chondrodysplasia punctate) [51]. In the presence of an established fat-soluble vitamin deficiency with coagulopathy assessment of a vitamin K_1 level should be considered.

The recommended Dietary Allowance for Vitamin K

Vitamin K	Males	Females
RDA* (India) [16]	70 mcg	60 mcg
RDA*(US) [17]	120 mcg	90 mcg
RNI**(UK) [18]	75 mcg	75 mcg
NRV***(Australia/New Zealand) [19]	70 mcg	60 mcg

*RDA** recommended dietary allowances, *RNI*** reference nutrient intake, *NRV**** nutrient reference value

Conclusion

Thiamine can be supplemented as part of a vitamin mineral supplement post bariatric surgery. Thiamine deficiency should be suspected and empirically replaced in any patient whose post bariatric surgery course is complicated by protracted vomiting. In thiamine deficiency, thiamine has to be supplemented with magnesium.

Copper can be supplemented as part of a vitamin mineral supplement post bariatric surgery with at least 2 mg of copper per day for BPD-DS and RYGB patients. Patients being treated for zinc deficiency should receive 1 mg of copper for each 8–15 mg of zinc as zinc replacement. Copper deficiency should be suspected in patients with neuropathy and normal vitamin B12 levels.

Selenium can be supplemented as part of a vitamin mineral supplement post bariatric surgery. Selenium deficiency should be suspected in patients with malabsorptive bariatric surgeries who have unexplained anemia, persistent diarrhea, cardiomyopathy or bone metabolic diseases.

Selenium can be supplemented as part of a vitamin mineral supplement post bariatric surgery to provide 8–15 mg of zinc. Zinc deficiency should be suspected in patients with hair loss, pica, significant dysgeusia, or in male patients with hypogonadism or erectile dysfunction.

Vitamin A, K, E needs to be supplemented alone or in combination with other fat-soluble vitamins after malabsorptive bariatric procedures. Routine screening for vitamin A deficiency is necessary which may present with ocular complications, Vitamin K needs should be suspected in coagulopathy. Symptomatic vitamin E deficiencies after bariatric surgery are rare.

Recommendations

- Vitamin A, K, E needs to be supplemented alone or in combination with other fat-soluble vitamins after malabsorptive bariatric procedures.
- Micronutrient replacements have to be done as a part of multivitamin replacement on a regular basis for all malabsorptive procedures. Similar replacements should also be supplemented after sleeve gastrectomy too. Specific deficiencies have to be carefully looked for and managed appropriately.

References

1. Osiezagha K, Ali S, Freeman C, Barker NC, Jabeen S, Maitra S, et al. Thiamine deficiency and delirium. Innov Clin Neurosci. 2013;10(4):26–32.
2. Thomson AD, Marshall EJ. The treatment of patients at risk of developing Wernicke's encephalopathy in the community. Alcohol Alcohol Oxf Oxfs. 2006;41(2):159–67.
3. Worden RW, Allen HM. Wernicke's encephalopathy after gastric bypass that masqueraded as acute psychosis: a case report. Curr Surg. 2006;63(2):114–6.
4. Sechi G, Serra A, Pirastru MI, Sotgiu S, Rosati G. Wernicke's encephalopathy in a woman on slimming diet. Neurology. 2002;58(11):1697–8.
5. Sutamnartpong P, Muengtaweepongsa S, Kulkantrakorn K. Wernicke's encephalopathy and central pontine myelinolysis in hyperemesis gravidarum. J Neurosci Rural Pract. 2013;4(1):39–41.
6. Herve C, Beyne P, Lettéron P, Delacoux E. Comparison of erythrocyte transketolase activity with thiamine and thiamine phosphate ester levels in chronic alcoholic patients. Clin Chim Acta Int J Clin Chem. 1995;234(1–2):91–100.
7. Manatakis DK, Georgopoulos N. A fatal case of Wernicke's encephalopathy after sleeve gastrectomy for morbid obesity. Case Rep Surg. 2014;2014:281210.
8. Lakhani SV, Shah HN, Alexander K, Finelli FC, Kirkpatrick JR, Koch TR. Small intestinal bacterial overgrowth and thiamine deficiency after Roux-en-Y gastric bypass surgery in obese patients. Nutr Res. 2008;28(5):293–8.
9. Aasheim ET. Wernicke encephalopathy after bariatric surgery: a systematic review. Ann Surg. 2008;248(5):714–20.
10. Becker DA, Balcer LJ, Galetta SL. The neurological complications of nutritional deficiency following bariatric surgery. J Obes. 2012;2012:608534.
11. Allied Health Sciences Section Ad Hoc Nutrition Committee, Aills L, Blankenship J, Buffington C, Furtado M, Parrott J. ASMBS Allied Health Nutritional Guidelines for the surgical weight loss patient. Surg Obes Relat Dis Off J Am Soc Bariatr Surg. 2008;4(5 Suppl):S73–108.
12. Bertinato J, L'Abbé MR. Maintaining copper homeostasis: regulation of copper-trafficking proteins in response to copper deficiency or overload. J Nutr Biochem. 2004;15(6):316–22.
13. Fiske DN, McCoy HE, Kitchens CS. Zinc-induced sideroblastic anemia: report of a case, review of the literature, and description of the hematologic syndrome. Am J Hematol. 1994;46(2):147–50.
14. Btaiche IF, Yeh AY, Wu IJ, Khalidi N. Neurologic dysfunction and pancytopenia secondary to acquired copper deficiency following duodenal switch: case report and review of the literature. Nutr Clin Pract Off Publ Am Soc Parenter Enter Nutr. 2011;26(5):583–92.
15. Balsa JA, Botella-Carretero JI, Gómez-Martín JM, Peromingo R, Arrieta F, Santiuste C, et al. Copper and zinc serum levels after derivative bariatric surgery: differences between Roux-en-Y Gastric bypass and biliopancreatic diversion. Obes Surg. 2011;21(6):744–50.

16. Kumar N. Copper deficiency myelopathy (human swayback). Mayo Clin Proc. 2006;81(10):1371–84.
17. Kumar N, Ahlskog JE, Gross JB. Acquired hypocupremia after gastric surgery. Clin Gastroenterol Hepatol Off Clin Pract J Am Gastroenterol Assoc. 2004;2(12):1074–9.
18. Griffith DP, Liff DA, Ziegler TR, Esper GJ, Winton EF. Acquired copper deficiency: a potentially serious and preventable complication following gastric bypass surgery. Obes Silver Spring Md. 2009;17(4):827–31.
19. O'Donnell KB, Simmons M. Early-onset copper deficiency following Roux-en-Y gastric bypass. Nutr Clin Pract Off Publ Am Soc Parenter Enter Nutr. 2011;26(1):66–9.
20. Naismith RT, Shepherd JB, Weihl CC, Tutlam NT, Cross AH. Acute and bilateral blindness due to optic neuropathy associated with copper deficiency. Arch Neurol. 2009;66(8): 1025–7.
21. Pineles SL, Wilson CA, Balcer LJ, Slater R, Galetta SL. Combined optic neuropathy and myelopathy secondary to copper deficiency. Surv Ophthalmol. 2010;55(4):386–92.
22. Shahidzadeh R, Sridhar S. Profound copper deficiency in a patient with gastric bypass. Am J Gastroenterol. 2008;103(10):2660–2.
23. Mechanick JI, Youdim A, Jones DB, Garvey WT, Hurley DL, McMahon MM, et al. Clinical practice guidelines for the perioperative nutritional, metabolic, and nonsurgical support of the bariatric surgery patient--2013 update: cosponsored by American Association of Clinical Endocrinologists, The Obesity Society, and American Society for Metabolic & Bariatric Surgery. Obes Silver Spring Md. 2013;21 Suppl 1:S1–27.
24. Papamargaritis D, Aasheim ET, Sampson B, le Roux CW. Copper, selenium and zinc levels after bariatric surgery in patients recommended to take multivitamin-mineral supplementation. J Trace Elem Med Biol Organ Soc Miner Trace Elem GMS. 2015;31:167–72.
25. Papp LV, Holmgren A, Khanna KK. Selenium and selenoproteins in health and disease. Antioxid Redox Signal. 2010;12(7):793–5.
26. Freeth A, Prajuabpansri P, Victory JM, Jenkins P. Assessment of selenium in Roux-en-Y gastric bypass and gastric banding surgery. Obes Surg. 2012;22(11):1660–5.
27. Prasad AS. Discovery of human zinc deficiency: its impact on human health and disease. Adv Nutr Bethesda Md. 2013;4(2):176–90.
28. Tuerk MJ, Fazel N. Zinc deficiency. Curr Opin Gastroenterol. 2009;25(2):136–43.
29. Schwartz JR, Marsh RG, Draelos ZD. Zinc and skin health: overview of physiology and pharmacology. Dermatol Surg Off Publ Am Soc Dermatol Surg Al. 2005;31(7 Pt 2):837–47; discussion 847.
30. Sturniolo GC, Montino MC, Rossetto L, Martin A, D'Inca R, D'Odorico A, et al. Inhibition of gastric acid secretion reduces zinc absorption in man. J Am Coll Nutr. 1991;10(4):372–5.
31. Sallé A, Demarsy D, Poirier AL, Lelièvre B, Topart P, Guilloteau G, et al. Zinc deficiency: a frequent and underestimated complication after bariatric surgery. Obes Surg. 2010;20(12):1660–70.
32. Ruz M, Carrasco F, Rojas P, Codoceo J, Inostroza J, Basfi-fer K, et al. Zinc absorption and zinc status are reduced after Roux-en-Y gastric bypass: a randomized study using 2 supplements. Am J Clin Nutr. 2011;94(4):1004–11.
33. King JC. Determinants of maternal zinc status during pregnancy. Am J Clin Nutr. 2000;71(5 Suppl):1334S–43.
34. Castillo-Durán C, Weisstaub G. Zinc supplementation and growth of the fetus and low birth weight infant. J Nutr. 2003;133(5 Suppl 1):1494S–7.
35. Gibson RS. Zinc nutrition in developing countries. Nutr Res Rev. 1994;7(1):151–73.
36. Gehrer S, Kern B, Peters T, Christoffel-Courtin C, Peterli R. Fewer nutrient deficiencies after laparoscopic sleeve gastrectomy (LSG) than after laparoscopic Roux-Y-gastric bypass (LRYGB)-a prospective study. Obes Surg. 2010;20(4):447–53.
37. Moizé V, Andreu A, Flores L, Torres F, Ibarzabal A, Delgado S, et al. Long-term dietary intake and nutritional deficiencies following sleeve gastrectomy or Roux-En-Y gastric bypass in a mediterranean population. J Acad Nutr Diet. 2013;113(3):400–10.

38. Thurnheer M, Bisang P, Ernst B, Schultes B. A novel distal very long Roux-en Y gastric bypass (DVLRYGB) as a primary bariatric procedure--complication rates, weight loss, and nutritional/metabolic changes in the first 355 patients. Obes Surg. 2012;22(9):1427–36.
39. Rojas P, Gosch M, Basfi-fer K, Carrasco F, Codoceo J, Inostroza J, et al. Alopecia in women with severe and morbid obesity who undergo bariatric surgery. Nutr Hosp. 2011;26(4):856–62.
40. Chaves GV, Pereira SE, Saboya CJ, Ramalho A. Nutritional status of vitamin A in morbid obesity before and after Roux-en-Y gastric bypass. Obes Surg. 2007;17(7):970–6.
41. Zalesin KC, Miller WM, Franklin B, Mudugal D, Rao Buragadda A, Boura J, et al. Vitamin a deficiency after gastric bypass surgery: an underreported postoperative complication. J Obes. 2011;2011: pii:760695.
42. Slater GH, Ren CJ, Siegel N, Williams T, Barr D, Wolfe B, et al. Serum fat-soluble vitamin deficiency and abnormal calcium metabolism after malabsorptive bariatric surgery. J Gastrointest Surg Off J Soc Surg Aliment Tract. 2004;8(1):48–55; discussion 54–5.
43. Dolan K, Hatzifotis M, Newbury L, Lowe N, Fielding G. A clinical and nutritional comparison of biliopancreatic diversion with and without duodenal switch. Ann Surg. 2004;240(1):51–6.
44. Brolin RE, Kenler HA, Gorman JH, Cody RP. Long-limb gastric bypass in the superobese. A prospective randomized study. Ann Surg. 1992;215(4):387–95.
45. Lee WB, Hamilton SM, Harris JP, Schwab IR. Ocular complications of hypovitaminosis a after bariatric surgery. Ophthalmology. 2005;112(6):1031–4.
46. Pereira S, Saboya C, Chaves G, Ramalho A. Class III obesity and its relationship with the nutritional status of vitamin A in pre- and postoperative gastric bypass. Obes Surg. 2009;19(6):738–44.
47. Dror DK, Allen LH. Vitamin E deficiency in developing countries. Food Nutr Bull. 2011;32(2):124–43.
48. Shearer MJ, Fu X, Booth SL. Vitamin K nutrition, metabolism, and requirements: current concepts and future research. Adv Nutr Bethesda Md. 2012;3(2):182–95.
49. Homan J, Ruinemans-Koerts J, Aarts EO, Janssen IMC, Berends FJ, de Boer H. Management of vitamin K deficiency after biliopancreatic diversion with or without duodenal switch. Surg Obes Relat Dis Off J Am Soc Bariatr Surg. 2016;12(2):338–44.
50. Van Mieghem T, Van Schoubroeck D, Depiere M, Debeer A, Hanssens M. Fetal cerebral hemorrhage caused by vitamin K deficiency after complicated bariatric surgery. Obstet Gynecol. 2008;112(2 Pt 2):434–6.
51. Eerdekens A, Debeer A, Van Hoey G, De Borger C, Sachar V, Guelinckx I, et al. Maternal bariatric surgery: adverse outcomes in neonates. Eur J Pediatr. 2010;169(2):191–6.

The manufacturer's authorised representative in the EU is Springer Nature Customer Service Centre GmbH, Europaplatz 3, 69115 Heidelberg, Germany. If you have any concerns regarding our products, please contact ProductSafety@springernature.com

Printed and bound by CPI Group (UK) Ltd, Croydon, CR0 4YY

29/04/2026

02099520-0001